Collaborative Community Mental Health Care

Edited by

Mary Watkins PhD, MN, RMN, RGN, Dip Nurs Ed
Head of Institute of Health Studies
University of Plymouth, Plymouth, UK

Nick Hervey PhD, BPhil, BA, CQSW
Mental Health Services Manager,
Southwark Social Services, London, UK

Jerome Carson BA (Hons), MSc, C Psychol
Lecturer in Clinical Psychology,
Institute of Psychiatry, London, UK
Honorary Principal Clinical Psychologist,
The Maudsley Hospital, London, UK

Susan Ritter MA, RGN, RMN
Lecturer in Mental Health Nursing,
Institute of Psychiatry, London, UK

A member of the Hodder Headline Group
LONDON • SYDNEY • AUCKLAND

First published in Great Britain 1996 by
Arnold, a member of the Hodder Headline Group
338 Euston Road, London NW1 3BH

Whilst the advice and information in this book is believed to be true and
accurate at the date of going to press, neither the authors nor the publisher
can accept any legal responsibility or liability for any errors or omissions that
may be made.

British Library Cataloguing in Publication Data
A catalogue record for this book is available from the British Library

Library of Congress Cataloging-in-Publication Data
A catalog record for this book is available from the Library of Congress

ISBN 0 340 54241 1

Typeset in 10/11 by Anneset, Weston-super-Mare, Avon
Printed and bound in Great Britain by J W Arrowsmith Ltd, Bristol

Contents

List of contributors

Jennifer Beecham BA(Hons)
Research fellow, Personal Social Services Research Unit, University of Kent at Canterbury, UK; and Lecturer, Centre for the Economics of Mental Health, Institute of Psychiatry, London, UK

Rob Brown BA(Hons), MA, CQSW, ASW
South London ASW Programme Director, CUBE, Croydon College, Croydon, UK; Mental Health Act Commissioner

Jerome Carson BA(Hons), MSc, C Psychol
Lecturer in Clinical Psychology, Institute of Psychiatry, London, UK

Joan Chandler BA.Soc(Hons) PhD
Principal lecturer in Sociology, University of Plymouth, UK

Maud Culhane CQSW
Team Manager, Wandsworth Social Services, Springfield Hospital, London, UK

Ruth Dixon BA(Hons) Dip Soc Admin, CQSW
Adviser, Mental Health, Hampshire County Council Social Services Department, Hampshire, UK

Leonard Fagin Méd(Arg) FRCPsych
Consultant Psychiatrist, Claybury Hospital, Essex; and Honorary Senior Lecturer, University College London, UK

Michael Farrell MRCP, MRCPsych
Senior Lecturer and Consultant Psychiatrist, National Addiction Centre, Institute of Psychiatry and The Maudsley Hospital, London, UK

Phil Fennell BA(Hons)Law, M.Phil, PhD
Senior Lecturer in Law, University of Wales, Cardiff, UK

Paramabandhu Groves BA, MB, BS, MRCPsych
Honorary Senior Registrar, National Addiction Centre, Institute of Psychiatry, London, UK

Debra Hall Dip COT, SROT
Head Occupational Therapist – Forensic Services, Maidstone Priority Care NHS Trust, Maidstone, UK

Frank Holloway MA, MB, MRCPsych
Consultant Psychiatrist, London; and Clinical Director, Community Directorate, Bethlem and Maudsley NHS Trust, London, UK

Martin Knapp BA(Hons), MSc, PhD
Professorial Fellow, Personal Social Services Research Unit, The London School of Economics and Political Science; and Professor of Health Economics and Director, Centre for the Economics of Mental Health, Institute of Psychiatry, London, UK

Elizabeth Kuipers BSc, MSc, PhD, C.Psychol, FBPsS
Reader in Clinical Psychology, Department of Clinical Psychology, Institute of Psychiatry, London, UK

Jo Lucas BSc, MSc, CQSW
Formerly Developments Director, MIND, Stratford, London, UK; now freelance consultant and trainer

Malcolm Peet MB, ChB, BSc, FRCPsych
Senior Lecturer, Department of Psychiatry, Northern General Hospital, London, UK

Shulamit Ramon BA, MSc, PhD
Course Director, Innovation in Mental Health Work, The London School of Economics and Political Science, London, UK

Sandy Robertson MA, MB, B.Chir, FRCPsych
Consultant Psychiatrist, Kidderminster General Hospital, Worcester, UK

Justine Schneider BA(Hons), MSc, CQSW,
Research Fellow, Personal Social Services Research Unit, University of Kent at Canterbury, UK

Michael Sheppard
Principal Lecturer, Department of Applied Social Science, University of Plymouth, UK

Geraldine Strathdee MRCPsych
GS, Community Psychiatrist, Head of Service Development, The Sainsbury Centre for Mental Health, UK

Kim Sutherby MRC Psych
Senior Registrar, The Bethlem and Maudsley NHS Trust, London, UK

Mark R Sutherland MA, LLB, Dip Ault Counselling
Chaplain The Bethlem and Maudsley NHS Trust, London, UK

Ben Thomas BSc(Hons), MSc, RMN, DipN(Lond) RNT, Cert Health Economics
Director of Clinical Services and Chief Nurse Advisor, The Bethlem and Maudsley NHS Trust; and Honorary Lecturer, Institute of Psychiatry, London, UK

Foreword

The mental health services are in a state of flux. The closure of mental hospitals in many parts of the world has been accompanied by a diversity of response in producing models for care in the community. Even within the United Kingdom, with Government publications exhorting us to conform to ever more prescriptive models of care, community care can take many forms.

Collaborative Community Mental Health Care reflects this diversity of response, and indeed accentuates it by inviting chapters from authors who write from many different perspectives. The result is a comprehensive work that covers a range of approaches to the subject, not all of which are consistent with one another. Here are to be found sober accounts of research from acknowledged experts, as well as expressions of impassioned polemic. The consensus has yet to emerge: and if it ever does, we will probably get a duller book.

The authors all appear to share an enthusiasm for recent changes and no one has much good to say about the mental hospital, nor do they dwell on the shortcomings of community care. It is worth remembering that the principles of psychiatric rehabilitation were laid down in the mental hospital era, and that a time when clinicians provided care for patients with severe, long-term disabilities – without counting the cost – had something to commend it.

However, we all do far more now, for less resource. The burden of care falls largely on the patient's family and other informal carers, and it is right that some of the chapters reflect research on how to involve families in care, as well as the contributions of voluntary agencies.

The editors have dealt with the diversity of approaches to community care by inviting chapters from authors from different disciplines, but do not doubt the need for all the present professions to be involved. However, it seems possible that our present combination of professions can only be understood by a social historian, and that the future will see a new profession of 'community carer', that will admit staff from a variety of backgrounds.

There are three other problems that face care in the community: how to ensure that the amount purchasers spend (from both health and social service perspectives) really reflects the need of particular areas; how to prevent what Frank Holloway and Jerome Carson describe as the ghettoisation of mental health care, as care is divorced from general health care; and how to organise services in such a way as to minimise burn-out of mental health staff. These problems remain to be faced: in the meantime, there is plenty to engage the reader in the 19 chapters which follow.

David Goldberg
Professor of Psychiatry
Institute of Psychiatry
London
1995

Introduction

The advent of information technology should have brought about huge advances in the management of health care, and yet even the collation of basic standardized statistics on mental health has been beyond us. In July 1841 the Association of Medical Officers of Asylums and Hospitals for the Insane in England pledged themselves to complete uniform statistical tables relating to their patients, but we have signally failed to emulate this small step. Recent researchers have found it nigh on impossible to collate information relating to the implementation of the Mental Health Act, owing to the widely varying data collection systems used in different health authorities. Figures relating to in-patient admissions cannot reliably distinguish readmissions from first contacts, and there is little agreement about what information we should be collecting.

Beyond information gathering lies the Gordian knot of information sharing, the focus of this introduction. If nothing else, the Ritchie Inquiry into the tragic history of Christopher Clunis should remind us yet again of the fallibility of human beings when it comes to sharing and passing on information. Such cases continue to haunt us like a grotesque game of Chinese whispers. Clunis is merely the latest in a depressing succession of social care inquiries which stretches all the way back to Maria Colwell. The thing they all have in common is the breakdown of information-sharing systems. For too long we have sheltered behind the bastions of professional identity and restrictive practice. This has distanced us from each other and from the users of our services, to their detriment. Of course there have been examples of good practice, but much of the time we have been living parallel lives. It is only in the last three or four years that many social service departments have begun to communicate effectively at a strategic level with other agencies such as the police, health authorities, and even with their own local authority colleagues in housing. There have been justifiable concerns about client confidentiality, but often this particular rubric has been hijacked to provide a convenient cloak for mediocre practice. The advent of client access to files in both local authorities and health authorities, after a great deal of wailing and gnashing of teeth, has generally been marked with a whimper rather than a bang, and the availability of this information has yet to really impact on, or empower, punters. In some countries such as Holland, for example, there is an expectation that users and their advocates have a much greater access to medical information and increased opportunities for a meaningful dialogue with the psychiatrist involved.

The chapters in this book highlight many exciting projects and theoretical approaches related to joint working in the field of mental health, and the major challenge facing us is to underpin these with really effective working agreements between agencies at a local level, incorporating the views of users and carers, and linking them to the dissemination and management of information. The Community Care Act has laid some of the groundwork for this by insisting on jointly agreed community care plans, implementation of the care programme approach (which has built on s. 117 of the Mental Health Act) and the adoption of a new, needs-led approach to planning services, but much of this has, as yet, been inadequately implemented.

The requirement for local authorities to publish information about their services in community care plans is crucial. For a client to recognize that his or her needs are not being met, or indeed for a social worker or community psychiatric nurse to record unmet need, all must know the breadth of existing provision. In many areas users and their carers remain largely in the dark about what is available, and many professional staff are poorly informed. This is the legacy of a previous era, when users of services were expected to be passive recipients of welfare. As the welfare rights movement demonstrated in the early 1970s, information is power. Many potential recipients of state benefits were unaware of their rights, but with access to information and help there was a huge uptake of benefits.

As health and local authorities expand the range of care provision by commissioning new services, users and carers should have the opportunity to make choices about the type of services developed and which ones they access. In the past, both service users and professional carers have been restricted in devising after-care plans, by their perceptions of what was available, and by the unwillingness of existing service providers to tailor what they offered to individuals' needs. The only way for this to change is for information about the potential range of services to be widely disseminated. This means new service models need to be publicized so that they can be commissioned and replicated elsewhere. It also means local authorities and other agencies have to encourage users and carers to take part in a dialogue about their needs, and how these can be met. New methods of sampling users' views will be needed. Many local authorities are now introducing new information technology systems, and in future assessments of individual needs will be aggregated, to see what the main areas of unmet need are. Already a steady demand for evening and weekend services is emerging, and the articulation of requests for a range of new provision, including specialized home care services, more informal drop-in services and a better range of sheltered employment opportunities.

In some areas authorities have sought root and branch solutions to information sharing, attempting to link health and local authority information technology systems. However the authors of such schemes are rightly concerned about the security of information, and they remain utopian. Most authorities are still struggling with more basic protocols relating to the consistent transfer of paper information when clients cross geographical boundaries. This is where joint agreements between agencies will be crucial. People who migrate across authorities will always cause difficulties. Some of these clients have already been failed by their local services, but the movement of others may be entirely without rationale. In future those responsible for clients on the supervision register will need some form of national information service to notify other authorities of their likely reappearance elsewhere. But for most psychiatric patients, jointly agreed local quality assurance standards are the way forward to strengthen the supportive network and ensure that information follows a patient when they move districts.

This book is an attempt to share information about current models of good practice in community-based care for people with mental health problems. In the past the confinement of large numbers of people in huge psychiatric hospitals was administratively convenient and created a separate community for the mentally ill. The sharing of information between hospital doctors and the community outside was poor. Good-quality community care means a very high quality of information sharing, and this is costly in terms of staff time and organization, especially as services become locally based and diversified. Of course we must make better use of new information technology, but real information sharing will only come with increased joint training and sharing of our different perspectives.

Nick Hervey on behalf of the Editors
1995

1 Teamwork among professionals involved with disturbed families

L. Fagin

A docudrama

The setting: A ramshackle old terraced house somewhere in East London, home to a community mental health team for the past ten years. The team consists of a group of mental health workers, a few of them based at the Centre, but most having shared responsibilities in other mental health facilities in the service. Ian Stevenson, the manager, has just arrived, and the building is dark, cold and empty. Outside, sirens from police cars wail by, superseding the constant rumble of slow-moving traffic trailing past as it aims for the City. As he closes the door, the telephone rings.

Whipping off his coat, he struggles to disconnect the telephone answering machine and drops into his chair.

Ian: Hello! Community mental health centre. Good morning.
Dr Baker: Ian, is that you?
Ian: Yep. Hello, John.
Dr Baker: I'm glad I found you. I've been very worried about one of my ladies I saw last night, Alison Birley, and I'd like to speak to you about it. Maybe your team can help.
Ian: OK. Shoot. (*He takes out a referral form and starts writing.*)
Dr Baker: She's 31, and lives very close to your centre. She's been having problems with her husband for some time, I suspect, but she's not been very forthcoming about it to me. She's been asking me for sleeping tablets and looks pretty washed out. I think she's depressed, because the last time I saw her she burst into tears, and told me she couldn't cope any longer. I know she's taken overdoses in the past and I'm concerned she might try again.
Ian: Has she got kids?
Dr Baker: Yes, three – two teenage girls and a five-year-old boy. I think social services were involved with them in the past, because the school had expressed worries about the girls' performance at school, and one of them was conferenced last year with suspicion of sexual abuse. I don't know what came of all that. I know the last child was unplanned, and she was depressed for some time after he was born.

Ian: What about the husband?

Dr Baker: I haven't seen much of him. I think he's out of work. He used to drive lorries until his firm went out of business. When he was working, he used to come in for sick certificates quite often, for migraine and tummy upsets. I suspect he drinks too much. He strikes me as not being very supportive. Social services suspected that he was abusing his eldest daughter, but they couldn't prove anything, and no action was taken.

Ian: Has Alison been seen before by mental health services?

Dr Baker: Not really. She only saw a psychiatrist briefly after her overdoses, and then after her last birth, probably for puerperal depression. I know she comes from a split family, and her mother received psychiatric care at some point. I don't think she was very happy as a child.

Ian: Do you think she wants help?

Dr Baker: I'm not sure. I think she feels she's at the end of the road, so she may accept it now. I told her I'd be talking to you, but she seemed a bit cagey, as if she were worried about the consequences. She didn't want to be seen as 'mental'.

Ian: Do you think we can involve the husband?

Dr Baker: I doubt it. I think she'd be frightened of approaching him about it. I don't think he knows she came to see me.

Ian: What did you do?

Dr Baker: I told her I would discuss it with you, and that probably you would be in touch. I started her on some of those new antidepressants, fluoxetine.

Ian: OK. I'll discuss it with the team at our next referral meeting and try and get Alison seen as soon as possible. Do you think a psychiatrist needs to be involved?

Dr Baker: I'd prefer it.

Later that week, at the referral meeting, Ian has given an account of the problem to the professionals gathered round the small conference room. They have already heard about another four referrals, and none have been allocated so far. All of them are urgent and in need of a response within a week.

Janet (senior social worker): I'm concerned about those kids. There's a chance that mum might be aware of continuing abuse, and her worry may be contributing to the presentation. Have you been in touch with social services?

Ian: Yes. The oldest girl had initially revealed to one of her teachers that her father had been approaching her sexually for at least five years. But when it came for her to disclose this to social services, she clammed up. The teachers think that mother would not allow anybody to intervene.

Janet: There's enough in the presentation to suggest the need to review the welfare of the children. I think we should reinvolve social services.

Joan (community occupational therapist): Is that wise? If we intervene heavy-handedly at this stage we probably wouldn't be able to help her. She's worried about statutory agencies already, and she might close ranks again.

Ian: I agree. The question is whether we should involve the husband at this point. Clearly he has a lot do with her unhappiness, and he should be part of our intervention.

Selwyn (*psychiatrist*):   I don't think that's going to get us very far at this stage either. She is already quite reluctant to accept an involvement with us, even on her own.

Frank (*community psychiatric nurse*):   Yes. I think we should go softly softly here, and arrange to see her pretty soon, on her own, preferably not at home, and when the kids are at school. She may benefit from seeing a female worker too.

This suggestion meets with the approval of the rest of the team, who nod assent.

Selwyn (*psychiatrist*):   But what about Dr Baker's request for her to be seen by a psychiatrist? Is that appropriate? She is, of course, on antidepressants, and there is a family history here.

Peter (*psychologist*):   I'm aware of that, but I think seeing a psychiatrist now is going over the top. It would be a confirmation that she's following in mother's footsteps. She's already concerned about being stigmatized. I think we can put these points of view to the GP, and I'm sure he'll understand. If later on we think she needs a psychiatric referral any one of us can pass this on for consultation. Meanwhile we can monitor her to see how she's responding to the fluoxetine, and let you and the GP know.

After some more practical discussion, a female psychiatric social worker is allocated to see her within the week.

A fortnight later, at the clinical team meeting, Gwen Samuels reports back her impressions of her assessment. The small conference room is crowded that morning, and the hustle and bustle of the High Road somehow gets through the closed sash windows.

Gwen (*psychiatric social worker*):   I can see why Dr Baker was worried. She's had quite an appalling history of abuse and rejections, and she obviously had difficulties in getting to trust me. Her father was a violent man, who took to drink after he came out of the Army. She was beaten up frequently as a child, and was sexually interfered with since the age of five until she left the family home at 15. Mother wasn't around much of the time for her, either because of her admissions to psychiatric hospitals or her liaisons with other men during and after she split up from her husband. Alison is the third of four children, and she suspects that her father also abused her younger sister, although Alison's never had the courage to speak to her about it. Mother was oblivious to what was going on, and still has no idea. Despite feeling unwanted, she still tries to make amends with her mum, is in touch frequently with her, but mum comes across as someone who is cold and rejecting, lonely and bitter, and now has serious arthritis to boot. So Alison is constantly at her beck and call, and gets little thanks for it. She thinks her father has remarried, and he is out of the picture. She still hates him, and can't even contemplate getting in touch with him again. I can tell you, all this was heavy going, not only because of what she was telling me, but also because I felt I had to be very careful with her. She was constantly expecting me either to know what was going on before she told me, or to be very disapproving of her.

Ian (*manager*):   I can quite see that. But what do you think precipitated the present crisis?

Gwen: Hold on. She told me more. She became increasingly distressed as the interview went on. I've seen her twice now. The first time I saw her for nearly two hours, and I was shattered after that. I wanted to go home and curl up in bed.

After leaving home, she led quite a chaotic lifestyle. She dabbled in drugs for some time, although she never tried the hard stuff. She had a couple of experiences of prostitution, just to survive. Her relationships were all stormy and abusive, and she never let anyone get too near to her. That is, until she got herself pregnant. The father of the child didn't want to have anything to do with the baby, and they split up before she was born. Alison was determined to have it, and thought that she would be able to provide the baby with all the love that was missing in her own life. Then her husband Ted came on the scene.

Peter (psychologist – with a hint of irony):   I suppose he was different then.

Gwen: Quite right. He was working as a hospital porter, and met her when she came up to antenatal classes. He didn't seem to mind that she was pregnant by someone else, and was very understanding. She said she was totally taken in by this, and fell in love with him. I think his background was pretty deprived too, although we didn't go into it very much.

Things went well for a couple of years. They got married, decided to have another baby, and Ted got an HGV licence and a job as a lorry driver, which was more lucrative, although it meant him being away from home often. Then things started to go wrong. She found out that Ted was seeing other women.

Janet (senior social worker):   Was this before or after the suspected abuse of the children?

Gwen: Oh, a long time before. Her two daughters were under three at the time, I think. She went berserk. She said her world felt like it had crumbled, she was already exhausted looking after her children, and became very depressed. She lost all sense of perspective, and took a small overdose, although she said she didn't really want to kill herself. The relationship deteriorated from then on. She got into uncontrollable rages whenever he was around, and Ted spent more and more time way. He started drinking, but still gave her money every week. The kids started to play her up, and she had no friends to share her problems with. She found it difficult to be intimate with anybody. The estate where she lives is very run down, graffiti and urine-stenched stairwells, that sort of thing.

She said she came to her senses after the overdose, and that her kids were the most important thing in her life, even if her trust in Ted had been shattered. They went on living together, but their sexual life went out the window, and he was never around. His drinking became quite heavy then, occasionally getting stroppy with her whenever they had an argument.

She found it very difficult to talk about the next part.

Janet: Was this about the abuse of the kids?

Gwen: Well no, not exactly. She started seeing this guy – she said it was mostly a sexual thing at first. The fact that Ted was away a lot of the time meant it was easy for them to meet at her flat, although Ted nearly caught them a couple of times. She said the man didn't mean much to her, but she felt she needed a life of her own. she said this with little embarassment, with a hint of anger. Inevitably, she became pregnant again, about six years ago. She didn't know what to do, initially decided to get rid of it, but she couldn't go through with an abortion. It was during her pregnancy, and after Ted lost his job through drink, that she now suspects the abuse started, although she was too full of her own problems at the time to realize. She broke down into tears at this point, and was quite inconsolable. She couldn't believe it was all happening again. After her baby was born she became quite depressed, and was seen by psychiatrists and treated with antidepressants. She couldn't get close to the baby at first, and had to be encouraged to look after him. The girls were out of her control, and she couldn't speak to them, although they were doing a lot of the housework and cooking by then, because Alison was too depressed and gave up. She then took another overdose, this time with serious intent, taking 30 paracetamol and all her antidepressants, spending some time in hospital.

And then the reports from the school raised concern about the girls...

Ian: You still haven't told us what prompted this referral.

Joan: (*community occupational therapist*) I'm surprised she hasn't come to our attention a long time ago.

Gwen: I think it's to do with the girls. Not only the realization of abuse. It's the fact that she now has no relationship with them, at least not enough for them to trust her, and that history seems to be repeating itself. She doesn't have the courage to confront Ted, and wants to leave him, but she feels trapped. It's come to the point where she can't keep up this illusion of independence and self-sufficiency.

Selwyn (psychiatrist):   She's revealed a surprising amount of painful information to you in only a couple of sessions. I'm feeling quite overwhelmed by it all, so I can imagine how you must have felt. Let's think about our approach for a while. What did you tell her?

Gwen: I told her I needed to discuss her problems with the team. She seemed to be a bit upset about the fact that the information would be shared with others, and she was particularly concerned that this revelation would not bring about an intervention by social services whereby she would lose custody of the children.

Selwyn: What did you say?

Gwen: I tried to reassure her, telling her that we worked as a team so that different professionals could arrive at a decision as to how best to help her, and she seemed happy with this.

Selwyn: Well, what do we do?

Frank: (*community psychiatric nurse*) I think she's made an important first step, trusting someone with her secrets, and clearly taking some risks. We should respect that. At the moment, she needs individual support, and time to build on her relationship with Gwen.

Janet: (*senior social worker*) I'm still concerned about those kids, though. I don't need to remind the team that we have statutory obligations in cases like these, and we would be seriously criticized if we hadn't considered intervention where child abuse is suspected.

Gwen: I'm pretty sure that her fragile confidence in me would be destroyed if we brought in the riot squad at this stage.

Joan: (*community occupational therapist*) What about using her own concern about her daughters as a lever?

Ian: (*manager*) What do you mean?

Joan: She must be worried sick thinking about what her daughters are going through, or may be going through, and would dearly like to do something about it. I was wondering whether there would be any way of getting her and the daughters together to talk about it.

Gwen: You must be joking! The way things stand between her and her daughters at this stage, I suspect they would find it very difficult to talk to Alison. They are more likely to talk amongst themselves, or to friends.

Selwyn: I disagree. The daughters seem to be worried about mum, they've had to take over at home to an extent, and look after her. I think Joan's idea deserves some thought. They could be brought in initially with the object of helping mum. They do have painful experiences in common, and this may be the best time to share them. But Alison would have to be counselled initially to prepare herself for making the first step. If she can confide her experiences to her daughters, they in turn may be drawn in by her openness, even if they have scores to settle with her. I think we can avoid the fear of blindly intervening statutory agencies if they have influence.

Gwen: Who do you suggest should approach the daughters?

Selwyn: Alison should do it, but perhaps she needs to talk to you about it first.

Gwen: OK, but if I do manage to get her to speak to them, and if they agree, and I still think those are two big ifs, I feel I would need a co-worker.

Ian: Who would be the most appropriate person to join you?

Peter (*psychologist*):   I don't think in this case it is relevant to think about a particular professional. We are talking here about a family that is on the point of disintegration. We've still only heard one side of the story. Who knows what Ted must be going through, even though our sympathies at the moment must lie with Alison. Perhaps what is more important here is to have a male co-worker, and prepare the ground for doing some family work if eventually we can get Ted to join the family meeting.

Janet (*senior social worker*):   I still think we have to anticipate the possibility of social work intervention and even legal action if there is enough evidence. If either or both of the daughters confirm this, I would not be happy just to plan a family meeting.

Peter (*psychologist*):   I'm also concerned that Alison is on antidepressants, especially when all her problems are clearly related to her present circumstances. What do you think, Selwyn?

Selwyn: Well, environmental stresses do not preclude the usefulness of antidepressants. But I must admit there is little evidence here that it is appropriate for her to be on them. There is always the possibility that she might impulsively take another overdose, although Dr Baker has put her on a drug with a reasonably safe profile. I think it would be prudent to talk to her GP and recommend stopping them. I think it is also important to involve Dr Baker in what we are doing, as he may be called in if there are future crises.

Ian: I think we've discussed matters as far as we can go at the moment. Although we have to take Janet's reservations on board, and be prepared to intervene if there is serious concern for the daughters' welfare, I believe that it is reasonable to plan to work with mother and daughters initially, and see what emerges from that approach. I'll arrange to have a male worker join Gwen, if Alison can convince the daughters. We may have to arrange another conference if there are further developments. I will let Dr Baker know what we have decided.

Discussion

608, the community mental health centre in Leytonstone, in East London, was opened in 1983, and the above fictitious example represents a not unusual referral. Working in multidisciplinary environments has opened opportunities for improvements in the quality of assessments, broadened the scope of our interventions, established better relationships with primary care and made the service more accessible to our patients, but at the same time it has highlighted some of the difficulties which professionals from different backgrounds have to face when attempting to work together with disturbed families.

In an attempt to discuss these difficulties I have broken them down into the following categories:

- professional/training issues
- organizational issues
- legal issues
- personal issues
- theoretical issues.

Professional/training issues

The disciplines represented in the team bring to it specific areas of expertise and responsibility. In mental health work, some professionals have more clearly defined roles than others. Thus, psychiatrists, social workers and community psychiatric nurses have professional responsibilities which are not shared with the rest of the team, whilst others, especially community occupational therapists, sometimes struggle to find clearly identified functions which set clear boundaries around their professional role.

Despite that, the range of problems presented to community mental health teams rarely falls within the boundaries of one professional group alone. In fact, most of the difficulties are psychosocial, determined by faulty personality development and unhappy relationships. Counselling skills, as well as expertise in working with couples and families, are at a premium in community mental health teams (CMHTs) and are likely to be dependent on individual choice of training.

The broader the range of skills available to the team, the greater the opportunities to respond to a wide variety of referrals, especially when families present complex problems that require joint professional work. CMHTs that stick to one theoretical approach, or have access to very limited areas of expertise, are thus handicapped when trying to offer comprehensive services to a community. The following are examples of skills and training experiences that have proved helpful to the team, and complement the work that can be done with couples and families:

- bereavement and HIV counselling
- psychosexual treatment techniques
- psychoeducational work with families of psychotic patients
- group therapies (analytical, task-orientated, psychodramatic)
- behaviour and cognitive therapies
- assertiveness training
- anxiety management
- counselling in sexual and physical abuse
- working with patients with eating disorders.

Whilst it is accepted that roles become blurred in day-to-day clinical tasks, specific professional responsibilities need to be negotiated and appreciated by the rest of the team. In the example quoted above, Selwyn, the psychiatrist, was consulted about the necessity for psychotropic medication, and Janet, the senior social worker, about the welfare of the children. Both professionals have statutory obligations to fulfil, and the dilemma is how much of these responsibilities can be delegated to other members. Teams which are unable to discuss policies beforehand can find themselves in endless discussions which can become pitched battles over sovereignty.

The process of delegation can become an opportunity for cross-fertilization and broadening of expertise. Selwyn, for example, can alert other professionals to the major symptoms of depressive disorder which may warrant more active psychiatric intervention. If, during the course of work with Alison, Gwen picks up an increase in suicidal ideation, such as marked sleep disturbances, unrealistic self-recrimination and feelings of hopelessness, psychomotor retardation and major inabilities in functioning, she should have the opportunity to arrange to draw in the psychiatrist to assess Alison's mental state and act accordingly. Likewise, Janet can make arrangements to supervise Gwen's involvement with Alison, liaise with school authorities, and have the team's backing to intervene if serious concern is raised over the children's welfare.

When the team is functioning well, Gwen can feel free to express her own limitations, especially if she has recently joined, or if for other reasons she feels anxious about taking extra responsibilities. This can only happen where there is an expectation of mutual support. It is helpful to make explicit an offer by senior members of the team to be available for informal consultation, as new members of the team may sometimes feel awkward discussing their difficulties in regular team meetings. These informal opportunities have the double advantage of increasing team bonding and cementing trust between members. Although they may be informal, and cross professional boundaries, they are an essential feature of team functioning. It is useful to discuss beforehand how this may affect supervisory intraprofessional arrangements, but in my experience if they are out in the open they rarely cause problems. Senior professionals can also be given room to approach each other if advice given in these informal consultations is contradictory.

Unfortunately, most teams find out about these problems after they have been set up, and don't anticipate them at the planning stage. This often leads to dissatisfaction in team work and lack of trust. Policies which are negotiated beforehand, written up as statements of team organization, and flexible enough to be reviewed at regular intervals, have the effect of offering a safe

structure for team members to operate within. Leeway must be given for professionals to exercise discretionary decisions in their work with clients,
respecting their areas of autonomy and expertise. Policies that are too rigid,
or that require members of the team to consult every decision, waste time,
are inefficient, create disgruntlement, and have the paradoxical effect of
deskilling professionals.

Management need to be aware of ongoing training needs for members of
the team, especially if there is a gap in service provision. Once again, if a list
of skills and services can be anticipated beforehand, it can be borne in mind
which professionals are required when appointments to the team are made
and what training will be necessary to fulfil as many demands as possible.
Team training can increase opportunities for joint work, and much can be
gained by inviting an outside expert to organize a course for all team members, for example in the management of psychosexual disorders. Likewise,
one of the team members may wish to organize in-house training in particular areas of therapy. The team psychologist, for example could train and
supervise behavioural approaches with clients, or join others in anxiety management groups.

Organizational issues

So what is a team? Who is a team member? How can we define its structure, mode of working and function? Bowen, Marler and Androes (1965)
define the psychiatric team as a 'process whereby various professionals who
make individual decisions concerning patients and who share a common purpose meet together to communicate and share knowledge from which plans
are made and thus future therapeutic decisions are influenced'.

This provides us with some insights. A team is not just a physical collection of individuals sitting together in the same room or even sharing a common administrative base. The team is a process, more than the sum of its
parts, and this dynamic nature implies continued change and fluctuations
which have to be accepted as part of its character.

Decision-making is not entirely dependent on the deliberations made within
the team, although it is likely to be influenced by them. Whilst each team member retains their own individuality, responsibility and accountability, the team
is used by everybody as an educational and supportive forum.

This notion destroys the prevalent myth that teams always need to arrive
at a consensus before carrying out a plan. No decisions can be imposed on
members against their will as a result of a majority vote. As mentioned earlier, each discipline carries with it areas of specific responsibility and skill,
which cannot be abrogated to the team as a whole.

In the example described above, we have tried to describe two main organizational issues which can affect team functioning:

* procedural pathways, which deal with the way in which referrals are
  received, discussed, allocated, reviewed and closed;
* team management matters, which deal with concerns about team structure,
  decision-making, documentation, leadership, responsibility and accountability. I am indebted to Øvretveit (1993) to whom I refer for more detailed
  descriptions and helpful suggestions.

Procedural pathways

Clients will arrive in the team by a variety of access gates, depending on local arrangements and team organization. Primary care referrals in the UK usually form the bulk of the team's caseload, but much will depend on the development of outreach efforts to other agencies, the possibility of self-referral and the degree to which the service is publicized and made easily accessible to the local community.

In the example quoted above, the GP was the first port of call for Alison, but the referral could have arrived via the educational services, if concern was expressed about the children at school and links had been established between the educational psychologist and the team. Alternatively, it could have been brought to the team's attention after a call from social services, if they were asked to intervene when sexual abuse was mooted, and if there were worries about Alison's mental health. Probation services may have been involved if matters had progressed to charges being made against Ted, and the family affected as a result, or the local drug and alcohol team may have been involved if Ted was referred for his alleged drinking problem. Finally, Alison or the children may have approached the service if open access was allowed and the team organized to take self-referrals. These different access points will shape the nature of the team's response, not only because of the individual who is presenting with the problem, but also because of the lines of communication that need to be established with referring agencies.

In dealing with disturbed families, one has to be aware that the emerging problem or crisis may only be an indication of overall family dysfunction, and the need to be cognisant of these contextual issues when discussing management. All too often the nature of the presentation clouds the underlying family dynamics which contribute to it, and agencies will think of individual rather than familial responses.

Efforts made to obtain adequate information at the point of referral save time and enable the team to make better decisions. This cannot be stressed enough. Dr Baker was well known to Ian, the team manager, who had made a point of spending time with all GPs likely to make referrals to the centre at the start of his appointment. This personal contact improves the quality of information Ian gets on referral. Ian prepared the GP for the sort of questions he would be asking so as to be able to present them to the team at the referral meeting. Team attachments to primary care, social services, probation services, etc., increase mutual awareness of inter-agency relationships, and foster possibilities of coordinated work and communication.

Sometimes it is not possible to obtain the necessary information from other agencies, especially if the patient refers herself to the team. It is useful at this stage to ask the patient to outline in writing what the nature of the problem is, and to give their permission to contact other agencies, if this is required. This raises the issue of what to do if the client refuses, and I deal with this in the section on legal issues.

The quality of the response will undoubtedly depend on the amount of information gleaned from all possible sources before it is discussed with the team. In this, the role of the manager/coordinator is crucial. Much of Ian's time is spent on the telephone, liaising with other agencies, and in this effort prior personal contact through visits were very helpful. We must not forget here the crucial role of the secretary, very much at the heart of team communications, and often the first voice a client or referrer will hear when approaching the centre. These calls are often anxiety-laden, emotional and distressing, and the secretary will need to handle them with sensitivity and forbearance. Some will say that teams will succeed or fail depending on the ability of the secretary as front-line person to respond to these calls, and I believe not enough time is spent supporting and acknowledging their contribution.

The *referral meeting* becomes the central common pathway into the team, and is the first opportunity for effective teamwork. Ian had already come to an understanding with the team that he would chair the meeting, briefly present all information obtained during the reception phase of the referral, record decisions made and liaise with clients and referrers once the outcome was clear. This is not an easy meeting for Ian to chair, particularly if there are many referrals to deal with that week, or if he is aware that staff are already under pressure and there is little room to take on new referrals.

Recent changes in the NHS (DoH 1989*a, b, c, d* and *e*; DoH 1991), especially those that put the team's functions on a contractual basis, have forced them to prioritize services and have clearer lines of demarcation when making decisions to allocate resources. As a result, Ian has been asked to establish priority criteria for team referrals. In the case of Alison, concern over her suicidal behaviour and welfare of the children placed the referral in the urgent category. Sometimes, however, priorities are much more difficult to define, especially with clients suffering from long-standing anxiety or neurotic conditions, which, whilst being disabling and distressing to both clients and carers, compete weakly for resources needed for patients suffering from chronic psychotic illnesses, self-damaging or aggressive behaviours and where the safety of children is threatened.

At the referral meeting the team decides whether the case should be taken up, and if there is enough information to take this decision. Despite Ian's best efforts, sometimes crucial information has not been obtained, and the core members who attend, usually the seniors from each professional group, can indicate other sources where it can be gathered. Are other agencies currently involved? Do they know about the referral to the CMHT? Is there scope for interagency work? How do we avoid duplication and overlap?

If the team agrees to accept the referral, the next stage is to allocate team members to make an *initial assessment*. Who is the best professional to undertake this task? Should it be a joint assessment, especially if there are complex factors in the presentation? Where should the assessment take place: at home, at the centre, at some other location? How urgent is the referral? Can it be placed on a waiting list? Allocation often depends on availability rather than professional expertise, and this can raise problems in busy teams. Effective caseload management, setting clear, realistic tasks, discussions on closure and regular audit meetings can help in releasing professional time to see more clients.

Despite the fact that sometimes referrals can be quite complicated, about eight to ten can be discussed every week in the 45-minute meeting.

Previously discussed policies have negotiated that when there are predominant social factors in the presentation, or where there is concern over welfare of children, a social worker should be involved in the initial assessment, accompanied by another team member, such as a psychiatrist or a community psychiatric nurse, if there are potential psychiatric symptoms or if patients are on medication that needs to be assessed. General practitioners tend to prefer to have a psychiatrist in the original assessment, but this is not always necessary. The involvement of a psychiatrist tends to confirm the expectation that a referral to a community *mental* health team means that the client is mad, a label which not only stigmatizes, but also imposes the illusion of a possible medical solution to the problem. Peter, the team psychologist, expressed his fear that Alison would see it in this way, especially with a history of mental illness in the family. Scott and Ashworth (1969) described how the 'shadow of the ancestor' tends to hang over families across two or three generations, and the devastating impact a diagnosis of mental illness can have on interpersonal relationships, closing down bonds of human relatedness. In the case where the team decides not to involve a psychiatrist, discussions and agreements have to be arrived at with the GP. This is again discussed in the section on legal issues.

The next stage of the pathway is at the time when the assessor(s) report back to the team at the *assessment meeting*. This is an opportunity, and not an obligation, for professionals to use a multidisciplinary forum to reflect on their findings.

If the assessment is straightforward, and the assessor feels comfortable about undertaking a piece of work with the client, multidisciplinary involvement is not necessary at this stage. In this situation, it would be inefficient and wasteful of team's resources to discuss the case at length, and the team has to feel able to entrust such decisions to each of its members. A common problem arises when assessors feel that the team expects ongoing work to be taken up by them following the assessment. We have found it helpful to make this expectation explicit, but at the same time it must not be an imposition if this arrangement is to be acceptable. From the client's point of view, it is obviously of benefit to continue to see the same worker and not have to change, but the assessor will have to make clear that this may not necessarily be so at an early stage in the assessment.

The *tasks* for the team at the assessment meeting are:

- to decide whether the referral is appropriate for continued involvement;
- to raise issues which may not have been explored adequately or sufficiently;
- to establish a strategy of action with clear goals and expectations;
- to offer further opportunities for review.

These decisions may involve other members of the team at a future time.

Opportunities for *review* can be offered in two formats. Once again it is important to clarify these beforehand.

- Each professional makes arrangements within their own line management to have supervision sessions in which they can discuss progress with their work. This is especially useful when the therapeutic relationship becomes entangled or stuck.

- If the mental health worker or supervisor feels that the case would benefit from multidisciplinary input, it is presented to the team, which allows a
broader perspective and an opportunity to get feedback or guidance about
issues beyond their professional expertise.

Finally, the allocated worker needs to make a decision on closure of the
case. This is usually the most difficult stage in the pathway and yet one that,
if effectively undertaken, not only ensures good practice but also the competent functioning of the team.

It is always tempting to find reasons why therapeutic involvement should
continue, especially if the tasks and strategy have not been clearly defined.
More often than not, new problems arise during the course of the intervention which urges a redefinition of therapeutic aims. Underlying this, one usually finds anxieties shared by both client and worker about separation and
loss.

Unless teams specifically aim to offer long-term psychotherapy, unresolved
issues in termination of therapy can obviously render the team ineffective
and useless, unable eventually to respond to future demand. Closure therefore needs to be anticipated early in the course of the therapeutic task and
communicated and shared with clients. A helpful strategy is to point out that
if future problems do arise, a new intervention can be discussed at a later
stage.

In this it is also important to bear in mind that usually the effectiveness of
the intervention cannot be gauged immediately at the time of the termination, and that sometimes it can take a while before improvements take place.
We are, after all, generally dealing with long-standing personality and relationship difficulties at points of crisis, often accompanied by disabling symptoms, and the team's strategy often needs to address these rather than the
protracted goals of character change. For many clients with severely dam-
aged personalities the team may have to be prepared to intervene at these
points of crisis, and act as a safety net, rather than promise long-term intervention.

Team management matters

Time spent on an agreed *management structure* for the team is time well
spent and, if successful likely to avoid many headaches at a later stage.
Professionals have an ambivalent attitude to teamwork. In mental health,
because of the nature of client work, associations with other professionals
help to contain the distress communicated to workers, as well as provide a
backdrop on which to discuss ideas. But it also threatens professional autonomy and independent decision-making. More specifically, in a field previously dominated by the medical hierarchy, it raises concerns that
multidisciplinary teams are just an excuse for ongoing medical feudalism outside the hospital framework.

This is particularly important when working with disturbed families. It is
uncanny to observe how often relationships reproduce family dysfunction in
poorly managed teams, especially if leadership issues are not adequately
resolved. This may be expressed in excessive stereotyping of particular professional groups, scapegoating of individual members of the team, gossiping,

innuendo and acting out behaviour. Adequate coordination of different services is essential to teamwork, and this needs an atmosphere of trust, safety and explicit acknowledgement of mutual interdependence which can only occur within an organization with a clear management policy.

The team manager or coordinator should be at the heart of such an organisation, and should be one that takes a lead on management matters. Underpinning this role is the ability to secure previously negotiated terms of reference for the team and levels and degrees of commitment from each of the team members. Teams will vary in their composition and the nature of their relationship with the manager.

At one end of the spectrum, is the *fully-managed formal multidisciplinary team* (Øvretveit 1993) (Fig. 1.1).

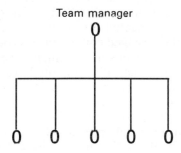

Fig. 1.1 Team members from different professions, fully managed by team manager

In this arrangement, professionals are employed as full-time members of the team and have direct lines of accountability to the manager, allowing clearer integration, task setting, coordination and decision-making. The manager is likely to carry a budget, will be responsible for setting team policies and for monitoring and evaluating team performance. The advantages to such teams is that they have a stable membership and a shared core ethos, an important feature when dealing with particular client populations. The disadvantages include a tendency for these teams to become self-centred, rigid in their functions, unable to change according to fluctuation in demands and their reliance on the manager's ability to be sensitive to the needs of different professional groups and sensitivities.

At the other extreme, teams can be composed of associated members only, whose loyalties and management structures lie with other agencies or professional departments, but gather around a coordinator for specific tasks.

These *coordinated formal multidisciplinary teams* (Fig. 1.2) are more difficult to manage. Responsibility and accountability can become confused, as coordinating and management functions are held by different individuals, who may be employed by separate authorities. There is no commitment for members to adhere to a team policy, and often much will rely on goodwill and understanding between managers and coordinators which can break down when problems of professional boundaries arise. Teams of this nature

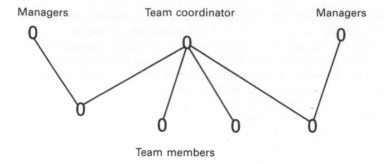

Fig. 1.2

will depend on availability of professionals unless negotiated previously with each team members's line management. These teams have the advantage of being highly flexible and respectful of professional autonomy.

A hybrid solution is the managed core team and coordinated or contracted associated team (Fig. 1.3). In this arrangement, the manager will be fully responsible for a group of specifically appointed professionals who form the core team, as well as a managerial role for professionals who are contracted to serve the team on a part-time basis. The manager has coordinating functions for associated members who commit time to team tasks according to prior agreement with professional superiors. The team can define its primary tasks to be undertaken by the core team, and have the flexibility to use associate and contracted members when other requirements are necessary.

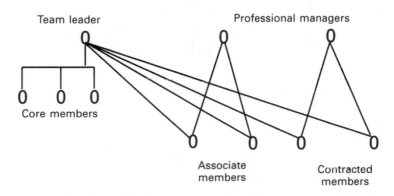

Fig 1.3

In all these team structures, issues about *responsibility and accountability* need to be addressed and clarified if they are to succeed. In the formally managed team, all professionals are responsible and accountable to the manager. This does not preclude the possibility of organizing professional advisors to supervise the clinical work of each team member, but in such a team advisors do not carry managerial functions. In hybrid teams, it is useful to discuss the distinction between managerial accountability and clinical lines of responsibility. Whilst each member may be managerially accountable to the manager or coordinator, in terms of adhering to team policy, ensuring allotted time to the team and following team's procedures, they can retain clinical responsibility for their own work, supervised through their own professional groupings. This tends to satisfy concerns about one discipline intruding on other professional territories.

I have already addressed issues about *leadership and decision-making*. Much time is spent expressing concern about who makes the final decisions when there is conflict and difference of opinion in multidisciplinary teams. In my experience, these issues rarely arise when members of the team are aware of other members' responsibilities and statutory obligations. It would be dangerous, however, to assume that teams do not require a formally designated leader, with specifically defined roles. The leader in community mental health teams is responsible for seeing that the team is functioning according to team policy, organizing and chairing clinical and business meetings, ensuring that tasks are being delegated and carried through, communicating and establishing ties with outside agencies, channelling complaints, monitoring and reviewing performance and finally keeping to budget. They are fully accountable for the work undertaken by those members they are asked to manage, and allowed to take disciplinary action if necessary. For those associate members whose management lines are elsewhere, the leader can discuss problems with each member before taking the issue to their line management when appropriate.

Legal issues

In the example quoted above, Dr Baker requested a psychiatrist to be involved. The team decided that this was not necessary, and for cogent reasons thought that it would be counterproductive at the assessment stage. The psychiatrist was involved in this decision. Who, then, retains medico-legal responsibility?

This issue can be further complicated if the team has previously committed itself to honour general practitioner's demands to have specific team members involved when they make referrals. Under current reforms to the NHS, GP fund-holders are likely to have an increasing stake in such decisions, which could undermine the ability of the team to determine who would be the best professional(s) to take on the case. If a tragedy occurs, questions would be raised about these resolutions in a coroner's court.

The team decided on the following policy to deal with this problem. Whilst continuing to offer GPs the option of making referrals to specific members of the team, an agreement was reached with GPs and the Family Health Service Authority to allow for team discretion and participation in decisions about allocation. When teams came to the conclusion that another team member should be involved the manager would discuss this with the referring GP to obtain his permission. If the GP was unhappy about the team's deliberations, an undertaking was given to comply with the GP's requests. Allied to this, an agreement was reached whereby GPs retained *medico-legal responsibility* for all cases referred to the team, even if a psychiatrist was involved. This was also vetted and agreed by the relevant Medical Insurance

Society. In turn, *clinical responsibility* for the work remained with each member of the team.

The tort of negligence is embodied in English law, whereby it is required for professionals to recognize and observe the limits of their professional training and competence and to satisfy themselves that those to whom they refer their clients are appropriately qualified and competent. There was no justification for the terms 'overall responsibility' or 'ultimate responsibility' (British Psychological Society 1985). This solution has been embedded in team policy and been adopted by other CMHTs in the UK. Arriving at this agreement has had the added advantage of making GPs more aware of the nature of teamwork in mental health, improving the quality of information given by GPs on referral, and including GPs in all stages of decision-making. These advantages are difficult to sustain when teams only operate on the basis of attachments to general practice and no reference is made to multidisciplinary team work where complex cases can be discussed.

Similar agreements have to be reached within the team, especially when statutory responsibilities for one of the team workers conflict with team decisions. Janet, the senior social worker, was understandably reluctant to skim over the possible danger to Alison's children with the possible threat of ongoing child abuse. The team has to accept that these obligations will occasionally have to supersede team resolutions, if it can find no way to make sure that these duties are being met.

I referred earlier to the situation when a self-referred client refuses the team access to other agencies, especially at the time of the initial contact. This can become complicated when, for example, the client is unhappy about a member of the team talking to the general practitioner or, if there are child-care issues at stake, involving social services. This could place mental health workers in invidious medico-legal and statutory complications.

Fortunately these situations are infrequent, but they are difficult problems to resolve, and do require unequivocal answers. The team decided that patients who ultimately refused GP contact could not be taken in for further work. Having said that, the client would be encouraged to understand the need to have appropriate medical backup and could be reassured that confidential information to the GP would be communicated only when the allocated worker considered this to be absolutely necessary. For example, the GP could be informed that their patient had contacted the centre for counselling without giving any further details, but the client would have to know that the mental health worker could involve the GP at a future date if his or her health was at risk.

In the case of refusal to contact social services, an explanation would be given to describe the statutory duties of the team, especially when children's welfare was at stake. This may involve the local social services department, but the fact that social workers form part of the team allows the possibility of an assessment being undertaken without having to make a referral elsewhere, and no further action would need to take place unless formal care proceedings are necessary.

Personal issues

Many failures of team functioning are blamed on faulty personalities. Clashes of temperament, proverbial chips on shoulders, resentment against authority figures, power battles, schisms and collusions are ever present in teams, as in any other organization or group. My experience is that these features tend to be acted out when there is uncertainty, when team members feel neglected or unheard or simply poorly managed and taken for granted. Unfortunately, the 'helping professions' have a poor record when it comes to making arrangements for looking after each other. When these basic needs are ignored, it is not unusual to see the team reproducing some of the pathology of their clients, especially when dealing with disturbed families (Brody and Haven 1957).

A sensitive manager knows when to alert team leaders to any stress which is unduly carried by any of its members, and then steps can be taken to ensure that something is done about it.

Not everybody has the capacity of working in teams. Some people are natural crew members. They enjoy the opportunity of sharing problems and will be stimulated by the opinions of others, as well as feeling comfortable in confronting and arguing their case. Others, however, will find it difficult to expose their work to others, and prefer individual supervision and clear boundaries around their skills and that of the rest of the team. This does not preclude their participation, and their styles need to be accommodated if they are to contribute to the gamut of opportunities offered by the service.

It is preferable to allow for an element of choice for individual members to define how they will fit in with team activities, rather than force them to work in a style which they find uncomfortable and threatening. Very occasionally one meets people who cannot work with others and who express their dissatisfaction in a destructive manner, either by not communicating or by taking individual decisions which fly in the face of team ethos. Usually appropriate supervision and clearly stated accountability can contain these problems, but managers and supervisors have to be prepared to accept when this fails and make separate arrangements for these professionals (Walldron 1983).

Another phenomenon that we have encountered is the lack of understanding of teamwork by professional managers. There are a number of reasons for this. Occasionally, outside supervisors and line managers have an anxiety that their staff may get lost in team activities, become too identified with the team structure, and disassociate themselves from their own professional group. They may also feel envious and excluded from the team, and unconsciously wish its dissolution. They are then likely to define the participation of the team member in a very restricted manner, either by rigidly controlling the time that is offered, or the type of work that they can undertake. At planning and review meetings they may play a negative role, undermining the team's achievements, or unnecessarily criticizing the operational characteristics of the team. Long, drawn-out and erosive battles may ensue if these difficulties are not tackled directly and squarely.

One way in which we have approached these difficulties is by having six-monthly away days. These meetings have two main aims. One is to have time to discuss matters of practical importance which can inform team policy, and set new agendas or directions for the service. For example, a day can be spent on how to improve accessibility for ethnic minorities, or establish priority criteria for allocation of work. The second aim is to improve team bonding, by training and sensitivity exercises which focus on particular problems in team functioning. Resolution of conflicts, interprofessional rivalries or difficulties with leaders can be explored in these sessions. Participation of outside managers also helps to integrate these distant members of the team. An occasional evening meal out can also work wonders!

Theoretical issues

Sharing a common philosophy of care is an oft-quoted aim of most multidisciplinary groups, but one that is usually difficult to define, and needs continuous restatement and revision. Most teams do not start with a prestated theoretical viewpoint, and tend to develop it over the years.

Multidisciplinary teams, practically by definition, attract professionals who are comfortable with the idea that the aetiology of mental disturbance is complex and multifactorial, and not subsumed to single causal explanations. Mental health problems are not considered synonymous with illness, and therefore a purely medical explanation is unsatisfactory in most cases presented to multidisciplinary teams. This should not, however, imply that every symptom can or should be explained by social, cultural or developmental factors either, and due recognition needs to be given to the needs of severely disabled individuals who require constant medical care and supervision because of recognized psychiatric disorders, such as schizophrenia or manic depressive illness (Fagin and Chapman 1986).

Underpinning this basic model is the conviction that symptoms cannot be seen out of context. Dr Baker's referral of a suicidally depressed mother could only be properly understood as emerging from disturbed family relationships, and interventions have to be geared to take this into account. Piecemeal solutions are likely to divert problems into other areas. On the other hand, developmental psychodynamic theories help us to understand the role of personal histories and background to the presentation.

Abusive relationships, for example, tend to be reproduced and regenerated in current circumstances. Abuse seems to be handed down through generations: victims often become victimisers or find relationships which mirror past experiences of humiliations and personal distress (Bentovim 1993). Teams are often placed in the dilemma of having to decide at what level they need to intervene: the personal or the familial. This is not necessarily an either/or clinical judgment. As in Alison's case, the team may have to deal with the personal before the familial can be tackled. Sometimes the urgency of the case requires a contextual intervention, especially if children are involved and in danger, leaving personal therapies as an option for a later time, when things have calmed down and a degree of commitment to long-term work is established. These decisions are often complex and require effective team discussion and open negotiation with the client. Team members with training and experience in personal psychodynamic theories contribute to the team's debate with those who have been trained in systems theories (Haley 1971) or those that use behavioural or cognitive interventions. This diversity of theoretical input informs the team and increases possible therapeutic options.

Current pressures on scarce resources have also influenced theoretical thinking. We have commented earlier on the difficulties for teams who have not been able to define criteria for closure of cases. Crisis theory (Caplan 1964) and brief, session-limited therapies (Weakland *et al.* 1974) have emerged as realistic options for busy community mental health teams. Offering brief, goal-centred interventions at times of crisis allows professionals to focus and reframe problems at a time when clients are most receptive to change, concentrating on the client's coping abilities, and reducing dependency on professionals.

Finally, we must not forget that many families referred to community mental health teams have to cope with serious mental illness, or that patients discharged from hospital may require familial interventions if care at home is to succeed. Effective care plan management, assertive approaches (Stein and Test 1985) and psychoeducational collaboration (Hogarty *et al.* 1986) between affected families and professionals require seamless coordination of services and teamwork if the needs of the seriously ill are to be met.

Summary

We have explored the nature of teamwork in a community mental health team working with disturbed families. Teams are complex groups which require nurture and constant attention if they are going to fulfil their functions adequately, especially if they are to avoid enmeshment with pathological family groups. In these conditions, teamwork can be a source of professional and personal satisfaction. If team matters are not properly addressed, however, at the least it can lead to disaffection and loss of commitment, at worst to personal stress and unhappiness.

References

Bentovim A (1993). Why do adults sexually abuse their children? *British Medical Journal*, **307**, 144.

Bowen W T, Marler D C and Androes C (1965). The psychiatric team: myth and mystique. *American Journal of Psychiatry*, **122**, 687–690.

British Psychological Society (1985). *Responsibility Issues in Clinical Psychology and Multidisciplinary Work*, London.

Brody W and Haven M (1957). Intra-team reactions: their relation to the conflicts of the family in treatment. *American Journal of Orthopsychiatry*, **27**, 349.

Caplan G (1964). *Principles of Preventive Psychiatry*. Tavistock Publications, London.

Department of Health (DoH) (1989*a*). *Working for Patients*. HMSO, London.

DoH (1989*b*). *Caring for People: Community Care in the Next Decade and Beyond*. HMSO, London.

DoH (1989*c*). *Working Paper No 1. Self Governing Hospitals*. HMSO, London.

DoH (1989*d*). *Working Paper No 2. Funding and Contracts for Hospital Services*. HMSO, London.

DoH (1990*e*). *Caring for People: Policy Guidance*. HMSO, London.

DoH (1991). *The Health of the Nation*, HMSO. London.

Fagin L and Chapman S (1986). Interdisciplinary Association of Mental Health Workers. Report of the policy group. *IAMHW Bulletin*, No. 4, 13–18.

Haley J (ed.) (1971). *Changing Families: A Family Therapy Reader*. Grune & Stratton, New York.

Hogarty G E, Anderson C M, Reiss D J, Kornblith S J, Greenwald P, Javan CD,

Manonia M J and the EPICS Research group (1986). Family psychoeducation, social skills training and maintenance chemotherapy in the aftercare treatment of schizophrenia. I: One year effects of a controlled study on relapse and expressed emotion. *Archives of General Psychiatry*, **43**, 633–642.

Øvretveit J (1993). *Coordinating Community Care. Multidisciplinary Teams and Care Management*. Open University Press, Buckingham.

Scott R D and Ashworth P L (1969). The shadow of the ancestor: a historical factor in the transmission of schizophrenia. *British Journal of Medical Psychology*, **42**, 13–32.

Stein L I and Test M A (eds.) (1985). *The Training in Community Living Model: A Decade of Experience*. New Directions for Mental Health Services No. 26. Jossey-Bass, San Francisco.

Walldron G (1983). *Interdisciplinary Work in Community Mental Health Settings*. Unpublished manuscript.

Weakland J H, Fish R, Watzlawick P and Bodin A M (1974). Brief therapy: focused problem resolution. *Family Process*, **13**, 141.

2 Integrating hospital and community services

M. Culhane

Introduction

This chapter is concerned with bringing together both the social care and the treatment aspects of services for adults who have mental health problems. My position as a team manager employed by a social services department, but based in a National Health Service setting has placed me in close proximity to the delivery of these services, and thus in a useful position to comment on some of the practical implications of government policies.

In the first half of this chapter the relevant legislative and policy framework is described, and background information on the development of services is provided. In order to bring this rather theoretical material alive and demonstrate its practical implications, the second half of the chapter considers the development and integration of services in one particular geographical area. There is a considerable emphasis on the work of community mental health teams as these are seen as increasingly important in the delivery of integrated and responsive mental health services. The terms 'user', 'client' and 'patient' will be used interchangeably throughout this chapter.

In recent years there have been two themes underlying government policies for the development of community care: that policies should be needs-led rather than service-led; and that the best way of meeting this objective is by the replacement of large psychiatric institutions with a flexible and relevant range of local alternative services (Hunter and Wistow 1987). The closure of the old long-stay psychiatric hospitals and the resettlement of many of their residents in smaller, community-based facilities has been paralleled by an increasing emphasis on the development of community-based services.

A number of policy documents were issued from the mid-1970s (Department of Health and Social Security 1975; House of Commons 1985; Griffiths 1988). These and other papers proposed major changes in the delivery of health and social care, and spelt out the need for closer cooperation between the NHS, social services departments and the voluntary sector.

The policy framework and other developments

Proposals set out in the Griffiths Report (1988) were further developed in the 1989 White Paper, *Caring for People – Community Care in the Next Decade and Beyond*. This White Paper aimed to establish the framework for good-quality local services and proposed key objectives which included the development of services away from a hospital setting. It focused on locally based provision, which as far as possible should be delivered to people in their own homes.

The National Health Service and Community Care Act 1990 has provided the legislative framework for the introduction of these changes. For political and practical reasons its implementation was delayed for over two years, but the key objectives remained as follows:

• to promote the development of domiciliary, day and respite services to enable people to live in their own homes wherever feasible and sensible;
• to ensure that service providers make practical support for carers a high priority;
• to make proper assessment of need and good case management the cornerstone of good quality care;
• to promote the development of a flourishing independent sector alongside good quality public provision;
• to clarify the responsibilities of agencies and so make it easier to hold them to account for their performance;
• to secure better value for the taxpayer's money by introducing a new funding structure for social care.

This legislation had some very important implications for mental health services. It aimed to improve and strengthen collaboration between health and local authorities in planning and providing services, and proposed that future change should be based on policy agreements rather than on the rather cumbersome joint planning structures previously in use. This proposal was seen as a way towards more flexible planning to suit local circumstances and methods of working. While local authorities were given the lead responsibility for the provision of social care, the expectation was that, as well as continuing to make direct provision themselves, they would develop purchasing and contracting arrangements to buy relevant services from the private and voluntary sectors. The promotion of a mixed market economy was seen as a way to promote healthy competition, ensuring both cost effectiveness and increased choice for users.

The 'duty' to ensure individual users' needs were properly assessed was given to local authorities, who were expected to involve relevant NHS staff and voluntary agencies in the assessment process. The Act put considerable emphasis on a needs-led rather than a service-led approach, and pointed out that user and carer consultation should be given high priority in both service planning and the delivery of services.

In a phased programme, beginning in April 1993, responsibility for the funding of residential and nursing home care was transferred from the Department of Social Security to local authority social services departments. The formula used for the transfer of these funds discriminated against those boroughs which had few existing private and voluntary establishments within their boundaries, which meant that such funding immediately became cash limited. The urgent need to find a means of limiting the rapidly expanding costs of residential care lay behind this particular change in the legislation. With the projected growth in the number of elderly frail people likely to need such services, this increasing cost looks set to continue (Thornicroft *et al.* 1993). By tighter assessment of need and a greater provision of domiciliary services, in order to keep people in their own homes, it was hoped that the cost of residential care could be kept down. The government also insisted that 85 per cent of the transferred money was to be spent in the private and voluntary sector, by which means it hoped to encourage the development of competition and thus more keenly priced services.

As already mentioned, a duty was placed on local authorities to develop systems of assessment and case management. The term was changed to 'care management' in 1991, in a Department of Health and Social Services Inspectorate guidance document (HMSO 1991) in order to emphasize that it is the care and not the person that is being managed.

The aim of the assessment and care management process was to ensure a comprehensive assessment of need and by care management to ensure the provision of relevant services. This was to include systems of monitoring and review to ensure their continuing appropriateness for as long as necessary. Local authorities were also enjoined to set up 'arms length' monitoring systems so that quality of service, both in the statutory and voluntary sectors could be ensured.

Guidance on the care programme approach was issued to health authorities which placed a responsibility on them for assessing, prior to discharge from hospital, the continuing health and social care needs of each patient. A named person (key worker) was to be appointed to ensure their needs were met.

As part of the 'Caring for People' initiatives a specific grant was made available to local authorities for the funding of services for people with severe mental health problems. This grant, while comparatively small, was clearly an effort to encourage joint planning as it was payable only on the basis of joint health and local authority initiatives.

An earlier piece of legislation which is of major importance in the care of those with mental health problems is the 1983 Mental Health Act. Its main emphasis is on the care of patients in hospital, with particular emphasis on those compulsorily admitted and detained. Of especial relevance to care in the community is Section 117 which relates to the after-care of those patients compulsorily admitted to hospital under treatment orders – Section 3 or 37 of the Act. Section 117 places a duty on both health authorities and social services to provide after-care services and, where appropriate, in cooperation with other other organizations. While this approach to discharge planning relates solely to detained patients, the care programme and care management approaches aim to apply similarly coordinated planning to the needs of a wider range of vulnerable people.

The legislation and recent guidance documents emphasize the importance of joint planning and multidisciplinary practice in the provision of health and social care services. The distinction between health and social care has been highlighted, but neither has been clearly defined. Onyett (1992) suggests that at practice level health and social care may be difficult to separate. He mentions a provider's amusing comment that the sole difference between a social bath and a health bath is that bubble bath goes into one and Dettol into the other!

Developments during 1993 have suggested that further legislative changes are likely to be made which may place a renewed emphasis on the importance of medication and the use of control in certain cases. The 1983 Mental Health Act is to be amended in order to incorporate a new power of supervised discharge which it is hoped will strengthen community care procedures and give sufficient power to certain professionals to provide care in the community to that minority of mentally ill clients who are unable to comply with voluntary care arrangements.

Development of social services departments

The functions and service provisions of the social services of England and Wales are enshrined in a statutory framework (Dobson and Culhane 1991). Major periods of legislation in the first half of this century laid the foundations of current services and legislation was enacted after the Second World War which gave the state responsibility for determining social policy and establishing social welfare systems, universal in character and free to all. The National Health Service was established and local authorities created three departments to provide services to vulnerable groups: Mental Health, Childrens' and Welfare Departments. In 1971, following the Local Authority Social Services Act 1970, these departments were merged into unified personal social services departments.

Democratically elected local authorities have responsibility for the organization of social services departments and for determining how government statute and policy are resourced and implemented locally. The funding of these services is a complex mix of local taxes and central government grant aid. Local variation in these, combined with discretionary elements in the legislation governing service provision, has led to considerable local variation in services.

Social workers, operating from district-based offices, have usually acted as the main gateway to the residential, day and domiciliary services provided by their local authority social services departments. Social workers' responsibilities include a number of statutory duties in relation to certain categories of clients, for example designated approved social workers have responsibility for assessments for compulsory admission to hospital under the 1959, and later the 1983, Mental Health Acts.

Until 1974 social workers based in hospitals were employed by the health authorities. Responsibility for their employment was then transferred to local authorities, thus enabling them to take on similar statutory responsibilities to their district colleagues and provide better integration of the social services provided to people as they moved into or out of hospital.

The Local Authority Social Services Act 1970 created social service departments with generic social workers expected to provide a service to all client groups. In recent years, a number of factors have created the need for a return to a greater degree of specialization. New laws have been enacted which have placed increasingly complex duties on social workers. The Children Act 1989 plus the implications of care management and the purchaser–provider split have led to major restructuring in social services departments, once again creating specialist departments focused on particular client groups.

Development of community-based mental health services

In recent years, and particularly over the past decade, sectorization of NHS psychiatric services has developed in England and Wales. 'Sectorization is the establishment of small geographical catchment areas with dedicated mental health staff providing care for all patients living in the area' (Johnson and Thornicroft 1993). While sectorization has occurred without central planning and with little evaluation, it is clear that it has advantages, such as accessibility to the community served and the development of close working relationships with primary care and other relevant local services. Certain services, such as the rehabilitation of long-term psychiatric in-patients, and the provision of out-of-hours emergency cover have generally been provided from a central base. For reasons of cost effectiveness, these and some other specialist services may, to a large extent, need to remain centralized. Careful planning will be needed to ensure effective links with sectors and the development of good referral and communication systems.

The following four service models for sectorized services have been described (Strathdee and Thornicroft 1992).

- *Model 1.* The Hospital Core Model, where the hospital forms the core of a system with closely coordinated facilities, such as day hospitals and mental health centres, located strategically in the community.
- *Model 2.* The Community Mental Health Centre Model involves the use of a community base within each sector which can provide a location for both acute and continuing care services and a base for outreach services with links to relevant voluntary facilities and social services.
- *Model 3.* The Integrated Primary Care Model postulates a method of working where most assessments, crisis interventions and out-patient work is carried out at health centres and in other primary care settings by members of the sector team. Team members would have specific liaison with general practitioners, social services and other relevant agencies. In-patient facilities would be provided on the hospital site.
- *Model 4.* The Assertive Outreach or Home-based Treatment Model may be most suitable for that core of hard-to-reach patients, unable or unwilling to attend at clinics or mental health services.

In practical terms the models of service actually developed are likely to contain elements from more than one of these.

Alongside the sectorization of services, other changes have to be taken into account. Service planning at the regional level of health authorities and service delivery at district level have undergone changes in relation to the purchaser–provider split introduced in recent years. There has been encouragement by the government for hospitals to develop into self-governing trusts. Where this has happened it is still too early for a full evaluation to be possible, and it is likely to be some years before the full effects can be seen and evaluated.

The voluntary sector

Where services to vulnerable adults are concerned, voluntary organizations in England and Wales have a long and honourable tradition. Nationally, an organization such as MIND, the National Association for Mental Health, has been a focus for both education and information, acting as a political pressure group, and providing advocacy services for users. The very nature of the focus and commitment available from such organizations has meant that they are frequently at the forefront of the development and setting up of locally relevant specialist services which, when successful, have received financial and other support from the statutory services. The National Schizophrenia Fellowship has a history of funding relevant research, and, by way of local groups, has provided much needed support to the relatives of sufferers. Typical projects developed and run by local MIND groups could include day centre or counselling services, and supported housing facilities. The funding of such organizations is a complex mix of charitable donations and funding by local and central government.

Recent legislative changes and the development of purchaser–provider splits in both health and social services have produced changes in the structures and functioning of many voluntary agencies. The arrangement for grant aiding by local government has been changed, and, alongside the private sector, voluntary agencies are being encouraged to develop day and residential services relevant to those users who fit the eligibility criteria of local authority social services and health authorities. In order to ensure that services remain relevant and good value for money, monitoring of these services by local authorities has been given high priority.

Voluntary organizations are often small and with rudimentary administration and support systems. In order to meet the challenge of their new role and deal effectively with interagency planning mechanisms they have been grouping together at a local level into alliances or partnerships.

Defining the service user group

Hospital- and community-based psychiatric services have been responsible for meeting virtually all the mental health needs in their geographically defined catchment areas. Services have to be provided for both those suffering from serious and chronically disabling mental illnesses, as well as those with milder forms of illness or short-term reactive crises.

Government policy documents and the recent community care legislation have made it clear that the priority group to be targeted should be the long-term mentally ill (LTMI), but whilst legislation has prioritized the seriously mentally ill, this grouping has not been specifically defined, apart from some operational definitions by health service providers outlined below.

Bachrach (1988) suggests that three parameters – diagnosis, duration and disability – are necessary in the definition of the LTMI.

Goldman (1981) defines the chronically mentally ill as follows:

* Diagnosis (DSM-111-R of):
  – schizophrenia and schizoaffective disorder 295.x
  – bipolar disorders and major depression 296.x
  – delusional (paranoid) disorder 297.x
* duration one year or more since onset
* disability sufficiently severe to cause serious impairment of functioning in one or more of the following areas:
  – family responsibilities
  – occupation
  – accommodation.

McLean and Liebowitz (1989) suggest that one or more of the following should be present:

* at least two years contact with psychiatric services
* the prescription of depot medication
* ICD diagnosis 295.x or 297.x
* at least three in-patient admissions in the last two years
* at least three day-patient episodes in the last two years
* DSM-111 'highest level of adaptive functioning in past year' rating of at least 5.

International Classification of Diseases (ICD), definitions of mental illness have been used in both Goldman's and McLean's examples. While these are health service definitions, Strathdee and Thornicroft (1992) suggest that as agencies form closer links in implementing community care a common language is needed in order to define service priorities. Their model, which is problem-orientated rather than diagnostic, has been drawn from Falloon (1988). Because of its potential usefulness in the planning and integration of services it is presented in full (Table 2.1).

Development of services in Wandsworth

The move towards care in the community, multidisciplinary working practices and close integration of services can be prescribed and encouraged by legislation and government policy documents, but in order for it to be successful, collaborative and innovative planning and consistent working together at all levels is necessary. Health authorities and social services departments are large, bureaucratic organizations, each with different planning, organizational and operational structures. While their tasks are governed by statute, social services departments are accountable to politicians at local government level and subject to considerable policy swings if the party in power changes. They also have major responsibilities in other areas of work, chiefly children at risk and in need of care. Health authorities on the other hand are subject to considerable involvement by central government, and are still in the process of dealing with the running down of many large, old hospital premises.

Table 2.1 A framework for interagency definition of severely mentally ill

Impairments	Disabilities	Handicaps
	Cognitive:	
Difficulties in thinking	Inefficient problem solving	Lack of friends
Interference with thought processes	Slowed learning	Unemployment
Distressing experiences of sight, sound or touch		
	Affective:	
Unusual, strange beliefs	Severe anxiety and fear	Limited leisure activities
Difficulty in movements and actions	Feelings of inadequacy	Poor housing and self-care
Decreased concentration		
	Behavioural:	
Loss of energy and drive	Low rate of constructive actions	Carer's burden
Reduced ability to solve problems		

Wandsworth is the largest of the inner London boroughs, with a population of 258 000. The 1991 census confirmed previous estimates that 20 per cent of the borough's population are of ethnic minority origin. This minority is mainly made up of Afro-Caribbeans, Africans and Asians, with a slight predominance of the former. The borough is bounded on one side by the river Thames, and while it contains a certain amount of industry is predominantly residential. There is a considerable amount of Victorian and Edwardian property, and a number of large high-rise council estates. While there are environmentally pleasant and affluent residential areas, in the north-east of the borough conditions are considerably more crowded, with a number of large council housing estates. This inner-city area of Battersea contains a number of electoral wards with high levels of social deprivation. Recent council policies of selling off housing stock have led to a certain amount of gentrification, but the concentration of deprivation and social problems in much of the area continues, with a resultant pressure on health and social services.

Psychiatric services for most of the borough are the responsibility of the Wandsworth Health Authority (WHA), with in-patient services provided at a Victorian hospital situated within the borough. A smaller area in the west of the borough has, in the past, been the responsibility of a neighbouring health authority. Recent changes in the structures of regional and district health authorities look set to continue with an increasing emphasis on the purchaser–provider split. Government policy has encouraged health authorities to apply to become self-governing, independent trusts. Change is now the order of the day and it is likely that health services in Wandsworth will undergo considerable restructuring.

Wandsworth Social Services Department is quite well endowed with mental health resources, including two day centres and four hostels. There is a strong local Association of Mental Health (MIND) responsible for running supported shared houses and a 'drop-in' day centre for the LTMI. There is some input to the mental health of racial minority groups via UNITY, a voluntary organization running a counselling service and hostels mainly for Africans and Afro-Caribbeans. The borough also contains several voluntary sector residential care homes.

The planning process

A strategic planning team consisting of senior managers from both the district health authority (DHA) and the local authority began meeting in June 1987. Their remit was to advise on the development of a local and comprehensive community service for the mentally ill in the borough of Wandsworth. In the autumn of the same year several teams were established at a more local level to report on service priorities. These teams consisted of DHA and SSD representatives, including front-line managers and practitioners, catchment area psychiatrists, general practitioners and representatives from the relevant voluntary sector organizations including housing associations and those with a brief for ethnic minorities.

Gaps in service and lack of knowledge of and access to services for both referrers and users were highlighted and reported to the strategic planning team by these short-life groups. A number of recommendations were made and planning schedules for their implementation set in motion.

The interim report of the strategic planning team (1988) recognized that achieving major changes in the focus, style, organization and standards of a service is a gradual process comprising numerous incremental, operational and strategic changes. It also requires constant encouragement, monitoring and review and all in accordance with an agreed set of principles, strategic aims and structure. Recognition of the resource implications of achieving the *process* of service development as well as the *outcome* was considered critically important. Whilst the hospital services remained it was recognized that resources could not be released from them and that budgeting finance was required to build up community services.

Six community mental health teams were to be established with appropriate multidisciplinary staffing. These teams would provide coordinated, integrated and continuing care in the community, and they would provide the focus for the mental health services for the population within each of their catchment areas. Improved outreach support to voluntary and other agencies supporting long-term seriously mentally ill clients was to be one of the aims of these teams.

A better range of day care services specifically orientated to the mentally ill was considered important to help reduce patient stay in hospital and where possible provide a more acceptable alternative to in-patient care.

Day facilities should include sheltered work schemes and, because of a well-recognized gap in the services, a patients' finance officer should be appointed to provide help and guidance with welfare benefits.

The provision of appropriate housing, properly managed and supported, was recognized to be a crucial and necessary resource for those long-term chronically ill who require a high degree of support, possibly for the rest of their lives. The model chosen for this was of houses, ideally clustered, managed by housing associations or voluntary agencies, with client care support provided by dedicated WHA nursing, occupational therapy and other support staff. This model was based on a scheme already existing in the borough, where the less seriously ill were supported in shared houses, owned and managed by housing associations and supported by workers employed by the local Association of Mental Health.

Throughout the planning process there was a clear recognition that the focus of the services should be on the long-term and seriously mentally ill. The report stated 'that due to the debilitating nature of long-term chronic mental illness many clients never make overt demands but slip further into isolation. These people require a highly pro-active, flexible and approachable service with resources dedicated to outreach work which encourages and sustains engagement' (Interim report 1988). It was noted that there were insufficient resources to allow for significant investment in services for the less seriously mentally ill.

In order to plan adequately for the relevant client group a definition of the LTMI was decided upon and a case register set up, to be updated on an annual basis in order to provide information for forward planning. To be included in the register a person had to be aged between 16 and 75 years, currently in contact with the psychiatric services, with first contact at least two years previously.

Development of community mental health teams (CMHTs) in Wandsworth

Of major significance in the development of community mental health teams (CMHTs) in Wandsworth was the example provided by the experience of the Doddington Edward Wilson (DEW) Mental Health Team (McLean and Liebowitz 1990). This was a specialist team appointed incrementally between 1984 and 1988. It was set up supernumerary to the hospital service, to attempt to reach a certain group of patients whose needs were not being met by the conventional catchment area teams. It had been discovered that 60 per cent of the admissions to the acute beds of the catchment area psychiatric hospital were readmissions of long-term patients. The support available during the much longer periods spent by these patients in the community was minimal compared with that available during hospital in-patient stays.

The multidisciplinary team functioned with an outreach model, and was based in small office premises on a large council housing estate in Battersea, in the north east of the borough, an area already mentioned for its concentration of social problems. In an attempt to minimize the stigma attached to mental illness, patients were seen at home, or in GPs' surgeries, and all patient activities were carried out in non-mental-health premises. The team planned to establish working links with relevant community agencies and facilities, and having established them aimed to maintain them. A major part of the team's strategy was to encourage and set up a series of social support groups, and where possible initiate these jointly with another agency. In order to provide continuity of care for these LTMI patients and prevent drop-out, systems for regular monitoring and review were implemented, with these continuing long-term even when patients were enjoying long periods of stability.

Although the team eventually lost its supernumerary status and became a catchment area team, projects its members had initiated, and much of its style of working, remained. It has provided a model from which other CMHTs being set up in the borough have been able to learn.

Liaison with housing and social services departments

The team's aims of establishing working links with non-mental-health community agencies bore fruit in a variety of ways. One example was the liaison group set up involving local authority housing department officers, hospital and area social workers and consultant psychiatrists from DEW and catchment area teams. The group met quarterly for one and a half hours, with the purpose of sharing relevant information and discussing tenants presenting behaviour problems so that, where possible, attempts could be made to lessen or resolve them. All those attending the meeting respected the confidentiality of the information presented.

This meeting was of value to the three agencies involved, and with almost the same format it continues in the Battersea area and has provided a model for similar meetings to be set up in other parts of the borough. While many clients are well known to the agencies concerned, and remain on the discussion list for long periods, new referrals can be picked up where the information suggests that investigation by health or social services may be helpful. The meeting provides a model of purposeful working together between the agencies involved, encourages good working relationships and the development and use of other relevant channels of referral and of information sharing.

Initiation of projects

Another example of a useful project initiated by the DEW team and which still continues to function is the Garfield Contact Group. Initially set up involving workers from the DEW team and from the local social services area team, Garfield is a weekly social group meeting for two hours over lunchtime in a local community centre.

This group, which also provides occasional outings has proved to be an extremely useful way of providing support to a number of LTMI socially isolated clients. Social groups or clubs have long been an important resource in the care of the LTMI, and at any one time several were likely to be in existence in Wandsworth. These had usually been set up and run by social services, or a health-authority-employed voluntary services officer. Garfield is jointly funded and run, with rent paid by the health authority, and the cost of refreshments and outings provided by the social services department. Regular input to the group is provided by a community psychiatric nurse, occupational therapist, and social worker demonstrating joint working in practice.

CMHT links with day care

Patmore and Weaver (1990) have suggested the importance for community mental health centres (CMHCs) of having an attached day centre or social club. This aided teams working with LTMI clients who, through attendance at the day centre, were able to form relationships with more than one worker. This enabled easier cover arrangements during periods when clients' key workers were on leave. Contact with clients attending the day centre meant their mental state and general level of functioning could be monitored in an ongoing and non-intrusive way and saved key workers time which could be used for other interventions. Where CMHTs do not have attached day centres, clubs like Garfield can have a similar function in allowing workers to keep contact with their clients. Given the high costs of day care and the varying rates of occupancy, such clubs can be an economic and effective use of resources and worker time in providing for certain social needs of the LTMI. As CMHTs have developed in Wandsworth it is now usual for their staff members to be involved in the setting up and running of such clubs.

Operational policies of CMHTs

Research in this country has suggested (Patmore and Weaver 1990) that many CMHCs tend to work with the 'worried well' and neglect the needs of the LTMI. CMHCs may differ somewhat from CMHTs in that the central base is the focus for the delivery of services. The staff group is usually multidisciplinary, but sometimes only includes limited input from psychiatrists. A number of factors need to be taken into account in order to ensure focus on the LTMI. Firstly, teams require a clear written and agreed operational policy, defining the target client group and outlining methods of assessment, allocation, monitoring and review. Secondly the importance of selecting clients from the known group of LTMI must be ensured via, for example, the caseloads of community psychiatric nurses (CPNs), and discharges from relevant psychiatric hospital wards. Links with GPs' surgeries, and 'walk in' clinics were seen as likely to attract the 'worried well' and did not often reach the LTMI. Thirdly, the practice of *ad hoc* self-allocation, in the absence of clear client eligibility criteria tended to encourage workers to select clients with problems which matched their personal skills and interests, and these were rarely the LTMI. It was also noted that the most successful teams had well-planned systems of management and accountability.

In Wandsworth CMHTs were developed on an incremental basis. As suitable premises became available in the community, conventional catchment area psychiatric teams moved into them, produced operational policies, and took on their new title of CMHT. Following on from the example of DEW where social workers were an integral part of the team, social workers moved into the CMHTs, although in the employ of the social services department and accountable to it. Apart from DEW, which covered a much smaller geographical area, the other two teams in Battersea had catchment area populations of around 32 000. Each team had the use of around 15 acute in-patient beds, with DEW having about half this number.

While a certain framework was imposed by the health authority, and teams were expected to follow the mental health unit's agreed strategy, each CMHT was encouraged to develop its own style in meeting the needs of its particular catchment area. A responsive and flexible attitude to referrals was recognized as important, and CMHTs ensured relevant agencies were provided with information about referral criteria and the services on offer. Following on DEWs earlier example, team members formed and maintained links with relevant community resources, for example a Family Welfare Association mental health day centre.

Working practices in CMHTs

While each CMHT was headed by a consultant psychiatrist, a coordinator, possibly the team's clinical psychologist, acted as budget holder and had responsibility for team coordination. The development of team work was considered extremely important, and when a CMHT was in the process of forming, a team or 'away' day was often part of the process. An outside facilitator was usual on such occasions, with the day being given over to reviewing practice and considering ways to improve team working processes and methods of work. The central plank of the CMHT was its weekly referral and review meeting, when, following assessment, team members met to allocate new referrals, and systematically review long-term cases.

While many cases were handled by way of office interviews, home assessments were common. If referral information indicated it might be useful, assessments could be carried out by two team members working in partnership. Team working was facilitated by the development of multidisciplinary casenote systems. In CMHTs where most members spend the majority of their working hours away from base, often in intensive and sometimes stressful client contact, the team secretary was of central importance. Informal mutual support and supervision was provided by way of shared case discussion and team working practices. CMHTs often supplemented this by a regular monthly visit from a psychotherapist, enabling a psychodynamic consideration of the needs of particular clients, and providing additional support and education for team members.

The development of relevant community groups had been an important part of the work of the DEW team. In line with this, the hospital's occupational therapy department developed a strong community focus. Gradually a series of social support groups had been set up, particularly in the Battersea area. Anxiety management and other therapeutic groups were run regularly. The continued development and coordination of groupwork in the area was handled by way of a regular meeting attended by CMHT representatives, and staff from health and social services involved in running groups.

Patmore and Weaver (1990) investigated 12 CMHCs and identified serious weaknesses in several, particularly in terms of lack of focus on the agreed target client group, the LTMI. Wandsworth's CMHTs are multidisciplinary catchment area psychiatric teams responsible for all mental health referrals within their area, although with access to relevant specialist services such as rehabilitation and forensic psychiatry. The CMHT is thus under pressure to prioritize the seriously mentally ill in line with the borough's community care strategy, which encourages a focus on the acute and long-term mentally ill.

Role of the key worker

Since 1991 district health authorities have been required to implement the care programme approach for patients with mental illness. Under the terms of the NHS Community Care Act a named key worker has to be appointed for all patients who require this approach and for whom a care plan has been drawn up. In Wandsworth the key worker was defined as the team member responsible for arranging the individual care plan in consultation with the multidisciplinary team and for arranging regular reviews. The key worker might be responsible for part or all of the specified care and could draw in other professionals or agencies in the light of the changing needs of the patient.

The move towards a key worker system in the developing CMHTs has meant a considerable change from the way patients have been dealt with by conventional psychiatric teams. In these the patient might have contact with several members of the team, for example a psychiatrist, a CPN or a social, worker but no one professional had a clear coordinating role. Having a named key worker means patient, relatives and outside agencies having one clear point of contact.

Patmore and Weaver (1990) have pointed out some of the drawbacks of key workers being too autonomous. They found some workers taking on tasks for which their training did not equip them. Clearly this is something which has to be recognized and addressed in CMHTs.

Multidisciplinary team work

CMHTs in Wandsworth comprise professionals from the following health service professions; psychiatry, community psychiatric nursing, psychology and occupational therapy. Social workers, employed by the local authority social services department, are integral team members, but are managed from outside the team. They also have some duties separate from it in providing a social services mental health emergency duty system.

Team members are responsible to their professional line managers for those tasks which are specific to their profession. However, in CMHTs with key working systems, considerable overlap can develop between the different professionals, and is necessary if clients are to have a satisfactory service. Joint working and consultation between different disciplines can enhance skills and provide support in this process. When specific needs arise, for example care management or knowledge of welfare benefits, joint training can be provided. Where team members engage in tasks which require new skills, outside supervision can be arranged, for example, where a CPN and social worker undertook to run a group for adult survivors of sexual abuse.

With the increasing shift of psychiatric services from hospital to the community the importance of flexible multidisciplinary working practices will continue to grow. Recent research in Wandsworth (Burns *et al.* 1993) noted the value of full utilization of the resources within the multidisciplinary team and suggested that a key worker approach could be useful even in relatively short-term treatments. Assertive, outreach ways of working are likely to continue to grow and develop in CMHTs in Wandsworth.

Development of care management in Wandsworth

In March 1991 Wandsworth Social Services Department was reorganized into specialist departments. The creation of a specialist mental health sector enabled the integration of hospital and community-based social workers and encouraged a more focused specialization in work with people with mental health problems, including the involvement of senior managers in joint planning as laid down by the National Health Service and Community Care Act 1990.

This Act has given local authority social services departments responsibility for setting up systems of assessment and care management, and transferred funds from the DSS to give them the responsibility for the funding of residential and nursing home care. In Wandsworth Social Services Department purchasing budgets for residential care have been devolved to team manager level, with social workers taking on care manager functions. It is recognized that in the case of work with the LTMI assessment is usually multidisciplinary and in Wandsworth a care management system has been agreed which allows not only social workers in CMHTs, but also any of the other disciplines, to take on the role of care manager.

While there are similarities between the care programme and care management approach, there are also differences, particularly in the care manager's responsibility to budget for packages of care. It remains to be seen whether the two approaches can be successfully integrated.

Conclusions

In recent years there has been massive change in the provision of health and social care. Structural and organizational change is set fair to continue as the major organizations attempt to rationalize their services. Under the NHS reforms in April 1991 district health authorities have been given the responsibility of improving the health of their resident populations. They therefore have to assess health needs and ensure that these needs are met by purchasing relevant health services from NHS providers and by close working with social services, family health services authorities and voluntary organizations. Local authority social services departments are having to develop an enabling role. In the process of developing an internal market, as well as purchasing and commissioning services from the private and voluntary sectors, health and social services are increasingly under pressure to change and adapt to the market economy and to ensure that services are relevant and cost effective. Consultation with users and carers and regular monitoring and evaluation of services is now an important part of the process.

Collaboration in planning and a shared strategy are of key importance in the development and integration of relevant and accessible services for people with mental health problems. The growth of services is an organic process, and while new ideas need to be tested out, successful services will only grow out of projects or services which over time prove both useful and cost effective.

References

Bachrach L L (1988). Defining chronic mental illness: a concept paper. *Hospital and Community Psychiatry*, **39**, 383–388.

Burns T, Beadsmoore A M, Bhat A V, Oliver A and Malhers C (1993). A controlled trial of home-based acute psychiatric services. *British Journal of Psychiatry*, **163**, 49–61.

Department of Health and Social Security (1975). *Better Services for the Mentally Ill*. Cmnd 6233, HMSO, London.

Department of Health (1991). *Care Management and Assessment: Managers Guide*. HMSO, London, p. 12.

Department of Health (1989). *Caring for People: Community Care in the Next Decade and Beyond*. HMSO, London.

Dobson, H and Culhane M (1991). Social work and the elderly mentally ill. In *Psychiatry in the Elderly* (eds. R Jacoby and C Oppenheimer). Oxford Medical Publications, Oxford.

Falloon I (1988). The prevention of morbidity in schizophrenia. In *Handbook of Behavioural Family Therapy* (ed. I Falloon). Hutchinson, London.

Goldman H, Gattozzi A and Taube C (1981). Defining and counting the chronically mentally ill. *Community Psychiatry*, **31**, 21.

Griffiths R (1988). *Community Care: An Agenda for Action*. HMSO, London.

House of Commons (1985). *Second Report from the Social Services Committee, Session 1984-85 Community Care*. HMSO, London.

Hunter D and Wistow G (1987). Mapping the organisational context. 1. Central departments, boundaries and responsibilities. In *Community Care in Britain, Valuations on a Theme* (eds. D Hunter and G Wistow). King Edward's Hospital Fund for London, London.

Interim Report of the Strategic Planning Team (October 1988). Services for People with Mental Illness in Wandsworth. Unpublished report, Wandsworth Health Authority.

Johnson S and Thornicroft G (1993). The sectorization of psychiatric services in England and Wales. *Social Psychiatry and Psychiatric Epidemiology*, **28**, 45–47.

McLean E and Liebowitz J (1989). Towards a working definition of the long-term mentally ill. *Psychiatric Bulletin*, **13**, 251–252.

McLean E K and Liebowitz J (1990). A community mental health team to serve revolving door patients: the Doddington Edward Wilson (DEW) mental health team 1984–1988. *The International Journal of Social Psychiatry*, **36** (3), 172–182.

Onyett S R (1991). An agenda for care programming and care management. *Health Services Management*, **87** (4), 180–183.

Onyett, S R (1991). *Case Management in Mental Health*. Chapman and Hall, London.

Patmore C and Weaver J (1990). *A Survey of Community Mental Health Centres. Good Practices in Mental Health, London*.

Strathdee G and Thornicroft G (1992). Community sectors for needs led mental health services. In *Measuring Mental Health Needs* (eds. G Thornicroft, C Bulwin and J Ling). Royal College of Psychiatrists, London.

Thornicroft G, Ward P and James S (1993). Countdown to community care. Care management and mental health. *British Medical Journal*, **306**, 768–771.

Acknowledgement

I would like to acknowledge many helpful contributions from colleagues in both Wandsworth Social Services Department and Wandsworth Health Authority.

3 Policy and finance for community care: the new mixed economy

J. Beecham, M.R.J. Knapp and J. Schneider

Introduction

There have long been many different providers of mental health care – particularly health and local authorities, charities and private therapists – and a multiplicity of funding routes. However, the reforms introduced by the 1990 NHS and Community Care Act promise to move the mixed economy of mental health care to new levels and in new directions. Market forces in particular are receiving their biggest boost for 50 years or more. There ought to be major implications for service users, staff and budgets if the government's expectations are realized.

The 1990 Act reinforces the importance of a mixed economy of health and social care in which increasing engagement with the independent sector is encouraged, in which service users and their carers have more influence over both their own service use and broader community care planning, and in which the balance of responsibilities between the NHS and local government is, if not actually resolved, at least clarified.

The aim of this chapter is to examine the implications of the mixed economy for mental health care. The community care reforms are introduced in the next section. We then present a conceptual framework for describing and analysing the developing mixed economy of mental health care. We then progress from the specific case of the voluntary sector, using data from a recent survey, to the complex interrelationships of services and funders for community care. Next we discuss the characteristics of markets with reference to mental health care, and explore the potential for joint commissioning. Our conclusions in the last section sum up the 'state of the mixed economy' in mental health care and highlight the developing roles for, *inter alia*, markets and joint commissioning.

The context – the community care reforms

One interpretation of the 1990 reforms would see them as the logical culmination of social, clinical and economic trends over the post-war decades (and earlier), with the Act pulling together a number of disparate elements and widely accepted though poorly structured intentions. An alternative view is that the 1990 Act was simply the extension into the health and social care arenas of Mrs Thatcher's zeal for market reform. Another interpretation is that the changes were the expedient, though delayed, reactions to a number of economic and social problems (and therefore also political problems) which had gathered considerable cumulative weight over the 1980s, including some well-publicized cases of neglect and rapidly escalating social security expenditure to support people in residential care and nursing homes.

The reality is probably some combination of all three interpretations. The 1990 reforms certainly included some clear continuations of good long-standing (though often only localized) health and social care practices, such as the better targeting of services on needs and the involvement of users in decision-making. The reforms also crystallized some more recent practices, such as care management. They were imbued with enough emphasis on privatization to satisfy most conservative voters and backbench MPs, whilst preserving the central ('enabling') roles of public sector agencies. But there is no denying that the organization and delivery of health and social care were weak in several areas:

- The community care system was dominated by perverse incentives and poor targeting, with the result that wasteful overlaps of agency responsibilities existed alongside yawning gaps in service responses to need.
- There was an enormous drain on social security revenue as a result of the access to residential and nursing home care without adequate assessment of care needs. By April 1993, the social security funding of these services (for all user groups) had reached £1568 million per annum (House of Commons Health Committee 1993).
- The burdens placed on family and other informal carers were uncompensated and inequitable. The General Household Survey showed that in 1990 there were 6.8 million carers in Great Britain, of whom 1.5 million (63 per cent of them women) spent 20 hours per week or more in caring activities (OPCS 1992).
- The rate of development of new or expanded community facilities was much too slow when compared with the speed of planned hospital run-down or the intended shift away from long-term residential or nursing home care. There were too few community-based alternatives to residential care, especially in the independent sector
- Many people with mental or physical disabilities or age-related needs were left with inadequate assistance, supervision and personal resources. Many of the growing numbers of homeless people in Britain's towns and cities provided dramatic evidence of the failings of community care.

The 1989 White Paper, *Caring for People*, sought to address these community care weaknesses, and the 1990 NHS and Community Care Act subsequently introduced the most sweeping changes to health and social care since the 1940s.

The reforms to community social care can be summarized as the encouragement of movement along four core strategic dimensions (Social Services Inspectorate 1992; Wistow *et al.* 1994). The first is the balance between institutional and community care. The 1990 Act explicitly encourages local authorities to shift the emphasis away from institutional in favour of community or domiciliary-based care, just as it also encouraged 'strategic shift' between in-patient and community-based treatment in the health service. The second strategic policy objective is to move the community care system away from supply-led, provider-dominated services to a system of needs-led, purchaser-dominated services. It is intended that services should be much more sensitive and responsive to the needs and preferences of users and their carers. The development of care or case management is being strongly encouraged to assist in this regard.

Alteration of the balance of responsibility for decision-making, funding and monitoring between the National Health Service and local government is the third element of the new community care policy. This change to the balance of responsibility should not be exaggerated, for it really only relates to those needs and services grouped under the 'social care' banner, but the change represents a clear attempt to improve collaboration and coordination in planning, commissioning and service provision. Thus far, it has mainly been achieved through the transfer of funds from the Department of Social Security to social services departments, the latter being given the lead role in community care. Jointly agreed annual community care plans and the development of joint commissioning are contributing in small but important ways.

The final dimension is the explicit emphasis on further development of the mixed economy of care: the encouragement of greater pluralism in provision, especially with markedly greater roles for private and voluntary agencies, and – over time, though certainly not yet on the main political agenda – the development of alternative sources of funding. Local authorities are rapidly replacing general grant aid to voluntary organizations with contractual links, floating off some of their own services to not-for-profit agencies, and grappling with the ideological and practical challenges of working more closely with the private sector. It is this fourth strategic dimension which is of particular relevance to this chapter.

The mixed economy of mental health care

A clear distinction can be drawn between the funding and supply dimensions of a mixed economy: between purchasing and providing (Knapp 1989). The two dimensions capture quite different responsibilities and forces, although it needs the combination of the two to reflect real world practice and potential future policy. The distinction is helpful not only for didactic reasons, but also when trying to stimulate or massage the mixed economy into a new shape through national and local policy initiatives, for it clarifies public authorities' fundamental objectives and can help to reduce the vested interests of providers. Central government has also stressed the benefits of purchaser–provider separation for the promotion of supply-side competition. Separating the principles of purchasing and providing enables a clearer distinction to be made between two sets of policy rationales: those behind supply-side subsidies to the voluntary sector, such as tax exemptions, grants or purchase of service contracts, and those rationales behind demand-side subsidies to consumers of voluntary sector services, such as income support payments or vouchers.

Four main provider sectors can be distinguished: public, voluntary, private and informal.

- The *public sector* includes local authorities, with responsibilities for social care, education, leisure, recreation and library facilities; the National Health Service, with its separate purchaser and provider units; and the Department of Social Security. Local authority social services departments are the pivotal agents of the new community care system.
- The *voluntary sector* comprises all those formal organizations which are independent of government and which, although they may earn profits, cannot distribute them to any owners or shareholders. Many, but not all, voluntary organizations have charitable status, conferring certain tax advantages and ensuring Charity Commission oversight. Closer monitoring comes through the contractual and inspection roles of local authorities.
- The *private sector* is profit-seeking and distributing, and constitutionally separate from government. In recent years, the private sector has become a much more important provider of services for all adult user groups, especially in residential care and nursing home settings.
- The *informal or household sector* is the fourth main provider group. It comprises a large number of individual carers (family members, neighbours and others) and some small groups of carers, but only such groups as have no formal constitution or set of rules.

On the other side of the new health and social care markets are the purchasers. We can distinguish a variety of different *purchasing routes* or *types of demand*. For example, we could distinguish the following six main routes:

- *Coerced collective demands*: where the public sector acts as purchaser on behalf of citizens, mandated by the electoral process. Funding comes predominantly from (coercive) central and local taxation, regulated through the democratic process. Health authority and GP fundholder purchases are the most important in mental health.
- *Uncoerced or voluntary collective demand*: voluntary organizations (and occasionally other bodies) use voluntarily donated funds to purchase services on behalf of donors for use by others. Donors do not have any real influence over *who* receives services. Organizations such as the National Schizophrenia Fellowship, MIND and the Mental After Care Association provide some services from donated funds.
- *Corporate demand*: funding or support in kind from private sector corporations or firms. For example, a company might provide counselling or other mental health care support or treatment to its employees.
- *Uncompensated individual demand:* payment for goods or services used by the payer, but not subsidized from social security or other transfer payments. An example is privately arranged sessions of psychotherapy.
- *Compensated individual consumption:* also payment for consumption by the payer, but now subsidized from transfer payments such as social security and housing benefit. For example, prescription charges are waived for people with low incomes, and there are income support payments for people accommodated in residential and nursing home care before April 1993.
- *Individual donation*: payment for goods and services to be used by someone else, payments being made directly to suppliers and not to voluntary

(or other) organizations as intermediary bodies (the latter being uncoerced collective demand). For example, families might pay for residential care for an elderly relative with dementia.

Cross-classifying the provider and purchaser dimensions produces a simple and informative representation of a pluralist welfare system (Table 3.1). The resultant 24-celled matrix is a stylized description of the myriad inter-relationships between demand and supply – between purchasers and providers – within the mixed economy of mental health care. Interestingly, every cell of the matrix can be filled with examples of mental health care provision and funding. The mixed economy before implementation of the 1990 Act already contained an array of transaction types which the new legislation seeks to develop and expand.

The same mixed economy matrix allows us to look at policy issues and trends. Arguably, the two most important policy changes now in train are: (a) the promotion of market forces, whether in an 'internal', NHS-dominated market or an 'external', local-authority-instigated market involving private and voluntary providers; and (b) the encouragement of the private and voluntary provider sectors to deliver more and different services. Both represent changes in the mixed economy of supply. A contrary policy shift – one which has diminished the mixed economy of purchasing relative to its position before implementation of the 1990 Act – was the rerouting of the funding of residential and nursing home care from demand-side to supply-side subsidies (and via local government rather than the Department of Social Security) from April 1993. Figure 3.1 ranges beyond mental health care itself, and illustrates how the framework locates some policy options. For example, the conventional post-war welfare state can best be summarized as public sector provision funded from taxation (coerced collective demand). User charges for local authority day care are located within the public provider column and uncompensated individual demand row.

The real world of the mixed economy is more complex than these summary diagrams, but even so we can see that the mixed economy in 1994 is already well developed. Most people confidently expect further evolution over the latter part of the 1990s, especially in relation to the sources or routes of funding. The real world is also more complex because of the blurred boundaries between provider types and funding types. For example, the not-for-profit organizations being established by some local authorities around floated-off former public sector facilities straddle the public/voluntary divide. Some self-help groups are partly formal voluntary organization and partly a loose grouping of informal carers. Innovative funding mechanisms involving the NHS and the private sector span two or more of the funding types. And, of course, most provider organizations have multiple funding sources.

The mixed economy framework therefore identifies a host of transaction types and policy issues, some of which are discussed below. We can also gather evidence from research completed within the Personal Social Services Research Unit (PSSRU) mental health programme to illustrate some of the issues. We now examine four aspects of the developing mixed economy of mental health: the funding of the voluntary sector services, the funding mix in community care, markets and joint commissioning.

Table 3.1 The mixed economy of mental health care: service examples

Purchase, demand or funding	Provision or supply of services			
	Public sector	Voluntary sector	Private sector	Informal sector
Coerced collective demand	NHS psychiatric hospital	MIND or other day care under contract to a local authority	Publicly funded placements in private nursing homes	Adult foster care
Uncoerced or voluntary collective demand	Voluntary organization payments for public sector training programmes	Self-help group paying for expert advice from larger voluntary organization	Purchases of goods and services by National Schizophrenia Fellowship or Alzheimer's Disease Society	Volunteers providing respite care organized through voluntary organization
Corporate demand	Private residential home payments for LA registration and inspection	Corporate donations to charities	Counselling offered to company employees	Employer-funded stress days: or redundancy payments for mental ill health
Uncompensated individual consumption	User charges for meals in LA day centre	Self-funding meal clubs run by voluntary organization	Payment for private residential care by resident	Exchanges in kind between neighbours
Compensated individual consumption	LA hostel funded by social security entitlements	Income support payments to voluntary homes	Housing benefit and other user subsidies for private housing	Attendance allowance used to purchase informal care
Individual donation (for use by others)	Volunteers working in NHS psychiatric hospital	Donations to the National Schizophrenia Fellowship	Volunteers in private residential homes	Intra-family transfers of resources and care

LA = local authority; NHS = National Health Service

Provision or supply of services

Purchase, demand or funding	Public sector	Voluntary sector	Private sector	Informal sector
Coerced collective demand	Welfare state	Contracting out by the public sector		Support for carers
Uncoerced or voluntary collective demand	National lottery			
Corporate demand		Encouragement of corporate philanthropy		
Uncompensated individual demand	User charges for public services	User-financed care insurance	Textbook markets	
Compensated individual demand	Vouchers for user-controlled care package purchasing			
Individual donation (for use by others)		Tax incentives for charitable donations		Reinforcement of the family

Figure 3.1 The mixed economy of mental health care: policy examples

Funding the voluntary sector

The permutations of care financing can be illustrated by focusing on one provider type, the voluntary sector. This sector is defined as comprising organizations which are formally constituted, independent of government, not distributing profits to those who control them, self-governing, primarily non-sacramental, not party political and benefiting to a meaningful degree from voluntarism (Brenton 1985; Kendall and Knapp 1994). Coupled with private (for-profit) agencies, the voluntary sector is held up in government policy as both an appropriate complement to traditional statutory services and increasingly as a direct substitute. The voluntary sector is certainly of some importance in the development of community mental health care as well as in other areas where social and health care are often indistinguishable. Recent legislation and guidelines on the implementation of community care indicate that voluntary organizations are to be involved as fully as possible (Department of Health 1989; Department of Health 1990; KPMG 1992). They are supposed to be consulted in formulating community care plans, they are to be enabled and encouraged by the public sector, and in England voluntary and private sector providers are beneficiaries of the ring-fenced special transitional grant monies (transferring former income support payments from social security to social services departments).

The mixed economy matrix suggests analysis of mental health care markets from the perspective of both purchasers (rows) and providers (columns). Table 3.1 gives examples of the activities of the voluntary sector both as purchaser or funder and as provider of services. However, most voluntary sector organizations would probably describe themselves as providers (of services, advocacy, research, information) rather than as purchasers or brokers of services on behalf of individuals or groups, and here we explore this dimension of the mixed economy.

A small survey of national voluntary organizations demonstrates the scope and scale of the voluntary sector as a provider of mental health services in 1990, prior to the community care reforms (Schneider and Pinner 1993). This information can be organized by looking at who funds the provision which the voluntary sector provides, based on the sixfold classification of purchaser types shown in Table 3.1. This does not include the many local voluntary organizations working in geographically limited areas which may have a different income distribution from that shown here. The survey also permits us to estimate the total annual income of UK voluntary organizations in mental health at about £40m in 1990. These national organizations employ about 1500 full-time equivalent staff and about 320 full-time equivalent volunteers. Compare this scale of operation to any local authority or health district, and it is clear that the voluntary sector in 1990 was relatively small in terms of personnel and income. Yet its role as a provider of services, funded by sources other than its own coffers, is large in relation to its size.

Twenty-two per cent of the income to the national voluntary organizations working in mental health came from individual donations (Table 3.2). A further 15 per cent came from collective and corporate sources, but a much larger proportion – 48 per cent – came from central funds, including government grants and social security allowances paid through service users' entitlements to housing benefit and residential care allowances, for example. Of course, statutory funding is usually conditional, being paid for specific services or functions, whereas donated income is generally not as restrictive, although receipt may require certain conditions to be fulfilled, such as registration of the organization as a charity.

These data go some way towards dispelling the myth that voluntary organizations are a limitless fount of resources in mental health care. For a large part of their total income in 1990 they were dependent on public sector funding. While the mixed economy of *funding* was already with us in 1990, it remains to be seen how far this will be further diversified by the community care reforms, and whether the main responsibility for mental health care will be shifted further away from public funders. The range and variety of voluntary functions, some examples of which are given in Table 3.1, are evidence of a mixed economy of mental health care *provision*, which with careful tending could continue to flourish, but which in terms of size may be the weaker partner in negotiations with commissioning authorities.

Table 3.2   Funding the voluntary sector

Type of demand	Source of income	Percentage income
Coerced collective demand	European Social Fund, central and local government grants, contracts and housing subsidies	19
Voluntary collective demand	Telethon	2
Corporate demand	Company donations, bank interest, endowments	13
Uncompensated individual demand	Business, fees and other operating income	15
Compensated individual demand	Rent, residential care allowance	29
Individual donation	Individual, in kind and undifferentiated donations	22

Will the terms of the NHS and Community Care Act be sufficient to preserve and promote the voluntary sector? Only, presumably, if public sector commissioners are sufficiently well informed and willing to manage the market. In relation to voluntary organizations, this means facilitating change in structures and funding mechanisms (from grants to contracts, minimizing transactions costs), making secure the existence of valuable but vulnerable providers (perhaps enlisting preferred suppliers, giving longer-term contracts, sharing capital investment), and maintaining standards and quality of care (through advice, training and secondment). If the mixed economy is to continue to develop, voluntary organizations (and other suppliers of care) must be neither smothered with bureaucracy nor starved of resources.

Funding mix and community care

By considering just one of the four provider sectors we have seen the multiplicity of funding sources which now exists. Each funding source takes time to negotiate and agree. But the voluntary sector should be placed in the broader picture of funding for health and social care in the UK. Figure 3.2 aims to describe the main *routes* by which money reaches providers such as the voluntary sector, to be found in the bottom left-hand corner of the diagram. If we focus on the local level, an even wider diversity of routes and interrelationships can be found between funders and providers. Again using research from the PSSRU we can illustrate the routes which finance can take *between* health authorities and describe some of the arrangements which ensured finance flowed to other provider agencies.

One of the four core strategic dimensions of the 1990 Act is the move from institutional to community-based care. The relocation of care from long-stay hospitals to the community (often involving some form of residential care) is one manifestation of this policy. Its implementation has involved the creation of new services to replace all those provided within the old hospitals and, in turn, this has meant the development of new alliances between agencies and new financing arrangements (such as 'dowries') with their own incentives and disincentives.

In the North-East Thames region, a financial transfer mechanism was developed to encourage district health authorities to develop community-based services allowing the closure of two long-stay psychiatric hospitals. The programme started in 1985 and has been the subject of a wide-ranging evaluation (Leff 1993; Knapp *et al.* 1993). The economic evaluation, undertaken by the PSSRU, describes the community services used by the former residents, calculates the associated costs and examines the cost-effectiveness of community care arrangements. An element of this work is inspection of the mix of service provision and funding and of the distributional effects of such a policy.

By 1992, service use data had been collected on 545 former long-stay patients one year after their discharge from hospital. We found that they used nearly 40 different *types* of services, such as accommodation facilities, day care, hospital care (short in-patient stays, out-patient appointments and day treatment), social work, community nursing and primary health care services (Hallam *et al.* 1995). This figure disguises the possible number of providers. The reprovision of hospital care has involved service providers from eight district health authorities and seven social services and other local authority departments. In addition, about 20 voluntary organizations and housing associations, and ten or more private organizations and individuals (mainly supplying residential facilities) provide care services.

There were three main ways in which finance moved between health authorities. First, regional health authority bridging finance was available to district health authorities, over and above their usual allocation, for both capital and revenue expenditure on community services. These reserve funds came not only from the region's own resources (see Figure 3.2) but, during the latter stages of the programme, were also supplemented with money from the sale of one hospital site to private sector developers. Regional resources already

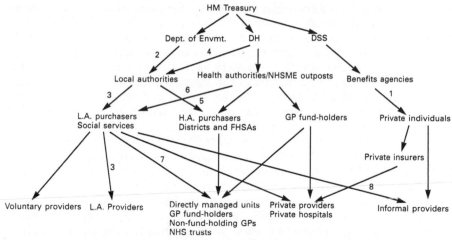

Notes
1 Social security funding via individual claimants
2 Annual revenue support grant
3 Purchaser–provider split is not currently operated
  across all local authorities
4 Special transitional grant and specific
  grants (e.g. drugs and alcohol)

5 Only when trusts or directly managed units provide
  social care
6 E.g. mental illness specific grant
7 E.g. local authority contracts
8 E.g. adult foster schemes

Figure 3.2 Principal funding routes in health and social care, 1994 (adapted from
Knapp and Wistow 1994)

devolved to district level moved from the hospital budget to the community budget via two further routes allowable under the financial transfer mechanism ('dowries'). We can distinguish the *intra*-district flow where, within the district providing hospital care, finance was transferred from the hospital budget to the community health budget to provide replacement services. *Inter*-district finance flows also occurred; the closing hospitals provided services to other districts, and repatriation of hospital residents was assured by transferring a sum of money for their care to their 'home' or receiving district.

Some districts, anxious to retain control of these resources, developed their own facilities but resources were also transferred to other agencies and providers. Regional policy did not stipulate a particular model of care, leaving districts to explore a range of possibilities and resulted in dowry monies being used to fund a diversity of care models. Here we can describe arrangements which illustrate some of the finance routes to providers shown in Figure 3.2. For example, the receiving district health authority might 'purchase' places in the social services psychiatric hostel or in an adult foster care programme. In the latter instance some of the money would also move into the informal sector where it was used to provide a 'top-up' payment to carers who also received money from clients' entitlements to social security benefits. Some of the resources transferred would also be used by the social services department to provide social work support and day care places for residents.

The development of consortia in this region has provided a route for money to move from health authorities to voluntary organizations. Originally, the availability of extra finance through social security care allowances may have been the incentive for health authorities to develop closer links with voluntary organizations, but these consortium arrangements also allowed health funding to enter the voluntary sector for building works or to cover extra revenue costs where higher levels of care were required than could be funded by client entitlements to social security benefits.

In North-East Thames, the voluntary sector played a large role as the *provider* of care – nearly a quarter of the sample of former hospital residents lived in accommodation managed by this sector, and nearly a fifth used voluntary sector day care. When we examined the funding implications of these services, our results reflected those found in the national survey (section 4 above): the role of voluntary organizations as *funders* of care was small. In fact they accounted for less than 6 per cent of the total care costs. Ninety-four per cent of the total costs of care, therefore, was funded by the public sector and this could be further disaggregated. Sixty-five per cent was funded by *coerced collective demand* (50 per cent by district health authorities and family health services authorities and 15 per cent by local government sources), and 29 per cent was funded by users, mainly *compensated individual consumption* through social security entitlements.

These activities, of course, pre-date the 1990 Act but they show how financial incentives, developed to support a specific policy directive, have encouraged greater diversity in service provision than previously provided in the hospitals. Since the implementation of the 1990 Act, public sector agencies involved in mental health care purchase services directly from provider units. Each of the provider units must ensure the service is acceptable to both the potential purchaser and the users. In mental health care these aims may not move in concert, for many users have long-term care needs which must now be satisfied by shorter-term contracts or purchasing (funding) agreements. In the next section we examine some of the implications of creating markets for mental health care and some of the pitfalls which must be avoided.

Markets

The creation of markets in health and social care has the potential to improve efficiency, encourage innovation and expand user and purchaser choice. These were the expectations of central government in framing its health and social care reforms. Public sector agencies have financial incentives to purchase the services which give greater value for money – better quality for a given price, or lower cost for a minimum quality attainment – and financial penalties await the unsuccessful. Competition between providers might be expected to push up quality and pull down prices. Greater participation by users and carers in decision-making should make the public sector more responsive to their needs and wants, and should also influence the types and qualities of services offered by providers. These are the government's expectations (Wistow *et al.* 1994). But a number of critics have raised ideological and political objections to markets. Is reliance on markets in mental health care sensible? There are numerous potential sources of difficulty – what the economist would call 'market failure' – each with implications for the ways in which public authorities perform their commissioning roles. They can be organized under three main heads: market structure, provider power and information difficulties (Knapp *et al.* 1994).

Market structure

There may not be sufficient competition between providers to produce quality and choice improvements or to allow purchasers to negotiate lower prices, whilst maintaining quality standards. Moreover, when one or more provider wields sufficient market power to determine the price, quantity or quality of a service, the market may not operate in the best interests of service users or taxpayers. One fear, therefore, is that there may not be enough independent residential and nursing homes, and certainly not enough domiciliary, day or respite services outside hospital settings to produce the competition – induced advantages which markets can produce. Today's providers may also be unable or unwilling to expand or diversify because the capital outlay is too high or because specialized labour is scarce. Initial heavy investment may commit providers to remain in business, giving them the incentive to undercut the prices of new entrants. We found that, over time, fewer former hospital residents in North-East Thames moved into residential care provided by the private sector (Hallam *et al.* 1995), and some of the homes opened in the early years of the reprovision programme are now concerned about their financial viability.

Provider power

In many areas of the country, therefore, public sector authorities need to encourage and assist new providers to overcome barriers to market entry if sufficient competition is to be created. But provider power over price, orientation or quality of service could also arise if markets become highly specialized, with only a few providers in each 'market segment'. Purchasers face a dilemma. On the one hand, they want to encourage service variety in order to extend the choices open to the designers of care programmes, care managers and users, thus presumably improving service targeting. But each different contract generates extra negotiation, management and monitoring costs for public authorities as well as for providers. On the other hand, if purchasers commission only standardized services in order to cut their transactions costs and open up the possibility of price competition, they may fail to address needs adequately, and providers' individual and distinctive contributions may be missed or destroyed.

Information difficulties

Mental health care is quite different from other so-called service industries like banking or insurance, even from local government services such as refuse collection, housing or grass cutting. Mental health care is also more complex than many other areas of health care in that there are more agencies with financial and service delivery responsibilities, and because the 'health gain' is often hard to observe and measure. To add to the complications, the characteristics of some users make it hard for them to participate in decision-making or to voice their opinions, and users who are very ill or heavily dependent cannot acquire market experience by 'shopping around'. Care is also a very personal service, and users should have a right to express their views on who provides their care. Users might invest heavily in personal relationships with carers, and might be unhappy about changes to contracts. Each of these features of mental health care makes it both difficult and costly to monitor provider performance, and consequently can be a source of market difficulties. Commissioners have to spend scarce funds to acquire information on existing and potential providers, and on the implications of provision for users. The challenge for commissioners or purchasers is to avoid incurring transaction costs in agreeing and monitoring contracts which exceed the efficiency savings from getting lower cost providers to deliver services. Do they again plump for the standardized contracting and commissioning procedures?

This may be one of the reasons why a number of local and health authorities prefer to work with the voluntary rather than the private sector, taking the view that they can spend less on monitoring services and contracts when the provider is a voluntary organization in which they have greater trust and confidence. Over the seven years that the reprovision programme has been in operation in North-East Thames it has been noticeable that voluntary organizations have widened their sphere of operations. Many of these organizations entered the mental health care market by providing 24-hour staffed residential care using the 'perverse incentive' offered by clients' entitlements to social security care allowances. Once they have cemented good relations, a local authority and voluntary organization might agree a contract to provide a day activity or employment programme. Districts have also allied themselves with voluntary organizations through consortia arrangements. Services have been developed where, within a consortium, health authorities have financed peripatetic support staff for people living in domestic housing. Residents' care is, however, *managed* by the voluntary organization. A similar proliferation of service provision has not occurred within the private sector.

The old style of public sector contracting-out – grant-funding of voluntary agencies, loosely-specified contracts for individual placements, and frequently the complete absence of strategic planning – was able to encourage or at least was not able to inhibit the development of a mixed economy. But the rate of development was gentle, and public authorities today need to develop much more specific skills. In particular, they need expertise and power to manage markets. This is where, for example, purchasing gives way to commissioning, for health and local authorities need to build up local 'competition policies' which coordinate the stimulation, regulation and encouragement of mental health care markets within an overall strategic framework. They must shape emerging markets to meet the needs of local populations, and this may also approach the market expectations of government (Forder *et al.* 1994, Wistow *et al.* 1994).

Joint commissioning

Local and health authorities have the chance to use commissioning to develop and encourage new forms of provision, engender competition and achieve the better targeting of resources on needs. They also have the opportunity to develop imaginative and affordable monitoring procedures which do not damage the desirable qualities of providers. At the macro-level commissioning is the responsibility of whole authorities, or large parts thereof, and can be conducted either singly or jointly by health and local authorities. Community care planning and population needs assessment are part of this macro-level activity. Micro-commissioning, by contrast, is the responsibility of psychiatrists, care managers or community teams. It involves individual needs assessments and the tailoring of central plans to local circumstances and people's potentialities, for example in relation to devolved budgets and spot purchasing (Knapp and Wistow 1993).

Commissioning can be interpreted as comprising a number of linked tasks, from agreement of a mission statement through assessment, service specification and contracting, to information feedback. In mental health care there are two main players – health and social services authorities – whose responsibilities for procuring care are often inextricably linked. Therefore good sense and the government have encouraged these two agencies to consider acting together wherever possible, perhaps by pursuing joint commissioning. Wertheimer and Greig (1993) have usefully characterized joint commissioning as comprising a number of features (a mixture of tasks and desirable attributes):

- 'money in the same pot', though not necessarily shared or merged financial systems
- joint decisions about how that money is spent
- a shared set of values in a climate of mutual trust
- joint commissioning as a means to improve outcomes for users and carers
- a commitment to improved quality in services
- an aim to achieve coherence at all levels of commissioning and purchasing, from macro-commissioning to micro-purchasing
- recognition that there will be gains and losses, and compromises to authority and autonomous decision-making powers, though not to their values
- individual organizations retaining the ability to discharge their statutory responsibilities in ways which enable them to retain accountability.

Because joint commissioning involves some pooling of resources and clarity about aims and methods, opportunities for it are more likely to arise when there are overlapping responsibilities or domains of activity, when health and local authorities are dependent on common (external or pooled) resources, and/or when one agency is heavily dependent on the other for funding or referrals. One of the service areas which has seen the development of joint commissioning initiatives is discharge planning for people leaving hospital (Henwood and Wistow 1993). Generally, macro-level joint commissioning is developing slowly but significantly, while at a micro-level there may also be opportunities for joint purchasing, with care managers pooling resources with fund-holding GPs, or operating from a single site to facilitate the joint micro-commissioning and monitoring roles in general.

The benefits of joint commissioning are that it can offer the opportunity for greater flexibility and coordination across agencies. There can be more effective use of available resources, reducing the likelihood of overlaps and gaps in service responses, and offering the potential for better targeting of resources on needs. From a procedural standpoint, joint commissioning improves the prospects of moving to clearer and more consistent eligibility criteria. It should raise mutual awareness, foster cooperation rather than competition, and weaken previous tendencies to shunt people and costs on to other agencies (Knapp and Wistow 1993). As yet, however, there is little such joint commissioning activity in the mental health area.

Summary

The aim of this chapter has been to examine the implications of the developing mixed economy for mental health care. The reforms encapsulated in the 1990 *NHS and Community Care Act* encompass changes to service delivery and service funding, and will have marked effects on the very structure and organizational culture in which these activities have taken place over the last 50 years. However, the mixed economy of care is not new. The different combinations of provider sectors and purchasing routes set out in Figure 3.1 are not textbook constructs but real-world arrangements in mental health care. They characterized the *pre*-reform system. We looked at the mixed economy of the voluntary sector and described the complex funding routes and the incentives and arrangements which underpin community care. It is interesting to speculate about how these may develop, in particular where funding links are apparently *absent* (Figure 3.2).

The introduction of a market in mental health care in itself will achieve little. Local and health authority personnel need to develop skills to influence market forces, to encourage greater participation by the independent sector and to support those whose services they wish to continue purchasing. To encourage informed debate by users adds another layer of complication – and cost – but it is vital if services are to be provided in sufficient quantity and of sufficient quality. Care managers and care programmers must also pass information between users and purchasers, bringing together the macro and micro elements of commissioning.

We concluded the chapter by discussing the emergence of joint commissioning. Activities jointly undertaken by the health and social services have had a patchy history, but experience suggests that *joint commissioning* is a promising way forward. Mental health services which straddle the traditional boundaries of health and social care can most easily be considered within joint purchasing and service delivery structures. Provision of long-term residential care, day care, respite care and non-custodial care for offenders with mental health problems might be appropriate examples (Lawson, 1993). Pooling of budgets at both macro- and micro-levels can give greater power to purchasers which, in turn, will encourage the development of a more diverse, more comprehensive and more coherent service. It is at this interface between health and social care that the many challenges posed by the developing mixed economy can be addressed.

References

Brenton M (1985). *The Voluntary Sector in British Social Services*, Longman, Harlow.
Department of Health (1989). *Caring for People: Community Care in the Next Decade and Beyond*. Cmnd 849, HMSO, London.
Department of Health (1990). *The Care Programme Approach for People with a*

Mental Illness Referred to the Specialist Psychiatric Services. Joint Health/Social Service Circular HC(9023/LASSL(90)11), Health Publications Unit, Heywood, Lancashire.

Forder J, Knapp M R J and Wistow G (1994). *Competition in the English Mixed Economy of Care*. Discussion Paper 975, Personal Social Services Research Unit, University of Kent at Canterbury.

Hallam A, Knapp M R J, Beecham J and Fenyo A (1995). Eight years of psychiatric reprovision: an economic evaluation. In *The Economic Evaluation of Mental Health Care* (ed. M Knapp). Arena, Aldershot, pp. 103–124.

Henwood M and Wistow G (1993). The buck stops here. *Health Service Journal*, **21**, October.

House of Commons Health Committee (1993). *Community Care: Funding from April 1993*. Third Report, Session 1992–93, HC309, HMSO, London.

Kendall J and Knapp M R J (1994). A loose and baggy monster: boundaries, definitions and typologies. In *An Introduction to the Voluntary Sector* (eds. J Davis Smith, R Hedley and C Rochester). Routledge, London.

Knapp M R J (1989). Private and voluntary welfare. In *The New Politics of Welfare* (ed. M McCarthy). Macmillan, London.

Knapp M R J and Wistow G (1993). Joint commissioning for community care. In *Implementing Community Care: A Slice Through Time*. Department of Health Social Services Inspectorate, London.

Knapp M R J, Beecham J, Hallam A and Fenyo A (1993). The costs of community care for former long-stay psychiatric hospital residents, *Health and Social Care*, **1**, 193–201.

Knapp M R J and Wistow G (1994a). Welfare pluralism and community care development: the role of local government and the non-statutory sectors in social welfare services in England. In *LEED Notebook*, vol. 19, Organization for Economic Cooperation and Development, Paris.

Knapp M R J, Wistow G, Forder J and Hardy B (1994*b*). Markets for social care: opportunities, barriers and implications. In *Quasi-Markets in Health Education and Social Care* (eds. W Bartlett and C Propper). School for Advanced Urban Studies, Bristol.

KPMG Management Consultants (1992). *Improving Independent Sector Involvement in Community Care Planning*. Report for the Department of Health, London.

Lawson R (1993). *Toolkit on Community Care for Purchasers*. North-East Thames Regional Health Authority, London.

Leff J (ed.) (1993). The TAPS project: evaluating community placement of long-stay psychiatric patients. *British Journal of Psychiatry*, **162**, Supplement 19.

OPCS (1992). *Office of Population Censuses and Surveys Monitor*. 17 November, HMSO, London.

Schneider J and Pinner J (1993). *United Kingdom Voluntary Organizations in Mental Health*. Discussion Paper 1002, Personal Social Services Research Unit, University of Kent at Canterbury.

Social Services Inspectorate (1992). *Getting it Together: Strategies for Implementation*. Department of Health, London.

Wertheimer A and Greig R (1993). *Report on Joint Commissioning for Community Care*. National Development Team, Manchester.

Wistow G, Knapp M R J, Hardy B and Allen C (1994). *Social Care in a Mixed Economy*. Open University Press, Milton Keynes.

4 Primary health care: roles and relationships

M. Sheppard

Primary health care in general. and GPs in particular occupy a focal position in the provision of mental health care. Primary care is frequently the setting to which people will turn first when seeking professional help for personal problems. Hence there is a high prevalence of mental health problems amongst attenders of primary health care (Skuse and Williams 1984). However, primary care is only one aspect of health and welfare services for people with mental health problems, while nonetheless having a critical role in the pathway to psychiatric care (Goldberg and Huxley 1980).

The pressure in both professional and official publications, for good interprofessional collaboration is, to a considerable extent, predicated on the wide presence of social and health problems in both health and welfare settings. Fawcett-Henessey (1987) identifies a core reason: that mental health and social care involve the skills of more than one profession and that each profession's skills should be harmonized with those of other professions in the interests of clients. However, mental health is, in many respects a contentious area, and the professions involved do not always make easy bedfellows. This is obvious in at least two interrelated ways: approaches to the issue of mental health and illness and the potential for interoccupational rivalry. The first is well known, involving a disparate antipsychiatric group of libertarian theorists (Szasz 1970), interactionist sociologists (Scheff 1966) and existentialists (Laing 1959), who questioned the very existence of mental illness and attributed much of its development as an idea to medical 'occupational imperialism'. Second, even amongst those accepting mental illness as legitimate there are differences of views, emphasizing, to a greater or lesser extent, biological social and psychological factors in the genesis, course, treatment and prognosis of mental health problems. Occupational rivalry is also evident: the professionalization of nursing has left nurses more reluctant to take the subordinate role traditionally expected by doctors; the expansion of community psychiatric nursing (CPN) has moved them into areas traditionally the preserve of social workers (Sheppard 1991*b*) and, perhaps most pervasive, there is a tradition of interoccupational rivalry between social workers and general practitioners (GPs).

The notion of 'teamwork' involves many elements. but one significant dimension involves the capacity to work collaboratively. which in turn recognizes the, often distinctive, contribution each participating professional may make. However, where the theoretical commitment of professionals is diverse, even conflicting, and occupational territory is, partly as a result, contested, collaboration may be more difficult than it may at first appear. This chapter, in focusing on primary care. will examine the often turbulent relationship between general practice and social work. This is undertaken because of the contentious nature of psychiatry and the potential for occupational rivalry generally. As a 'case example' the very difficulty of the relationships between these occupations may throw into sharp relief the potential for disruption generally, and the ways in which these may be avoided. In doing so it will focus on primary care as part of the web of health and welfare services, involving not just the examination of relationships within the primary health care setting, but between it and other settings.

Care management and provision

Before proceeding further, it is worth outlining the main changes in the organization of health and welfare services resulting from the National Health Service and Community Care Act 1989. Because these changes are so fundamental, it is only by understanding these that the significance of previous research may be understood.

The central distinction in health and social care is between purchaser and provider. In the health service this has taken the form of trusts purchasing from provider services and, in some cases, budget-holding GPs who purchase services on behalf of their patients. The presence of budget-holding GPs is patchy as amongst many in the profession there has been considerable resistance. The purchaser–provider split in social care is evident in the development of care management and care provision, distinct (though not completely differentiated) roles which are manifested primarily through the organization of social care. The local authority has responsibility for purchasing and developing services to meet local need. This is done at the level of organization through senior management which is responsible for the development of appropriate resources. At the individual level of the client this is undertaken by care managers, frequently but not exclusively social workers, whose responsibility will be to assess need, identify appropriate services and review their provision. Care provision, it is intended, will be, to a considerable degree, carried out separately through provider units to whom care managers will refer clients. The differentiation is not complete, because, for example, a care manager may refer to a provider unit for specialist assessment (assessment being a major part of care management), and the care manager may themselves be a provider, for example in the provision of therapeutic help. As with health care, social care is to involve a mix of publicly and privately provided services (including the voluntary sector), although it is intended that there will be a considerable increase in the latter. The local authority is to undertake an enabling role in a mixed economy of care, encouraging the development of services appropriate to local need, and ensuring the best possible quality in these services.

The central thrust of the reforms, therefore, is that of a needs-led service within a mixed economy of care responding to the limits of available finances. In both health and social care it is intended that the money will follow the client. However. this review is both tentative and schematic. It is too early to tell how these services will develop and there will be local variations. It would also be wrong not to recognize with some cynicism, that the purchaser–provider distinction is both a response to the the limited available finance (some would say underfunding) of health and social care, and a desire to devolve responsibility to local areas and even individual professionals.

Mental health in the community: primary care and social services

GPs and social workers share, to a considerable degree, a common concern with mental health problems in the community. They are a major social affliction: Goldberg and Huxley (1980) suggested a point prevalence of between 90 and 200 per 1000 at risk for areas including rural and urban locations, as well as different countries. The most frequent mental health problems are minor mood disorders, involving various combinations of depression and anxiety, while the major psychotic syndromes are rare. Female rates are roughly twice that of male rates. The single most common problem in random community samples is depression (Weissman and Myers 1978a and b; Brown and Harris 1978), where female rates are particularly high. However, the psychiatric services do tend to see those with most severe problems. According to Goldberg and Huxley (1980) severity is a major influence on referral. Wing (1976), using the Present State Examination (PSE), found that the most severe problems were present in 20 per cent of out-patients and 59 per cent of in-patients, but none of his community sample. Cooper (1966) found that while 4 per cent of GP patients suffered some psychosis, 25 per cent of out-patients and 72 per cent of in-patients suffered schizophrenia and affective psychosis.

Primary health care, therefore. has a strategic position in two respects: it has a focus on health problems in the community, and it is an important 'staging post' between the community and specialist treatment. There is, furthermore, evidence that most people with marked mental health problems. and the majority with mild ones, do consult their GP (Wing 1976; Brown and Harris 1978). Research using the General Health Questionnaire (GHQ) shows that rates of psychiatric morbidity vary, but not by very much, Sims and Salmons (1975) identifying a rate of 30.8 per cent at one extreme and Marks et al. (1979) finding a rate of 39.7 per cent. Other studies have identified rates of morbidity between these figures (Goldberg and Blackwell 1970; Goldberg et al. 1976; Skuse and Williams 1984).

The diagnostic capacity of GPs is, however, very variable. Shepherd et al. (1966) and a number of subsequent studies, have shown treatment in general practice frequently to be haphazard and inadequate. Marks et al. (1979) found four significant factors related to GP accuracy: interest and concern (such as empathic manner and asking questions about home and family); conservatism (related to personality and interview style); psychiatric focus (the doctor's interest in psychiatry); and time pressures. Those with a low bias (tending to avoid making psychiatric assessments) tend to be high-status doctors, those with leisurely office hours and racial homogeneity in their patient group (and, in America patients, with private health insurance). Those with high bias show the opposite characteristics (Goldberg and Huxley 1980). Studies by Johnson (1973, 1974) showed that few patients were offered psychotherapy, that despite the correlation of stress factors with mental health problems no attempt was made to contact social agencies nor modify these factors, very few patients found their intervention helpful and limited use was made of antidepressants. Even amongst good doctors, Johnson concluded, knowledge about and interest in psychiatry was limited.

A number of studies, not all using standardized instruments, have concluded that mental health problems are widely present amongst social work clients in area teams (Corney and Briscoe 1977; Corney 1979, 1984a; Huxley and Fitzpatrick 1984, Fisher *et al.* 1984). Of those using standardized instruments, Corney (1984) found about two-thirds of adult social work clients aged 65 or under in both GP attachment and local authority settings suffered mental health problems, overwhelmingly minor affective disorders, mainly anxiety and depression. Cohen and Fisher (1987) including older clients, found that, depending on the 'cut off' point, 35 or 52 per cent of clients had a mental health problem and that it was present in over half of these six months later. The study, furthermore, showed that about three-fifths of relatives of clients were rated positive. Using the PSE, Huxley *et al.* (1987) found a morbidity rate of 25 per cent in their sample of local authority and attached social workers' clients, which increased to 53 per cent when 'threshold' cases were included. Isaac *et al.* (1986), in a small study of children in care, found that over half the mothers and a third of fathers were GHQ 'positive', and that data for short-term (less than three months in care) and 'long-term' (over one year in care) cases was almost identical. Quinton and Rutter (1984) found 78 per cent of mothers of children receiving care a second time had mental health problems, compared with 21 per cent of a matched group.

Social workers do not always recognize mental health problems in their clients. Corney (1984) found social workers in both settings tended to underestimate the extent of mental health problems in clients by about a half, as did Cohen and Fisher (1987). Although rates of detection increased where both CTP and social work assessments were used, false positives also increased markedly. Huxley *et al.* (1987) found social workers' 'recognition rate' of mental health problems to be 66 per cent, higher than they expected. and that they were at least as accurate as the GHQ.

Research on social work–GP relations

The extensive presence of mental health problems amongst both GP and social work clients provides a strong prima facie case for collaboration. Research on social work–GP relationships is patchy and generally not specifically focused on mental health, but does gives cause for concern. GPs' comments about social work can be dismissive in the extreme: social workers were characterized, in one study of mine, as being an occupation of 'young girls' with little life experience, as having a rather inflated view of their own professional expertise and a slow and frequently obstructive approach to the referrals (expectations?) of GPs themselves (Sheppard 1987). Fisher *et al.*'s

(1984) research found that amongst social workers the good GP was seen as the exception, social workers considering that GPs were reluctant to communicate and frequently used social services as a dumping ground for awkward patients. 'Atrocity stories' in relation to individual practice, which are told at the expense of the doctor's competence, have been found to circulate amongst social workers (and health visitors) (Dingwall 1977).

Three approaches to collaboration can be gleaned from research, as follows.

Contact and collaboration when separate

One rural study of GP referrals (Sheppard 1983) showed GPs had a limited conception of social work, using social services as a resource-mobilizing extension of the health services. Referrals showed a bias towards the elderly, problems of (physical) ill health and requests for practical help. This use of social services in a predominantly rural area is also evident in urban areas. Where social workers are based in a social services department and separate from primary health care, doctors are likely to refer predominantly practical problems and those in need of welfare services (Corney and Briscoe 1977). While this reflected an appropriate use of home care and occupational therapy services, this was less the case for social work, which includes psychotherapeutic as well as wider environment work with social and emotional problems, well known to be prevalent in primary care (Shepherd *et al.* 1966: Eastwood and Trevelyan 1972: Lamberts 1979). The stigma attached to referral to social services, their opaque, intimidating nature and bureaucratic structure and image may affect referral. However, doctors themselves seemed to have a limited understanding of social workers' roles and skills, and in the absence of a clearer understanding they may have fallen back on criteria based on their own training and experience to decide when to make referrals.

The poor quality of communication was emphasized in a further study (Sheppard 1985). Referrals from GPs, according to social services workers, frequently lacked sufficient background information about personality and social relations (though not health) while a fifth of referrals were made *without the prior agreement of the patient*, so that social services' involvement was often greeted by clients with some surprise. Contacts with general practitioners subsequent to referral were very limited: in one-third of cases no contact was made at all, and in a further half of cases only one contact was made. Social workers rather than GPs initiated contact, but they did not greatly involve them in case management. Overall, when contacted, it seems GPs could be helpful in case management, but that conflict was reduced by a technique of 'avoidance': GPs whose view of social work was generally regarded as poor made few referrals, and when referring, social workers tended not to contact them during intervention.

However, there may be some disjunction between GPs' stated views about social work and their actual practice. A study of the views of members of primary health care teams in both rural and urban environments found considerable occupational differences, and views within each occupation were complex and variable (Sheppard 1986). Health visitors had a more 'professional' image of social workers, compared with a more 'agency apprentice' model more frequently held by district nurses and GPs. Furthermore, over half the GPs – more than health visitors or district nurses considered liaising with health workers and counselling individuals and their family in mental health cases to be poorly performed by social workers. However, most GPs – surprisingly in view of other research – felt social workers performed compulsory admission assessments adequately. Overall, all health groups felt social workers performed practical help on the whole adequately or well. However, GPs attached greatest importance to social work involvement with problems related to child abuse, learning difficulties, financial, housing and delinquency difficulties. Overall, there were differences of view between occupations which suggests that perceptions of social work are as much a property of the occupation perceiving it as of social work itself, and that claims to 'occupational territory' may be significant in this respect.

GPs and Community Mental Health Centres

The obvious reference point for GPs seeking specialist care for those with mental health problems is the psychiatrist (Goldberg and Huxley 1980). However, with the advent of community mental health centres (CMHCs), an alternative reference point, frequently not headed by psychiatrists, and involving other occupations such as social workers and community psychiatric nurses, is available. However, even here it appears that GPs relate primarily to specialist doctors, although this relationship is not necessarily direct and is certainly complex. Sheppard (1992a) found processing of GP referrals was marked by its medical emphasis: once referred by a GP an individual was considerably more likely to remain within the ambit of the medical profession, by allocation to a specialist doctor, despite the availability of non-medical personnel as alternatives. They were, furthermore, more likely to be considered to suffer more severe mental health problems and to be treated with drugs. When referred from the CMHC for further help, GPs' referrals were considerably more likely to receive in-patient care. The availability of specialist non-medical services did not, therefore, lead to a greater use of these services. Although we cannot be definitive, it is certainly plausible that doctors, whether GPs or specialists, felt more comfortable working with members of their own profession, and that this significantly influenced the direction of referrals.

This limited capacity to relate to other professions was reflected in the interaction of GPs with social workers and CPNs in the same CMHC (Sheppard 1992b). Two main themes were evident from this study: that CPNs contacted GPs far more frequently than social workers and that GPs initiated contact with both these professional groups far less frequently than either of them. Social workers' contacts tended to be more purposive than CPNs, involving a greater degree of collaboration with GPs in case management, while CPNs contacted GPs more frequently for simple provision and exchange of information. The evidence pointed to the possession, by CPNs, of a concept of team which transcended work settings, hence allowing more frequent contact between specialist and primary health care setting. This was not one possessed by social workers, who were welfare workers working within a health setting rather than health workers *per se*. The pattern of communication also suggested an assumption of team leadership on the part of GPs when dealing with non-medical personnel in a health setting, leaving other occupations with two alternatives: either to collude with this assumption or to limit the amount of collaboration which might prove damaging to the client's interests.

GPs do appear able to distinguish referrals to CMHCs for compulsory admission and other referrals (Sheppard 1992c). By comparison with other GP referrals, compulsory admission referrals were characterized by five triggers: patients tended to have a definite disorder, a psychotic condition; previous contacts with the psychiatric services; problematic behaviour occurring in a familial or wider context; more frequent tendency to be women. Other referrals were less severe, more frequently neurotic, more frequently had emotional and relationship problems and received considerably more advice and psychodynamic support. However (Sheppard 1992d), although GP referrals for compulsory admission were generally appropriate in terms of the presence of a mental health problem, they appeared, relative to other, frequently lay, referrers to be rather 'trigger happy', and to be so in particular at the expense of women. GP referrals were significantly more frequently informally admitted or not admitted at all, and GPs seemed at times incapable of distinguishing between the need for treatment and the need for compulsory treatment. This is particularly important because of implications for civil liberties. Furthermore, they often appeared unaware of the potentially positive implications of social support available to the subject. These factors further emphasize the limited medical perspective used, and that awareness of social perspectives is of significance.

The specific emphasis on women appears particularly worrying, raising a question about the extent to which GPs were using compulsory admissions as a means for the social control of women (Sheppard 1991a). Approved social workers, with an 'injection' of a psychosocial perspective appeared to play a part in diverting the women from compulsory admission, but even they appear not to have been free from patriarchal assumptions.

Attachment schemes

Two alternative forms of social work–primary health care collaboration have been tried: *liaison schemes*, where a social worker visits the practice at prearranged times to pick up referrals or discuss cases, acting largely as an intermediary between social services and primary health care; and *attachment schemes*, in which a social worker takes referrals from a general practice and works, part or full-time, in primary health care (Clare and Corney 1982). Liaison schemes appear to have had little impact on the pattern of referral to social services or relationships between social workers and GPs. Attachment schemes, which have been extensively studied consistently report a wholly more positive outcome (Foreman and Fairbairn 1968; Goldberg and Neill 1972; Clare and Corney 1982). A greater range of work more appropriate to the role and skills of social workers has been evident, particularly in relation to the use of more pychodynamic skills (Corney and Briscoe 1977; Briscoe *et al.* (1983). Clients' views about their practice, incorporating this wider range of skills have been very positive (Corney 1981). Social workers themselves have felt positive about the setting and the helpfulness of their work (Rushton and Briscoe 1981) and a similar view was expressed in a (small) group of GPs who had attachments (Williams and Clare 1979).

Social work help is likely to be greatest in relation to primary health care with neurotic problems, which are the most prevalent mental health problems in this setting. Studies of effectiveness of social casework methods have yielded variable results. A controlled study of attached social work with chronic neurotic clients (Cooper *et al.* 1975; Shepherd *et al.* 1979) found that in both clinical and social adjustment scores social work clients improved significantly more than the control group receiving routine help at one year follow-up. The reduction in use of psychotropic drugs and referral for psychiatric help indicates that it was a partial alternative to specialist services. However, Corney (1984*b*) found no significant differences between depressed women receiving attached social work help and a group not receiving this help. This study did suggest that a particular group, women with chronic problems and poor social support, do benefit from social work, particularly when given both counselling and practical help.

It has proved possible, indeed, to identify many of the ingredients leading to successful attachment schemes (Corney 1980). Access to adequate facilities, particularly a room in the health centre, is of considerable significance. This provides them with a base to conduct their work, indicates a sense of permanence or identification with the surgery to patients and encourages the social worker themselves to spend more time at the health centre. Second, they are more successful where the social worker has had the opportunity to 'educate' primary care workers, and particularly GPs, about their role and skills. This requires time to be spent at the health centre where each occupation may learn about the others' roles and skills and where a coordinated approach to treatment may develop. Third, where an individual attached social worker handles all the cases themselves, greater confidence develops. The doctor prefers developing trust in the individual concerned rather than social workers in general and it facilitates case discussion. Fourth, a high level of commitment is necessary by all participants, including the GPs and social worker: without such commitment the schemes are likely to founder on indifference. Fifth, the choice of social worker is important: an ability to work independently, a feeling of professional security and an ability to relate to other professionals is important. Finally, the organization of the practice is important: attachments are more successful where adequate opportunities for informal contacts as well as formal meetings are available.

It is possible, however, to be overoptimistic about prospects for attachment schemes. A wide study, comparing the views of GPs who had experienced attachment schemes with those who had not, found little or no differences in their views about social work (Sheppard 1987). This may be because GPs accurately assessed social workers to have had little impacton their patients (see, e.g. Corney 1984*b*). Alternatively, social workersmay well have had an impact, one supported by consumer studies (Corney 1981), and the GPs involved failed to appreciate their contribution. On the latter assumption GPs appeared as a very homogeneous group who are highly resistant to changes in their views. Furthermore, the results suggested that attachment schemes reported in published research are not representative of such schemes generally, as this wider survey of general practices showed social workers based in primary care for relatively short periods each week.

The prognosis seemed gloomy: for occupational culture, characterized by negative stereotypes held by GPs and social workers about each other, may be so pervasive that, except on relatively rare occasions, attachments will not affect GPs' perspectives.

Causes of collaboration problems

The difficulties encouraging effective use of, and communication and collaboration between, GPs and social workers are surprisingly consistent, regardless of national boundaries (Mizrahi and Abramson 1985; Falk 1978; Wilson 1976; Huntington 1981).

Fisher *et al.* (1984) considered that the separateness of social and health services is responsible for much of the difficulty experienced by social and health workers in working together. In particular, no professional worker is likely to have a comprehensive understanding of the resources available in services other than his/her own – indeed this may be the case with their own service. Furthermore, no professional is likely to possess detailed knowledge of the social priorities and policy adopted by other services, or the ways in which workers in other professions set about the tasks of defining needs, problems and interventive techniques. Indeed it is arguable that the continual reorganization of both local authority and health services in recent years has considerably exacerbated this situation. This explanation, which emphasizes organizational context, would suggest that problems of collaboration could be resolved by placing the relevant professionals in the same setting. Such an explanation is consistent with attachment schemes.

However, Sheppard (1992*b*) has suggested that other factors may play a part. In contrast with social workers, community psychiatric nurses. despite being situated in a setting (CMHC) separate from GPs (primary care), were able to maintain contact with GPs in the overwhelming majority of cases, whether or not referred by the GP themselves. This suggested CPNs were better tuned to the information needs of GPs than social workers. Some of this may be due to the similarity in setting – both were concerned primarily with health issues. However, nurses have a clear concept of themselves as health professionals, part of a group of such professionals which would include GPs. Social workers would not normally see themselves as health professionals *per se*, but as welfare professionals who are based in a health setting. This could lead social workers to define themselves as external specifically to health care responsibilities, leading to less concern with long-term health concerns beyond their own intervention. Furthermore, CPNs' training and team involvement with doctors may well have an impact. Even when not working from the same base they may possess a concept of 'team' which transcends work setting. CPNs' behaviour, unlike social workers', was consistent with this transcendent team concept. The provision of information by CPNs in cases not referred by GPs, for example, suggested a greater awareness than amongst social workers of GPs' responsibility for continuing care.

These observations are consistent with work derived from the sociology of occupations suggesting that the problems are deep rooted (Mizrahi and Abramson 1985; Huntington 1981). These relate to the 'assumptive worlds' of different occupations – what Douglas (1971) calls the deep rules of the occupations, which are unspoken and so much a part of everyday work that they are not generally expressed. A number of these are of considerable significance. Social workers and GPs are increasingly *competing for the same occupational territory* (in this respect similar to social work and CPNs) (Sheppard 1991*b*). Social work has traditionally emphasized a personalized service to individuals, related to their psychosocial functioning. Hence, BASW (1977, p. 19) defined social work as 'the purposeful and ethical application of personal skills ... directed towards enhancing personal and social functioning of an individual, family group or neighbourhood'. The search by general practice for recognition as a specialism within medicine has led to a claim to similar territory: hence an increasing body of medical literature defines general practice as 'primary and continuing care' including developmental psychological and social components of patient care with a focus on the 'whole person' or 'total family' (Huntington 1981).

This is allied to a *demand for dominance* and executive authority as a condition of other occupations being allowed to work within what is regarded by doctors as their occupational territory. In particular, articles about 'teams' and 'teamwork' written by non-medical members are frequently replete with democratic imagery – interdependence, collaboration, cooperation. Writings by general practitioners about the primary health care team are characterized by an assumption of the doctor's unchallenged and unchallengeable authority, regardless of the problem confronted (Conn *et al.* 1973). Any attempt to assert greater equality and challenge this automatic right to leadership is likely to be regarded as an act of professional hostility towards medicine.

The *dominant frames of reference* by which GPs and social workers address problems are quite different. GPs tend to adopt a 'biophysical' frame, involving an emphasis on disease, pathology and its treatment, contrasting with the predominantly 'psychosocial' frame of reference in social work which emphasizes the psychosocial context (and definition) of problems and which is suspicious of pathological models of human problems. Medical training emphasizes knowledge and skills required for the study and treatment of disease, while psychosocial aspects of health and disease are ignored or minimized. Many social work educational establishments reject a 'medical model' with its focus on pathology and disease. The concepts used by the different occupations, as a result, are quite different, inhibiting ease of communication. This has a consequence, furthermore, for the focus of work: while GPs focus on individual patients, social workers lay emphasis on relationships within the family community and society as a whole.

The *predominant value orientation* of each occupation differs significantly. While, for example, 'respect for persons' provides the guiding value for social work; the corresponding value in medicine is 'respect for life'. This can lead to conflict where, for example, an elderly person wishes to remain in their own home, even though this threatens their life and they would be safer in residential care. Furthermore, the assumptions about humans and society dominant in each occupation leave social workers more likely to identify causes of problems in the social environment and GPs to focus on the individual. The disadvantage suffered by the clientele of welfare agencies is more likely to be attributed by GPs to a lack of moral fibre in individuals rather

than to socioeconomic factors more prevalent in social workers' understanding of their clients' predicament.

A further dimension relates to the *possibilities for oppressive practice*.
Social work has in recent years increasingly emphasized the importance of
being aware of the possibility of oppression by professionals in relation to
disadvantaged groups and antidiscriminatory and antiracist training is deeply
embedded in the educational process (CCETSW 1991). Such training, challenging individual and institutional discrimination can only be properly
founded on a clear understanding of the social world derived primarily from
the social sciences. While this forms a central part of social work education
this is not the case with other health professionals. The potential for conflict
arises where one group, without necessarily having any intention of so doing,
acts in a discriminatory manner, and is challenged about it. While the discriminatory behaviour of a number of caring professions, including social
work (Broverman *et al.* 1970), has been remarked upon, and this is clearly
related to moralizing about behaviour (Rees 1978) this has been particularly
the case with the medical profession including GPs (Littlewood and Lipsedge
1982). The problem appears in medicine's successful expansion of its empire.
Doctors are consulted on a wide variety of matters, which are frequently
beyond the scope of medical education. Medical advice can, as a result, frequently have the force of moral imperative. In relation to women, for example, this leads to doctors behaving as social control agents in three ways.
First, GPs frequently use their medical-moral language to offer advice
based on the conventional wisdom of their social milieu, adjusting women
to a life located in the home, maintaining an unrewarding and demoralizing
existence (Barrett and Roberts 1978). Second, drugs are prescribed for
psychological conditions far more frequently for women than men. Valium
is a case in point, frequently prescribed for problems such as loneliness
and marital discord, yet its prescription is frequently related to an individual's ability to live up to social ideals, and the physician's judgments are factors in a pseudo-objective diagnosis (Cooperstock 1978). Third, GPs may
more easily resort to the route of compulsory admission for women as compared with men in order to deal with mental health problems (Sheppard
1991*a*).

Alternative models for collaboration

Given these problems, what alternative models for collaboration may be
developed and what are their implications? We can examine this in terms of
choice of setting involving three dimensions: the possibilty of professional
autonomy and independence, the opportunity for collaboration and the
extent to which a specialist or generalist role may be adopted. In the following discussion the term 'team' is not restricted to particular settings, but
can involve interprofessional collaboration across different settings.

A traditional social services model

This bases GPs in primary health care and social workers in local authority
district teams. This may involve two forms. The first is a liaison scheme, in

which a delegated social worker visits the health centre/surgery at regular intervals to take referrals and discuss cases, but where the decision whether to allocate referrals rests with the social services managers, and they may be given to any social worker. An alternative is complete separation, where the GP is in a position no different from that of any other referrer. This has certain advantages in terms of professional independence, for the primary health care team is one where, in general, and traditionally, GPs dominate. It is their territory, and their practice and there is a danger that social workers may find themselves in a subordinate role. Social workers, second, may have the advantage of working more regularly with other social workers. This may help foster their sense of a clear professional identity and also aid the development of skills. In a discipline like social work, which relies less on formal knowledge, and more on the use of a flexible imaginative intelligence applied to practice situations, a close relationship with professional colleagues can be highly significant, giving greater opportunity for formal and informal case discussion from which practice learning may take place. A social service base, furthermore, provides the opportunity to specialize, or to be a more generalist worker (although recent legislation points increasingly to a separation of adult and child care workers). This flexibility allows team development and individual practice in a way deemed to be more appropriate for the needs of the local area. While generalist and specialist social work offer different advantages, both may be developed in a setting where the identity and skills of social workers are paramount.

Attachment model

Here the social worker is part of the primary health care 'team', usually including health visitors and district nurses as well as GPs (and possibly CPNs, although under these circumstances clarity about role and skills will be required) (Sheppard 1991a) and they are based, for part or all of their working week, at the health centre/surgery. Here the issue of professional independence is more problematic. In a setting which GPs frequently regard as primarily their territory, and where they assume leadership of the team, it may be difficult for the social worker to exert adequate control over the content and nature of their practice. The GP may see the social worker as 'their' worker. This can have the advantage of acceptance by GPs of the presence and contribution of the social worker, but may also implicitly present the social worker as subordinate to them. It may also be difficult to assert properly a clear social work role independent of the more limited preconceptions of GPs themselves. Of course, this does not necessarily follow, and many of the more successful schemes are characterized by mutual respect and professional tolerance. However, while GPs remain the dominant profession in the primary care setting, the risk to professional independence and integrity remains.

The opportunity for collaboration is considerably greater with the attachment model. This arises primarily from the physical presence of both social workers and GPs in the same building: the opportunity for contact is far greater than is available when the two occupations are based in separate settings. Collaboration may occur at at least two levels. First, it can involve the opportunity for detailed and informal as well as formal case discussion, in which the work and contribution of the two occupations may be examined and fully developed in relation to any particular case. Second, it can involve actual joint work, or a division and pacing of tasks which allows both professions to 'dovetail' their practice. This collaboration relates to a third dimension: the development of understanding of the role and contribution of the two occupations. It is both predicated and based upon such collaboration. If collaboration is to be efficiently achieved, it must be based on a mutual recognition by each professional of the specific role and skills of the other occupation. However, this recognition is, to a considerable degree, fostered by closer working relations based upon working together.

The opportunity exists, at the primary health care level, for both a generalist and specialist approach. Primary care provides the opportunity to work with all ages and different client groups, with a wide range of problems. This generalist work will differ from district teams (local authority) work, since the latter will reflect the nature and pace of referrals to that setting. Furthermore, it is primarily in the district teams that the statutory tasks of social work, such as child protection, are undertaken. Social workers may focus in particular on mental health issues, and only accept referrals which involve such issues. In doing so, however, their work will largely reflect the level in the pathway to psychiatric care at which they operate. While the primary care setting provides access to the greatest number of mental health problems, the emphasis in this setting is on minor or neurotic problems particularly depression and anxiety. The skills required are the ones related to these, rather than psychotic problems.

Specialist mental health model

This will very much reflect the local provision for mental health. Social workers may, for example, be hospital or CMHC-based, and the setting will affect the nature of the work undertaken. The degree of collaboration with GPs is likely to be less than in primary care settings, because of the physical separation of the two occupations and the opportunity for day-to-day contact does not exist. However, prospects for collaboration are greater than where social workers are based in district teams, since they will be working within a health setting, with which GPs have a greater identity and a clearer idea of the range of tasks. Social workers, furthermore, are likely to benefit from the positive effect on GPs' perceptions of their closer contact with other medical professionals (psychiatrists). CPNs have shown that a transcendental team concept is possible when working within a CMHC. Of course the more limited opportunities for collaboration with GPs must be weighed against the greater opportunity for collaboration with specialist mental health professionals.

The issue of professional independence differs from both social service and attachment models. Mental health settings have traditionally been dominated by doctors, and this remains the case with many teams. However, and particularly with the development of CMHCs, a more democratic team approach has developed, in which no one occupation predominates and the contribution of each profession to any particular case varies according to the problem confronted (Sheppard 1991*a*). There has, even in settings traditionally dominated by doctors, been a greater recognition of the multifactorial nature of mental health problems, and consequently a wider recognition of the social work contribution than in other health, particularly primary care, settings. The result is both a clearer understanding of the social work role and skills and a greater opportunity for social workers to exert control over the nature and range of work undertaken.

The mental health setting is, by definition, a specialist one. However, this is not straightforward. First, the focus on a particular client group can blind us to the generic nature of problems within this client group. A good example of this is maternal depression. Mothers, particularly working-class and with three children aged under 14 or single mothers with a child under six, are at high risk for depression (Brown and Harris 1978). However, this is closely related to a range of social deprivations: poverty, poor housing, lack of access to resources and so on (Moss and Plewis 1977). Furthermore, child care problems are closely related to maternal depression – developmental, emotional and behavioural problems, and problems of parenting, including child abuse (Sheppard 1994). Specializing in 'mental health problems' therefore, can also involve work on child care problems. Second, the nature of mental health problems confronted will differ according to setting. A hospital-based social worker is likely to confront psychoses to a greater degree than a CMHC-based worker, who will probably see more of these than a primary-care-based worker (Sheppard 1991*b*; Goldberg and Huxley 1980). CMHCs are likely to see more minor mental health problems than hospitals or, indeed, primary care.

Thus the nature of collaboration between social workers and GPs will vary according to the setting for each profession. While the GP is necessarily based in primary care, social workers may be based in different settings with consequences for collaboration. What are the 'generic' qualities to be encouraged for good collaboration, regardless of setting?

Democratic imagery

Although doctors, by virtue of their longer training, may wish to regard themselves as invariant team leader, this is likely not to be accepted by other team members conscious of their own professional skills. This is the case not simply with social workers, but other professionals like CPNs and psychologists. Adequate team work and dovetailing of professional skills is unlikely to survive resentments built up by dominant–subordinate relationships perceived as unfair by non-medical professionals.

Frames of reference

There should be an awareness that quite different frames of reference are adopted by different professionals. This requires some understanding both of the training undertaken and expectations prevalent within different occupations. For example, the predominant 'scientific' paradigm of medical training differs from the humanist perspective prevalent in social work, and unless professionals are aware of these differences it may be easy to dismiss or undervalue the contribution of other professionals. Equally, the context for practice, with a strong emphasis on the legal origins of social work responsibilities and accountability vested within a managed hierarchy, contrasts with the 'individual practitioner-professional' emphasis and ideology in general practice.

Capacity for tolerance of frames of reference

The lack of consensus concerning the nature, cause and management of mental health problems is likely to be reflected in the different emphasis adopted by different professionals. However, there is a limit to the extent to which outright conflict can be accommodated within any team. Extremes of view, such as purely biological versus purely labelling perspectives on mental illness will carry with them such potential for conflict that teamwork is unlikely to be maintained in any real sense. There must, therefore, be some common ground between the different team members. However, there must also be tolerance of differences of emphasis and a preparedness to accept that, while consensus may be sought, it will not always be achieved.

A realistic understanding of the nature and limits of professional skills

The complexity of mental health problems is such that no single profession, and certainly no single professional, can possess all the skills required. The risk of failing to recognize one's own limitations is great. GPs who claim they carry out social work, or that they undertake psychotherapy or counselling, are usually greatly overestimating their skills. Their training does not prepare them for this, and, indeed, their scientific paradigm may be inimical to the development, let alone manifestation, of such skills. Advice based on lay prejudice should not be confused with psychotherapy. Likewise however, social workers may possess an 'oversocialized' view of human nature and problems. Such a view, regarding human nature and problems as entirely the result of social influences, inevitably means dismissing the importance of biophysiology. If doctors should recognize the limits to their psychotherapeutic skills, then some recognition by social workers of the significance of biology is necessary for any kind of constructive relations with doctors.

Awareness of the nature and role of different professions within the team

This is most obvious in the rather limited use – outside attachments – made by GPs of social workers, with an emphasis on practical tasks. The role of the GP in providing continuing care and doing so with an emphasis on biophysiology contrasts strongly with the more episodic-periodic nature of social work involvement which emphasizes psychosocial explanations and intervention. Furthermore, the contexts in which they work may differ: GPs will generally focus primarily on the individual patient; social work may focus beyond the individual to the family or wider environment. Indeed, for social work, prevention may involve working with communities rather than more traditional individual or family work. Without a clear understanding of roles, proper use is unlikely to be made by one professional of the other, providing the seeds for frustrations, quite possibly to the detriment of client interest.

Recognition that the 'lead' role by any professional may depend on the problem confronted

At base, this is fairly simple: if, for example, a GP claims more expertise in the identification and management of disease, particularly, for example, through the use of drugs, and disease is the problem, then case management should be led by them. The same could be said about psychosocial problems with social work. However, illness is frequently accompanied by psychosocial problems. The lead role may depend on the relative importance of each. Where an illness is, for example, accompanied by minor practical problems, the GP will take the lead. Where psychosocial problems are at the fore the reverse can be the case. Difficulties may arise where a more equal balance between illness or psychosocial problems exist, or differences about the definition of the problem arise. It is here that two central principles must be adopted – equality and tolerance. Tolerance of the other professional's view is necessary and an equal working relationship would allow each to pursue case management in their own area of expertise. Compromise may be critical here, although in the real world there are bound to be some occasions where disagreement is too great for compromise. If teamwork is to survive it will be necessary to accept such tensions.

Preparedness to inform and contact and knowledge of other professionals' information needs

Where professionals are located in different agencies with different cultures and priorities this can easily fall by the wayside. Development of a 'collaborative culture' could considerably aid communication, and this could be encouraged by relatively simple organizational procedures, such as pro-forma letters from social workers to GPs informing them of their involvement and, at case closure work undertaken. Of course this is relevant to GPs also.

The social organization of collaboration

While it is clear from earlier remarks that fundamental changes are occurring in the organization of health and social care, the relevance of these issues for collaboration will nonetheless remain, largely because of their deep-rooted nature involving differences of ideology and expectation between GPs and social workers.

From the standpoint of GPs, the possibility of holding budgets does offer opportunities for collaboration with social work. Most obviously, they could decide to use part of their budget to engage a social worker as a member of the practice in a form of 'attachment', the advantages of which have been outlined. There are, however, pitfalls. The most obvious lies in the 'employee' status of the social worker which would inevitably place them in a position subordinate to the GP. This contains the seeds of frustration which accompanies assumptions about team leadership held by many doctors. GPs' capacities to assess client needs furthermore, will depend on their frames of reference. If an assumption of leadership is accompanied by an insistence on defining the nature of, and response to, the problem, this would limit the social worker's freedom to assess and respond to problems in areas where they are likely to possess considerably more professional knowledge than GPs. The capacity to help clients through multidisciplinary work, it is suggested, requires a degree of professional independence and interprofessional equality. Otherwise a profession may impose its own – limited – frame of reference on all situations, to the detriment of the client.

Of course, these problems may not arise. It is likely that GPs prepared to commit a significant amount of money to a practice social worker will already have a strong commitment to, and belief in, the usefulness of social work. However, the problem is really a structural one. Primary health care is primarily the terrain of doctors: it is they, and not other professionals such as health visitors, social workers and district nurses, who are partners. A more equal form of professional relationship rests, in the last analysis, not simply on a more democratic ideology of interprofessional relations, but on a more egalitarian structure within which these relationships operate. In the end, this requires primary health care not to be partnerships simply of GPs, but, rather that either all participating professionals are partners, or all are equal employees of health or social services.

From a social services standpoint the relationship between GPs as referrers and social workers as care managers or providers is central. While the key role of the GP in identifying core social needs is recognized, the social security changes mean that GPs will no longer be able to admit to residential and nursing homes in the independent sector – and much else in that sector – without prior referral to social services (NHS Management Executive 1992). In one study (Leedham and Wistow 1992), it was widely agreed that GPs should adopt the role of initial referrer, providing basic identification of needs, and that the lead role in assessment should subsequently be taken by the care manager. This is a view echoed in the Foster/Laming letter issued in September 1992 from the Department of Health.

However, specific tensions could well arise, first because of the GPs' role as the patient's advocate and the rationing aspects of the assessment and care management process. Second, conflict could arise where GPs' perceptions of their patients' needs differ from those of care managers or where care managers consider GPs to have given insufficient weight to the carers' needs relative to those of the patient (Leedham and Wistow 1993). Such potential conflicts are entirely consistent with the issues of interprofessional relations discussed earlier. In view of this, it is perfectly clear that these issues will be as relevant in the future as they have been in the past. The models adopted – and it is possible for more than one to be adopted in any one locality – and the generic qualities of good multidisciplinary collaboration will be much the same as already outlined.

Conclusion

This chapter has focused on interprofessional collaboration between social workers and general practitioners. The lessons to be learned from this are, however, more widely applicable. The principal components of good multidisciplinary arrangements will be as relevant to CPNs, health visitors, district nurses and psychiatrists as they are to GPs and social workers. Of course multidisciplinary work is often not simply about professional dyads, and the complexity of relationships will grow along with the number of involved professionals. This, however merely serves to emphasize still further the importance of these components.

References

Barrett M and Roberts H (1978). Doctors and patients: the social control of women in general practice. In *Women, Sexuality and Social Control* (eds. C Smart and M Smart). Routledge and Kegan Paul, London.

Briscoe M, Winny J, Chandler V, Mulgrew K, Williment S and Rushton A (1983). Long term social work in a primary health care setting. *British Journal of Social Work*, **13**, 559–578.

British Association of Social Workers (BASW) (1977). *The Social Work Task*. BASW, Birmingham.

Broverman I, Broverman D, Clarkson F, Rosenkrantz P and Vogal S (1970). Sex role stereotypes and clinical judgements in mental health. *Journal of Consulting and Clinical Psychology*, **34**, 1–7.

Brown G W and Harris T O (1978). *Social Origins of Depression*. Tavistock, London.

Central Council for the Education and Training of Social Workers (CCETSW). *Rules and Requirements for the Diploma in Social Work,* second edition. CCETSW, London.

Clare A and Corney R (1982). *Social Work and Primary Health Care*. Academic Press, London.

Cohen J and Fisher M (1987). Recognition of mental health problems by doctors and social workers. *Practice*, **3**, 225–240.

Conn H, Rakel R and Johnson T (1973). *Family Practice*. Saunders, London.

Cooper B (1966). Psychiatric disorder in hospital and general practice. *Social Psychiatry*, **1**, 7–10.

Cooper B, Harwin B, Depla C and Sheppard M (1975). Mental health in the community: an evaluative study. *Psychological Medicine*, **5**, 372–380.

Cooperstock R (1978). Sex differences in psychotropic drug use. *Social Science and Medicine*, **12b**, 179–186.

Corney R (1979). The extent of mental and physical ill health of clients referred to social workers in a local authority department and a general practice attachment scheme. *Psychological Medicine*, **9**, 585–589.

Corney R (1980). Factors affecting the operation and success of social work attachment schemes to general practice. *Journal of the Royal College of General Practitioners*, **30**, 149–158.

Corney R (1981). Client perspectives in a general practice attachment. *British Journal of Social Work*, **11**, 159–170.

Corney R (1984a). The mental and physical health of clients referred to social workers in a local authority department and a general practice attachment scheme. *Psychological Medicine*, **14**, 137–144.

Corney R (1984b). *The Effectiveness of Attached Social Workers in the Management of Depressed Female Patients in General Practice*. Cambridge University Press, Cambridge.

Corney R and Briscoe M (1977). Social workers and their clients: a comparison between primary health care and local authority settings. *Journal of the Royal College of General Practitioners*, **27**, 295–301.

Dingwall R (1977). 'Atrocity stories' and professional relationships. *Sociology of Work and Occupations*, **4** (4), 371–396.

Dohrenwend B and Dohrenwend B (1974). Social and cultural influences on psychopathology. *Annual Review of Psychology*, **25**, 417–452.

Douglas J D (1971). *American Social Order: Social Rules in a Pluralistic Society*. The Free Press, New York.

Eastwood M R and Trevelyan M H (1972). Relationship between physical and psychiatric disorders. *Psychological Medicine*, **2**, 363–372.

Falk H (1978). Social work in health settings. *Social Work in Health Care*, **3** (4), 395–403.

Fawcett-Hennessy A (1987). The future. In *Recent Advances in Nursing* (ed. J Littlewood). Churchill Livingstone, Edinburgh.

Fisher M, Newton C and Sainsbury E (1984). *Mental Health Social Work Observed*. George Allen and Unwin, London.

Foreman J and Fairbairn E M (1968). *Social Casework in General Practice*. Oxford University Press, London.

Goldberg D and Blackwell B (1970). Psychiatric illness in general practice: a detailed study using a new method of case identification. *British Medical Journal*, **11**, 429–443.

Goldberg D and Huxley P (1980). *Mental Illness in the Community: The Pathway to Psychiatric Care*. Tavistock, London.

Goldberg D, Kay C and Thompson L (1976). Psychiatric morbidity in general practice and the community. *Psychological Medicine*, **6**, 565–569.

Goldberg E M and Neill J E (1972). *Social Work in General Practice*. George Allen and Unwin, London.

Huntington J (1981). *Social Work and General Medical Practice. Collaboration or Conflict*. George Allen and Unwin, London.

Huxley P and Fitzpatrick R (1984). The probable extent of minor mental illness in the clients of social workers: a research note. *British Journal of Social Work*, **14**, 67–73.

Huxley P, Korer J and Tolley S (1987). The psychiatric 'caseness' of clients referred to an urban social services department. *British Journal of Social Work*, **17**, 507–520.

Isaac B, Minty E B and Morrison R M (1986). Children in care – the association with mental disorder in the parents. *British Journal of Social Work*, **16**, 325–339.

Johnson D (1973). Treatment of depression in general practice. *British Medical Journal*, **2**, 18–20.

Johnson D (1974). A study of the use of antidepressant medication in general practice. *British Journal of Psychiatry*, **125**, 186–192.

Laing R D (1959). *The Divided Self*. Tavistock, London.

Lamberts H (1979). Problem behaviour in primary health care. *Journal of the Royal College of General Practitioners*, **29**, 331–335.

Leedham I and Wistow G (1992). *Community Care and General Practitioners*. Working paper no. 6, Nuffield Institute for Health Studies, University of Leeds.

Leedham I and Wistow G (1993). Just what the doctor ordered. *Community Care*, **747**, 7th January 22–23.

Littlewood R and Lipsedge M (1982). *Aliens and Alienists*. Penguin, Harmondsworth.

Marks J, Goldberg D and Hillier V F (1979). Determinants of the ability of general practitioners to detect psychiatric illness. *Psychological Medicine*, **9**, 337–353.

Mizrahi T and Abramson J (1985). Sources of strain between physicians and social workers. *Social Work in Health Care*, **10** (3), 33–53.

Moss P and Plewis I (1977). Mental distress in mothers of preschool children in inner London. *Psychological Medicine*, **7**, 641–652.

NHS Management Executive (1992). *General Practices and 'Caring For People'*. HMSO, London.

Quinton D and Rutter M (1984). Parents with children in care: current circumstances and parenting. *Journal of Child Psychology and Psychiatry*, **25** (2), 211–229.

Rees S (1978). *Social Work Face to Face*. George Allen and Unwin, London.

Rushton A and Briscoe M (1981). Social work as an aspect of primary health care:

the social workers' view. *British Journal of Social Work*, **11**, 61–76.

Scheff T S (1966). *Being Mentally Ill*. Aldine, Chicago.

Shepherd M, Cooper B, Brown A C and Kalton G W (1966). *Psychiatric Illness in General Practice*. Oxford University Press, London.

Shepherd M, Harwin B G, Depla C and Cairns V (1979). Social work and the primary care of mental disorder. *Psychological Medicine*, **9**, 661–669.

Sheppard M (1983). Referrals from general practitioners to a social services department. *Journal of the Royal College of General Practitioners*, **33**, 33–40.

Sheppard M (1985). Communication between general practitioners and a social services department. *British Journal of Social Work*, **15**, 25–42.

Sheppard M (1986). Primary health care workers' views about social work. *British Journal of Social Work*, **16**, 459–468.

Sheppard M (1987). Dominant images of social work: a British comparison of general practitioners with and without attachment schemes. *International Social Work*, **30** (1), 77–91.

Sheppard M (1991a). General practice, social work and mental health sections: the social control of women. *British Journal of Social Work*, **21**, 663–683.

Sheppard M (1991b). *Mental Health Work in the Community: Theory and Practice in Social Work and Community Psychiatric Nursing*. Falmer Press, London.

Sheppard M (1992a). G.P. and informal group referrals to a community mental health centre: an examination of the pathway to psychiatric care. *Social Work and Social Sciences Review*, **3**, 3.

Sheppard M (1992b). Contact and collaboration with general practitioners: a comparison of social workers and community psychiatric nurses. *British Journal of Social Work*, **22**, 419–436.

Sheppard M (1992c). General practitioners' referrals for compulsory admission under the Mental Health Act, I: comparison with other GP mental health referrals. *Psychiatric Bulletin*, **16**, 138–139.

Sheppard M (1992d). General practitioners' referrals for compulsory admission under the Mental Health Act, II: the process of assessment. *Psychiatric Bulletin*, **16**, 140–142.

Sheppard M (1994). Maternal depression, child care and the social work role. *British Journal of Social Work*. **24**, 33–51.

Sims A and Salmons P (1975). Severity of symptoms of psychiatric outpatients: use of the general health questionnaire in hospital and general practice placements. *Psychological Medicine*, **5**, 62–66.

Skuse D and Williams P (1984). Screening for psychiatric disorder in general practice, *Psychological Medicine*, **14**, 365–377.

Szasz T (1970). *Ideology and Insanity*. Penguin Books, Harmondsworth.

Weissman M M and Myers J K (1978a). Rates and risks of depressive disorders in a US urban community. *Acta Psychiatrica Scandinavica*, **57**, 219–231.

Weissman M M and Myers J K (1978b). Psychiatric disorders in a US urban community: 1975/6. *American Journal of Psychiatry*, **135**, 459–462.

Williams P and Clare A (1979). Social workers in primary health care: the general practitioners' viewpoint. *Journal of the Royal College of General Practitioners*, **29**, 554–558.

Wilson L (1976). The social worker in general practice. *Medical Journal of Australia*, **1**, 664–666.

Wing J K (1976). Preliminary communication: a technique for studying psychiatric morbidity in in-patient and out-patient series and in general population samples. *Psychological Medicine*, **6**, 665–671.

5 Day care and rehabilitation services

F. Holloway and J. Carson

Both professionals and lay people tend to adopt a short-term view of illness. There is an expectation that it should respond rapidly to specific treatments that are prescribed by the doctor. In reality many physical and psychiatric illnesses take a chronic course and the sufferer and carers have to experience long-term disability. To understand the impact of chronic illness it is useful to make a distinction between the underlying impairments associated with the illness, the consequent disability and the resulting social handicap that is produced (WHO 1980).

Impairment, disability and handicap

The basic impairments of mental illness result in symptoms (e.g. hallucinatory voices; delusional beliefs; 'negative' psychotic symptoms such as slowness, underactivity and social withdrawal; low mood; the physical concomitants of anxiety and depression) and a range of abnormalities in psychological functioning, for example poor attention and concentration. Typical disabilities resulting from a mental disorder include poor interpersonal skills, difficulty coping with finances and inability to work and carry out domestic chores. The social handicaps associated with a long-term mental illness include the stigma of a mental illness diagnosis, poverty, unemployment, lack of social support and homelessness. These handicaps may be compounded by adverse personal reactions to illness, such as depression, despair and loss of motivation for self-help. Long-term mental illness induces similar feelings of hopelessness amongst professional and lay carers (Wing and Morris 1981). These problems will be made worse by any social disadvantages that precede the appearance of illness. It is, however, perfectly possible to experience the impairments of a severe mental illness (for example systematized delusions), without exhibiting obvious disability or social handicap.

Key principles of rehabilitation

Despite significant advances in social and psychological treatment we cannot, at present, abolish the impairments underlying chronic mental illness.

Tackling the disability and social handicap associated with long-term psychiatric disorder is the province of rehabilitation (Shepherd 1991). Psychiatric rehabilitation has been defined as 'the process of helping a ... disabled person to make the best use of his (*sic*) residual abilities in order to function at an optimum level in as normal a social context as possible' (Bennett 1978). It is an endeavour that demands multidisciplinary working and multiagency cooperation. Effective rehabilitation must be based on a thorough and holistic assessment of the needs of the patient and their carers, taking full account of their views (MacCarthy *et al.* 1986) and strengths. (See Chapter 9 for a fuller discussion of the assessment of long-term clients.) One constant dilemma of rehabilitation is the tension between respecting the wishes of the service user and allowing them to 'rot with their rights on' when their choices are objectively wrong for themselves or dangerous to others.

The aims of a mental health rehabilitation service will be: (1) to improve functional and interpersonal skills; (2) to ensure that people can successfully occupy as wide a range of social roles as possible (e.g. family member; worker; homemaker; sexual partner; friend); (3) if necessary to provide supportive environments that allow maximum possible independence despite any residual disability; and (4) to offer continuing care. The focus should be on improving the quality of life of the patient/client and decreasing the burden on carers. A number of authors have identified the key features of good rehabilitation services. Table 5.1 summarizes the recommendations of Anthony *et al.* (1982), Bachrach (1992) and Pilling (1991).

Rehabilitation is often confused with resettlement, which is the preparation and placement of people with long-term disabilities into new, and often less dependent, living settings. Psychiatric rehabilitation differs from the rehabilitation of physical disorders in that it is likely to be a continuing process. In contrast with resettlement, successful rehabilitation does not cease once the patient has left hospital.

Rehabilitation services and research into the care of the long-term mentally ill have concentrated on the needs of people with a diagnosis of schizophrenia. It is usually assumed this experience is readily applicable to patients suffering from other mental illnesses. This assumption is unlikely to be the case, particularly for people disabled by anxiety, somatization and personality disorders for whom the traditional rehabilitation model of skills training is unlikely to be relevant (Watts and Bennett 1983).

Development of rehabilitation services

Active rehabilitation for mental illnesses dates back to the era of 'moral treatment' in the early nineteenth century. 'Humanity, reason and kindness animated [the] philosophy' of moral treatment (Porter 1987). In practice this meant care in small, well-staffed asylums where residents were encouraged to engage in normal social activities, with an emphasis on productive work and an expectation of return to pre-existing social roles on discharge. However asylums fell into a 'long sleep' that was to last in Britain for a century, until in the early 1950s active rehabilitation of inmates was introduced (Bennett 1983). Two factors were important: an emphasis on discharge when-

Table 5.1 Key principles for psychiatric rehabilitation services

Anthony et al. (1982)	*Pilling (1991)*	*Bachrach (1992)*
Functional assessment of client's skills	Based on client's rights to full citizenship	Orientated towards individual need
Client involvement in rehabilitation	Client involved in all decisions	Pays attention to the patient's environment
Individual rehabilitation plan	Clients integrated into their natural community	Utilizes patient's strengths
Direct skills teaching to clients	Promote development of normal patterns	Active involvement of patient in their care
Environmental assessment and modification	Maximize independence – build on assets and supports	Aims to restore hope in patient and their carers
Follow-up of clients in real-life environments	Service based on assessment of individual need	Emphasis on the value of occupation
Rehabilitation team approach	Service evaluated for accessibility, acceptability, equity, cost-effectiveness and comprehensibility	Addresses social life and recreational needs
Evaluation of desirable outcomes	Service comprehensive	Is an ongoing process
Consumer involvement in policy and planning	Service coordinated within and between agencies	
	Service to encourage continued personal development of clients	

ever possible and a renewed focus on the role of work as a medium for rehabilitation. Subsequently the introduction of antipsychotic treatment, the rise of the district general hospital psychiatric unit and the realization that institutional care could be damaging to inmates led to the overoptimistic conclusion that appropriate treatment (both social and medical) could abolish long-term disability altogether (Lavender and Holloway 1992). In many areas effective rehabilitation services that had developed within psychiatric hospitals languished. Community care services lacked adequate systems for rehabilitation and aftercare (Brown *et al.* 1966).

Unfortunately, the assumption that long-term disability would be abolished by community-orientated care proved to be incorrect. Although very long-term follow-up of patients with schizophrenia has suggested that improvement in mental state and social functioning will often occur (Harding *et al.* 1987*a*), continuing disability remains common in patients who have been hospitalized as a result of affective illness (Lee and Murray 1988) and schizophrenia. So-called 'minor' psychiatric disorders also often take a chronic course (Goldberg and Huxley 1992). Increased understanding of the nature of psychiatric disability and experience gained from the continuing programme of mental hospital closure has led to a rediscovery of the role of rehabilitation (Shepherd 1991). In the USA, 'psychosocial rehabilitation' has developed quite separately from mainstream psychiatric services (Bachrach 1992). Rejection of the (mythical) 'medical model' is common in contemporary community-based services for people with long-term mental health problems. In contrast these services are often profoundly influenced by the principles of normalization or social role valorization (Wolfensberger 1983), which focuses on the ethical importance of valuing individuals with disability.

Despite its enormous influence on service development and provision (Ramon 1988; Brown and Smith 1992) the principles upon which normalization are based have received surprisingly little critical evaluation (Carson *et al*. 1992; 1993). Only one published study has attempted to evaluate day services from a normalization perspective (Wainwright *et al*. 1988), using the PASSING (Program Analysis of Service Systems' Implementation of Normalization Goals) assessment (Wolfensberger and Thomas 1983). The evaluation identified very different issues from a study of the same unit that used a 'needs assessment' technique based on a more traditional illness model (Holloway 1991*a*).

Role of rehabilitation in mental health services

Rehabilitation should be an aspect of all mental health services. The acute in-patient unit and residential, day care and community services should be aware of the long-term needs of their clients. These needs include control of distressing or disabling psychiatric symptoms; pharmacological, psychological and social methods of relapse prevention; general health care; promotion of independent living skills; the support and education of carers; crisis intervention; accommodation; structured day activities and opportunities for meaningful occupation; leisure opportunities; and the development of supportive social networks (Lavender and Holloway 1992).

Since so many clients of mental health services have long-term problems the need for specific 'rehabilitation' services within a locality is unclear. Concern over the possible 'ghettoization' of people with a mental illness and other forms of disability has led to emphasis on the use whenever possible of generic community resources for long-term support. However there is a well-documented tendency for community services to drift towards providing for people with short-term 'problems of living' and dealing with crises. A focus for long-term care therefore seems to be necessary. One option is the 'continuing care team' that supports patients with the most severe disabilities (Holloway, 1991*b*). This team would have to be supplemented by a range of resources, including day care and residential facilities.

The rest of this chapter is devoted to the role of day care: other important aspects of long-term care are discussed in Chapters 9 (Interventions with long-term clients), 12 (Interventions with Families), 14 (Long-term medication) and 15 (Daily living skills for clients in the community).

Overview of day care

History of day care

The first recorded psychiatric day hospital opened in Moscow in 1933, apparently in response to a lack of in-patient beds (Field 1967). The unit provided work-orientated rehabilitation and acted as a half-way house between hospital and community. The first day hospitals in the West were opened in 1946 by Cameron in Montreal, Canada, and Bierer in London (Goldman 1989). At that time, psychiatric care was almost entirely based within the mental hospital. It was argued that day hospital treatment would produce less risk of institutionalization and less stigma, allowing the patient to remain in contact with family and friends. It was also hoped that day hospital care would be cheaper than 24-hour care in hospital. Day hospitals rapidly established themselves in Britain (Farndale 1963).

Many early day hospitals followed Bierer's original therapeutic community model (Bierer 1959). This was based on the assumption that much mental illness was caused by faulty or inadequate relationships and that treatment should therefore be of 'an experiential or situational nature' using the social group. Therapeutic community principles have had a profound effect on the development of day care in Britain (Holloway 1988). However, other units followed a more traditional 'medical' model, with the day hospital functioning as an ordinary ward with the exception that the patients went home at night. Day hospitals that developed in association with large mental hospitals often took on the role of providing support to psychotic former long-stay patients who had been discharged as part of the new pattern of 'community care'.

Government policy for day care

Initially mental health day care was provided solely by the health service. Following the foundation of the National Health Service (NHS) in 1948 local authorities were given responsibility for preventative and after-care services. However this was never made a statutory obligation. Local authority day care was non-existent before 1960 and services were only developed on any scale following the establishment of social service departments in 1971 (Vaughan 1983).

The government White Paper *Better Services for the Mentally Ill* (DHSS 1975) outlined an ideal system of day care for Britain. Local authority social service departments were to provide 60 places per 100 000 population in day centres. These were to cater for clients' long-term needs for shelter, occupation and support and to provide respite for families. Day hospitals were to provide a short-term treatment-orientated service under medical supervision, with a norm of 30 places per 100 000 population. Day hospitals and day centres were to be supplemented by employment rehabilitation services and the voluntary sector, which would focus on offering low-key 'drop-ins' and social clubs. In the event the bulk of long-term day care is still provided by the NHS, and it is very doubtful that the neat distinction between treatment and long-term care can readily be made. Day centre clients and day hospital patients with long-term mental illnesses have very similar needs (Holloway 1991*a*, 1991*c*), although day hospitals tend to have much higher staffing levels.

Norms are now no longer fashionable, but the 'Better Services' pattern of care remains British government policy. The community care White Paper *Caring for People* (DoH 1989) stated that health authorities were resonsible for 'health' aspects of care whilst the social services authorities were responsible for the bulk of care in the community. Both authorities must take on the role of 'purchaser' of services, with a variety of statutory, private and voluntary sector providers competing for service contracts. The implementation of these policies will have a profound effect on the future provision of day care and other 'rehabilitative' services (Holloway 1990), which do not fall neatly on either side of the artificial health/social care divide.

Day care and mental health services

The development of day care in Britain has been aptly described as 'disordered' (Vaughan 1983). There are gross disparities in the availability of day places. Day hospitals, local authority day centres and voluntary sector facilities cater for similar client groups with markedly differing staffing, in terms of numbers of staff and their professional background, and degree of backup from the psychiatric services. Confusion remains as to what day care actually is, what its legitimate functions are and how these functions are best carried out.

There is no recognized training for staff working in day care. Local authority workers may have a social work background and may go on to receive generic social work training. The majority of staff within day hospitals have either psychiatric nursing qualifications or training in occupational therapy. The background of voluntary sector workers is very heterogeneous. Although individual counselling and assessments of daily living skills may be carried out, most day activities involve groups of attenders. Staff therefore require considerable groupwork skills to be effective as day care workers.

A number of core functions of day care can be identified (Holloway 1988):

- an alternative to in-patient admission for people who are acutely psychiatrically ill and cannot safely be maintained as out-patients
- a service of support, supervision and monitoring during the transition between in-patient care and living at home
- a site for brief intensive therapy for people with personality difficulties, severe neurotic illnesses or in need of short-term focused rehabilitation
- a source of long-term support and structure for people with long-term disabilities.

In addition to these 'clinical' functions, a day unit may act as an information resource, a centre for training staff who provide community care and a focus for potentially fragmented community services. The role of the day unit

as a mental health resource centre is potentially important but as yet uneval-
uated.

While we go on to review a number of controlled studies of day care in
the next section, it is helpful to note some of the typical problems encountered in evaluating day care identified by Milne (1987). Milne found that
most day care programmes have vague or unstated goals, the programmes
tend to be based around staff interests rather than the needs of users, specific therapeutic groups may not be carried out proficiently and programmes
are rarely systematically evaluated.

Acute day care

The potential for a day hospital to act as an alternative to admission to the
in-patient ward has long been recognized (Harris 1957), and *Better Services
for the Mentally Ill* assumed that the day hospital would offer 'acute' care.
A number of controlled trials have been carried out in Britain and the
United States of America that have shown such 'acute' care to be clinically
feasible and at least as good in terms of outcome as traditional in-patient
treatment (Wilder *et al.* 1966; Herz *et al.* 1971; Dick *et al.* 1985; Creed *et al.*
1990).

There are problems in interpreting the research literature. Firstly, all studies have adopted a 'black box' approach to day care: it is very difficult to
get a feel for what actually went on in the day unit during the study. Secondly,
all studies have excluded a high proportion of patients presenting for admission (up to 80 per cent), because they were too ill for day care, required
admission for social reasons (e.g. lack of community support), were too well
for in-patient care, or because they fell outside certain diagnostic or age criteria set by the researchers. Thirdly, the research appears at odds with the
bulk of clinical practice, certainly in Britain where true 'acute' day care is
rarely provided. Some units that do take in 'acute' patients and maintain a
rapid patient turnover do so by admitting patients in psychosocial crisis who
would not now generally gain admission to hard-pressed inner-city in-patient
units.

Two studies by Creed and colleagues (1990; 1991) go some way to identifying the ingredients of successful 'acute' day care. They carried out parallel studies of acute day care in two settings: a well-staffed day hospital that
had a long-standing philosophy of acute care and a policy of discharging
patients who were becoming 'chronic'; and a less well-staffed unit that had
previously catered for patients who were less acutely ill or required rehabilitation. In the first service 80 per cent of the patients randomly allocated
to day care were successfully engaged with treatment whilst in the second
unit only 54 per cent could be engaged, largely because severely disturbed
behaviour could not be tolerated. Even in the first unit 40 per cent of the
patients could not be allocated to the study because they were too obviously
disturbed, were detained under the Mental Health Act or lacked adequate
social support. Creed *et al.* (1990) concluded that given the right setting
roughly 40 per cent of all patients presenting for admission to their inner-
city psychiatric unit could satisfactorily be managed in a well-staffed day unit
without any recourse to admission. The research evidence therefore suggests

that acute day care might become a useful complement to in-patient beds and community support services, but that adequate resourcing and committed staff are essential.

Transitional day care

Many day hospitals offer transitional care for patients who have just been discharged from the in-patient unit. Some occupational therapy departments offer a rather similar day treatment programme for former in-patients. Day care has been shown to be a useful adjunct to policies of 'brief in-patient care', where in-patients are rapidly discharged from the ward but offered the option of continuing daytime support (Endicott *et al.* 1979; Herz *et al.* 1979; Hirsch *et al.* 1979). 'Brief-care' can be further supplemented by providing a low-key residential setting on the same campus as the in-patient/day hospital psychiatric unit (Gudeman *et al.* 1985). However one controlled study of patients with schizophrenia or severe affective disorder who were stable at the time of discharge showed no clinical advantage from a structured 'transitional treatment programme' lasting 6–12 weeks over an out-patient follow-up group (both patient groups continuing to receive medication) (Glick *et al.* 1986). There is also a suggestion that simple transitional care will be less appropriate for the 'revolving door' patient who comes into hospital with pre-existing social handicaps. These patients probably require long-term assertive community management (Stein and Test 1980).

One issue that is never addressed by the proponents of acute and transitional day care is that of dependence on the setting. Clinically it is common for patients who engage with day settings to become dependent on the unit, which becomes an important part of their social world. This may even be seen as a necessary part of the process of therapy, particularly for patients who have long-term disabilities. The effect of dependence is to make people reluctant to accept discharge plans when staff feel that the time has come for the attender to move on. The problem may be obviated by excluding admissions who have long-term problems (scarcely practical in the inner city) or, possibly, by rigidly enforcing limits on the length of stay in the day unit.

Short-term treatment and rehabilitation

Day care and the 'neurotic' patient

Day hospital care provides no additional benefit to the generality of patients referred for a psychiatric opinion by their general practitioner to the out-patient department who suffer from 'neurotic' illnesses (Tyrer and Remington 1979). However there is an obvious role for a day unit in providing short-term, focused treatments for patients who cannot satisfactorily be managed in out-patient settings but who do not require in-patient treatment (Dick *et al.* 1991).

Some day units provide intensive psychotherapy, usually on group-analytic lines (Newby *et al.* 1987). The therapists are often specially trained nursing staff who receive supervision from a consultant psychotherapist. There is little evidence for the effectiveness of this form of day treatment, although Dick and Wooff (1986) reported success in terms of decreased service utilization and increased self-satisfaction amongst a group of patients who had engaged in a 12-week therapy programme that involved small groups, community meetings, Gestalt therapy, 'video feedback' and art therapy. Interestingly a subgroup of patients who engaged in therapy, who were retrospectively diagnosed as having a borderline personality disorder, showed markedly increased service utilization during the follow-up year. Sims *et al.* (1993) studied symptomatology and social relationships in a cohort of referrals to Tuke House, a psychotherapeutic day unit in Leeds. The drop-out rate from the study was high, but patients who complied with treatment showed a significant improvement in symptoms after a 12-week treatment course. Improvement in social relationships was only found at 18-month follow-up, by which time patients' level of symptoms had again worsened. Psychotherapeutically-orientated day units are likely to exclude people with severe disabilities, either as a matter of policy (Sims *et al.* 1993) or by the selective dropping out of less articulate and less well-motivated clients (Bender and Pilling 1985).

Day hospital rehabilitation

Day treatment has an obvious role in improving the social competence of patients who lack social and functional skills as a result of long-term mental illnesses (Holloway 1988). Components of social competence include socialization skills (the ability to relate to others); self-care and home management skills; ability to use community facilities; work skills; and literacy and numerary skills. The focused short-term cognitive and behavioural interventions discussed in Chapter 9 may readily be offered in a day facility. Although it has eloquent advocates who have developed an impressive array of behavioural interventions (Liberman 1988), there is surprisingly little research evidence underpinning 'rehabilitative' day care. The 'skills training' approach is particularly prominent in the USA, whilst in Britain the practical difficulties that are encountered in generalizing gains in skills to other settings are emphasized (Shepherd 1991).

Falloon and Talbot (1982) described a model day treatment programme that attempted to meet the stated needs and goals of attenders, which were felt to fall into three broad categories: socialization; work; and the relief of symptoms. Specific treatments, with a strongly behavioural focus, were developed to meet these needs. These included social-skills training groups, a work training programme and specific group and individual treatments targeted at psychiatric symptoms and behavioural problems. Considerable success was reported in meeting the goals defined by attenders of the programme, which was supplemented by the provision of medication and adequate after-care. Table 5.2 lists some targeted interventions that may usefully be provided within a day care setting.

Studies have claimed that day units that focus on attenders' achieving specific behavioural goals are more successful than units with a less structured approach (Austin *et al.* 1976; Milne 1984). However this research has been methodologically flawed (Holloway 1985). Only one controlled study of day

Table 5.2 Targeted interventions that can be offered in a psychiatric day unit

- Needs assessment
- Training in basic living skills
- Social skills training
- Work skills training
- (Behavioural) family therapy for schizophrenia
- Cognitive–behavioural treatments for delusions and hallucinations
- Educational programmes about schizophrenia and its treatment
- Cognitive–behavioural treatments for anxiety and depression
- Bereavement counselling
- Group psychotherapy
- Case management/care management

hospital rehabilitation for patients with chronic psychotic illnesses living in the community has been carried out. This found no overall differences in outcome after one year of treatment between patients who received day care and those who only received standard out-patient management (Stevens 1973). Interestingly the author of that study noted that some patients did particularly badly in the day hospital because they found that the group therapy that was offered was ineffective and disturbing.

Improving social networks

A further issue that needs to be addressed by rehabilitation services is the patient's social network. People with a long-term mental illness have impoverished social networks that often consist entirely of family members (Mueller 1980). Relationships tend to be non-reciprocal, with aid flowing from carer to patient. A variety of approaches have been developed to improve the quality and quantity of social networks. Family management approaches are reviewed in Chapter 12. Where the immediate family has become depleted and exhausted by the burden of care, attempts have been made to engage the patient's entire social network (Schoenfeld *et al.* 1986), including relatives, friends co-workers and significant others. Residential and day care provide an artificial social network: many day care attenders are specifically motivated to attend by the social contact that is offered (Holloway 1989). Rehabilitation services should be encouraging people to use generic resources, such as local pubs, cafés, sports centres and libraries, and fostering the development of new social networks. Befriending schemes may also be valuable. At their best the contrived relationships that develop are indistinguishable from natural friendships.

Problems with short-term day care

The problem of dependence, which was discussed above in relation to 'acute' day care, is also relevant to a rehabilitation setting. A contrasting problem with a short-term approach to day treatment is the process of engagement with services. For patients with severe psychiatric disabilities, who often have problems developing any form of trusting relationship, this may be a very laborious and prolonged process. Difficulties that have been encountered in generalizing skills gains acquired in group or individual treatment to 'the environment of need' have led to interest in 'in vivo' training (see Chapter 14) within the patient's natural environment. One innovative approach to rehabilitation is a day service that dispenses with a building but runs sessions in a variety of settings (e.g. local church halls, adult education facilities, sports halls). More users can be helped by this flexible deployment of resources than within a traditional day unit. Moreover there is reason to doubt the quality of much of the "rehabilitation" work that goes on in day units (Holloway, 1991*a*). Although there is a general agreement that programmes should be tailored to individual need, many units slot attenders into already existing treatment groups. Assessments are often haphazard and staff have often not been adequately trained for the work and are rarely adequately supervised.

The future of short-term day hospital treatment is unclear. In the current managerial and financial climate units will only survive if they can persuade purchasers of services that they are deploying proven and cost-effective treatments to an appropriate client group and achieving acceptable outcomes and adequate through-put of clients/patients. One attractive option is the development of a 'mental health resource centre', which is readily accessible to the local community (particularly the local GPs), carries out rapid assessment of need and then offers a flexible programme including specific targeted interventions, such as anxiety management programmes, bereavement counselling, social-skills training and the family management of schizophrenia. Such a centre could become the hub of an active network of community care services, closely integrated into the local system of 'care management'.

Day care and long-term support

Day care has an important role in providing long-term support for people with severe psychiatric disabilities (Holloway 1988). From the users' perspective a day unit offers somewhere to go, away from wherever they live. This may provide respite from a fraught family situation or alternatively from complete social isolation. Hopefully the unit is physically comfortable and warm. A free or cheap meal is generally provided. Practical help with day-to-day problems, such as financial difficulties and welfare benefits, may be available. Attenders may derive comfort and support from getting to know people who have similar problems to their own, and staff may be viewed as a major source of emotional support. Others, particularly people with the more severe disorders, find great benefit in the availability of 'company without intimacy' (Mitchell and Birley 1983). Most day settings offer some form of occupation or recreation, which in some facilities amounts to a highly structured programme of sheltered work. Studies of attenders' views of day care confirm that the availability of occupational and recreational activities is highly valued (Holloway 1989).

From a social-psychological viewpoint, day care plays a role closely akin to the 'latent' psychological functions of work. In addition to its obvious role in providing people with financial rewards (the 'manifest function') work provides a structure to one's time, enforces activity, offers social relationships outside the home and produces external goals for achievement (Jahoda 1981). The value of projects that actually provide work is discussed later in this chapter.

Despite its significance the role of supportive long-term day care has not been much researched. An important multicentre controlled trial of day treatment compared with out-patient drug management of patients with chronic schizophrenia found that day care improved attenders, social functioning (Linn *et al.* 1979). However only some units were able to reduce the frequency of psychotic relapse amongst attenders. Successful units were characterized by an accepting low-key atmosphere, a key-worker system, slower patient flows through the unit and an emphasis on occupation and recreation rather than 'therapy' (Linn *et al.* 1979). The findings of Wing and Brown 1970) in their classic study of in-patients with schizophrenia in three mental hospitals are relevant in this context. They identified a number of important characteristics of a good-quality long-term care setting. These included regular staff–user meetings, a key-worker system, good communication within staff hierarchies, high staff morale and positive attitudes of staff towards patients. The factor that was most clearly related to the development of the 'negative' symptoms of schizophrenia was 'time spent doing nothing': this in itself is a powerful argument for a day care service that makes positive demands on users with psychotic illnesses.

A number of studies have been carried out on the needs of day care attenders who have a long-term mental illness (Pryce *et al.* 1983; Wykes *et al.* 1985; Brugha *et al.* 1988; Brewin *et al.* 1988; Holloway 1991*a,c*). This research suggests that no substantial distinction can be drawn between the needs of day hospital and day centre attenders. Although some day hospitals may be more effective in meeting need than local day centres (Brewin *et al.* 1988) this is not necessarily the case (Holloway 1991*a*). The key to an effective day service is regular multidisciplinary review of service users (Wykes *et al.* 1985): successful day units draw on the expertise of other agencies in order to ensure that their clients' needs are met (Holloway 1991*a*).

Many people with long-term mental illnesses, particularly those who live alone, find evenings and weekends very difficult. Voluntary organizations can be particularly successful in providing informal 'drop-ins' which can complement more formal day care services. A low-key and unstructured 'drop-in' may attract clients who are reluctant to engage in more formal day care, satisfying the need for 'company without intimacy' (Mitchell and Birley 1983). Voluntary sector facilities are often able to involve clients in the running of the unit.

The Fountain House model of psychosocial rehabilitation

The importance of engaging users in the running of their day unit has recently become widely accepted. User involvement was always a key feature of day facilities that operated along therapeutic community lines. It is also one of the elements of the influential 'clubhouse' model, which was pioneered by John Beard at Fountain House, New York (Beard *et al.* 1982), and has subsequently spread across North America and into Europe. A handful of 'clubhouses' have opened in Britain, although evaluation of these units has not yet been reported.

'Clubhouse' attenders are members of the club. Membership brings certain rights (access to the facilities) and responsibilities (contribution to the running of the clubhouse). Staff have a facilitative role, and members take responsibility for the running and maintenance of the clubhouse. Work groups provide catering, domestic and clerical services to the clubhouse and arrange the social and recreational activities that are offered. The aim is to provide a range of opportunities for members, so that everyone can contribute, whatever their current level of ability. A vital element of the clubhouse philosophy is that members should feel wanted and needed rather than the recipients of help that they require. There is a strong emphasis on the value of productive work.

The Fountain House programme has a number of components. These include a prevocational day programme (essentially the activities required to run the facility), a transitional employment programme, evening and weekend activities, outreach to members who have inexplicably stopped attending, a thrift shop and a clubhouse newspaper (Beard *et al.* 1982). In addition, Fountain House holds leases on flats, which provide access to housing for members and a base for skills training for patients moving out of the local mental hospitals. (Future leases depend on access to affordable rented accommodation.) In contrast with many community mental health projects, Fountain House actively acknowledges the value of medication in maintaining the stabilty of members. When signs of relapse are identified, members are encouraged to seek help from the relevant clinic or hospital.

The transitional employment programme (TEP) is a key element of the programme. It involves placing members into 'entry level' jobs, initially in a part-time capacity, which require minimal training or job skills. These placements are underwritten by a guarantee that in the absence of the member the job will be filled by other Fountain House personnel, if necessary a staff member. TEP placement may result in permanent employment for the member.

No controlled trial has been carried out comparing referral to a clubhouse with an alternative form of long-term care. There must be doubts about the capacity of a clubhouse to engage people with severe psychiatric disabilities. However the validity of this model, at least within a North American context, is demonstrated by a continuing expansion in clubhouse numbers. Certainly it provides a provocative contrast to the generality of mental health day care, which tends to view attenders as recipients of care rather than active participants.

Role of work

Employment is nature's best physician and is essential to human happiness. (Galen, AD 172: quoted in Harding *et al.* 1987*b*).

No other technique for the conduct of life so firmly attaches the individual to reality as laying emphasis on work; for work at least gives him a secure place in a position of reality, in the human community.

(Freud 1930)

The general psychological importance of work is shown most clearly by the impact of unemployment on mental health (Warr and Jackson 1985). Jahoda's (1981) conceptualization of the 'latent' and 'manifest' functions of work, which was discussed above, was developed during her research into the impact of unemployment during the recession of the 1930s, when demoralization and despair gripped whole communities. Warner (1985) has hypothesized that the significantly better prognosis for schizophrenia in Third World countries is in part due to the reduction in handicap provided by readier access to work opportunities for people with a mental illness in non-industrialized societies.

The history of psychiatric rehabilitation strongly emphasizes the value of work for people with a severe mental illness, although 'the integration of work into systems that treat severe mental illness is limited, sporadic and inadequately addressed' (Harding *et al.* 1987*b*). Work-related activities were a key feature of rehabilitation within the psychiatric hospital (Bennett 1983) and played an important role in early community care programmes (Bennett 1970). However, sheltered work fell into disfavour and was frequently stigmatized as exploitative and dehumanizing. The pendulum is now swinging back. Work is again recognized as an important component of any comprehensive mental health service (Pilling 1988).

Research into the role of work in the rehabilitation and long-term support of people with severe mental illnesses has been reviewed by Pilling (1988). There is evidence that work has a protective function, both in the prevention of readmission (Anthony *et al.* 1972) and in reversing the development of 'negative' psychotic symptoms (Wing and Brown 1970). Work training programmes developed for people with a physical disability require adaptation, notably in offering longer periods of training (Cornes *et al.* 1982). Success in resettling people who have been through work rehabilitation depends on the social skills of the trainee (Watts 1978): there is some evidence that (at least within a work context) these skills can be developed (Miles 1972). Long-term work projects have to take account of the nature of psychiatric disability: the importance of structure, supervision and clear task identification have been emphasized (Wadsworth *et al.* 1962). Perhaps most encouragingly attenders report a number of benefits from such programmes. In one study 70 workshop attenders were interviewed using a 69 item questionnaire that asked about their work history, job satisfaction, relations with staff and issues around the protective nature of work (Carson *et al.* 1991). Some 90 per cent liked the work atmosphere, 88 per cent enjoyed being with others during the day and 58 per cent enjoyed working with other people who had mental health problems. Although 59 per cent aspired to obtain open employment only 17 per cent believed that they would eventually be able to do so.

Ideally a range of work-related provision is required. Simple advice and encouragement that people make use of mainstream provision for the unemployed, including job clubs and work training schemes, will suffice for many people who are not severely disabled by their illness. Work assessment may be offered: this will involve identifying the current level of occupational functioning and may include assessment of interests and aptitudes. Sheltered work schemes are particularly important, and many innovative projects have opened in recent years. These may be complemented by sheltered placements in open employment. The Fountain House transitional employment programme is a particularly well-structured form of sheltered placement. However, work is not a panacea for mental illness. Some people are too disabled or unmotivated to engage in the structure and commitment required for a successful work project. For people who are less disabled, the prospects of open employment are strongly dependent on the economic situation: people with disabilities are disproportionately affected by recession and high levels of unemployment.

Conclusion

This chapter has discussed the history of psychiatric rehabilitation and current thinking about the role of rehabilitation in mental health services. Day care and work services have also been reviewed. Unfortunately there is no blueprint available for the ideal system of rehabilitation and community support for people with a long-term mental illness (Holloway 1988). Services should develop according to local assessment of need, the availability of resources and local priorities.

However, a number of principles are clear. Interagency working is vital, both at the level of the purchaser of services and between service providers on either side of the artificial and unhelpful health/social care divide. Help that is offered should be based on a thorough and valid assessment of need. The wishes of service users and carers are of prime importance, although these may at times may have to be overridden. Given the fragmentation of community care services it is important to have at the heart of any system of long-term care a team whose task is the welfare of people with long-term and severe mental illnesses. The 'continuing care team' will aim to provide a coordinated package of support, orchestrated by a key worker or case manager (Holloway 1991*b*). This team should be able to access a range of day and work services that offer a variety of activities, social groups and therapeutic approaches.

References

Austin N K, Liberman R P, King L and De Risi W J (1976). A comparative evaluation of two day hospitals. *Journal of Nervous and Mental Disease*, **163**, 253–262.
Anthony W A, Buell G J, Sharratt S and Althoff M E (1972). The efficacy of psychiatric rehabilitation. *Psychological Bulletin*, **78**, 447–456.
Anthony W, Cohen M and Fargas M (1982). A psychiatric rehabilitation treatment program: can I recognize one if I see one? *Community Mental Health Journal*, **18**, 83–95.
Bachrach L L (1992). Psychosocial rehabilitation and psychiatry in the care of long-term patients. *American Journal of Psychiatry*, **149**, 1455–1463.
Beard J H, Proust R N and Malamud T J (1982). The Fountain House model of psychiatric rehabilitation. *Psychosocial Rehabilitation Journal*, **5**, 47–53.
Bender M P and Pilling S (1985). A study of variables associated with under-attendance at a psychiatric day care centre. *Psychological Medicine*, **15**, 395–402.

Bennett D H (1970). The value of work in psychiatric rehabilitation. *Social Psychiatry*, **5**, 224–230.

Bennett D H (1978). Social forms of psychiatric treatment. In *Schizophrenia: Towards a New Synthesis* (ed. J Wing). Academic Press, London.

Bennett D H (1983). The historical development of rehabilitation services. In *Theory and Practice of Psychiatric Rehabilitation* (ed. FN Watts and DH Bennett). Wiley, Chichester.

Bierer J (1959). Theory and practice of psychiatric day hospitals. *Lancet*, 901–902.

Blake R, Millard D W and Roberts J P (1984). Therapeutic community principles in an integrated local authority mental health service. *International Journal of Therapeutic Communities*, **5**, 243–273.

Brewin C R, Wing J R, Mangen S P, Brugha T S, MacCarthy B and Lesage A (1988). Needs for care among the long-term mentally ill: a report from the Camberwell High Contact Survey. *Psychological Medicine*, **18**, 457–468.

Brown G W, Bone M, Dalison B and Wing J R (1966) *Schizophrenia and Social Care*. Oxford University Press, London.

Brown H and Smith H (1992). *Normalization: A Reader for the Nineties*. Routledge, London.

Brugha T. Wing J K, Brewin C R, MacCarthy B. Mangen S. Lesage A and Mumford J (1988). The problems of people in long-term psychiatric day care. An introduction to the Camberwell High Contact Survey. *Psychological Medicine*, **18**, 443–456.

Carson J. Luyombya G. Wilder J. Barrow S and Boyle M (1991). Job satisfaction? *Health Service Journal*, **101**, 21.

Carson J, Dowling F. Luyombya G, Senapti-Sharma M and Glynn T (1992). Normalization . . . and now for something completely different. *Clinical Psychology Forum*, **49**, 27–30.

Carson J, Glynn T and Gopaulen J (1993). The influence of normalization on psychiatric services. In *Dimensions of Community Care* (eds. M Weller and M Muijen). Harcourt Brace Jovanovich, London.

Cornes P, Alderman J, Cumella S, Harradence J, Hutton D and Tebbutt A G (1982). *Employment Rehabilitation: The Aims and Achievements of a Service for Disabled People*. Manpower Services Commission, HMSO, London.

Craft M (1958). An evaluation of treatment of depressive illness in a day hospital. *Lancet*, 149–151.

Creed F, Black D, Anthony P, Osborn M, Thomas P and Tomenson B (1990). Randomized controlled trial of day patient versus in-patient psychiatric treatment. *British Medical Journal*, **300**, 1033–1037.

Creed F, Black D, Anthony P, Osborn M, Thomas P, Franks D, Polley R, Lancashire S, Saleem P and Tomenson B (1991). Randomized controlled trial of day and in-patient psychiatric treatment 2: comparison of two hospitals. *British Journal of Psychiatry*, **158**, 183–189.

Department of Health and Social Security (1975). *Better Services for the Mentally Ill*. HMSO, London.

Department of Health and Social Security (1989). *Community Care in the Next Decade and Beyond*. HMSO, London.

Dick B M and Wooff K (1986). An evaluation of a time-limited programme of dynamic group psychotherapy. *British Journal of Psychiatry*, **148**, 159–164.

Dick P, Cameron L, Cohen D, Barlow M and Ince A (1985). Day and full time psychiatric treatment: a controlled comparison. *British Journal of Psychiatry*, **147**, 246–250.

Dick P H, Sweeny M L and Crombie I R (1991). Controlled comparison of day-patient and out-patient treatment for persistent anxiety and depression. *British Journal of Psychiatry*, **158**, 24–27.

Endicott J, Cohen J, Nee J, Fleiss J L and Herz M I (1979). Brief versus standard hospitalization. For whom? *Archives of General Psychiatry*, **36**, 706–712.

94 *Day care and rehabilitation services*

Falloon I R H and Talbot R E (1982). Achieving the goals of day treatment. *Journal of Nervous and Mental Disease*, **170**, 279–285.

Farndale W A J (1963). The British day hospitals. In *Trends in Mental Health Services* (eds. H Freeman and W A J Farndale). Pergamon Press, Oxford.

Field M G (1967). Soviet and American approaches to mental illness. In *New Aspects of Mental Health Services* (eds. H Freeman and W A J Farndale). Pergamon Press, Oxford.

Freud S (1930; republished 1985). *Civilization and its Discontents*. Pelican Freud Library, vol. 12. Penguin, Harmondsworth.

Glick I D, Fleming L, DeChitto N, Meyerkoff N, Jackson C, Muscara D and Good-Ellis M (1986). A controlled study of transitional day care for non-chronically ill patients. *American Journal of Psychiatry*, **143**, 1551–1556.

Goldberg D and Huxley P (1992). *Common Mental Disorders*. Routledge, London.

Goldman D L (1989). The forty year evolution of the first modern day hospital. *Canadian Journal of Psychiatry*, **34**, 18–19.

Gudeman J E, Dickey B and Evans A (1985). Four year assessment of a day hospital-inn program as an alternative to hospitalization. *American Journal of Psychiatry*, **142**, 1330–1333.

Harding C M, Brooks G W, Ashikaga T *et al.* (1987*a*). The Vermont longitudinal study II. Long-term outcome of subjects who once met the criteria for DSMIII schizophrenia. *American Journal of Psychiatry*, **144**, 727–735.

Harding CM, Strauss JS, Hafez H and Lieberman PB (1987*b*). Work and mental illness. *Journal of Nervous and Mental Disease*, **175**, 317–326.

Harris A (1957). Day hospitals and night hospitals in psychiatry. *Lancet*, 729–730.

Herz M I, Endicott J, Spitzer R L and Nesnikoff A (1971). Day versus in-patient hospitalization: a controlled study. *American Journal of Psychiatry*, **127**, 1371–1382.

Herz M I, Endicott J and Gibbon M (1979). Brief hospitalization: Two year follow-up. *Archives of General Psychiatry*, **36**, 701–705.

Hirsch S R, Platt S. Knights A and Weyman A (1979). Shortening hospital stay for psychiatric care: Effect on patients and their families. *British Medical Journal* (i), 442–446.

Holloway F (1988). Day care and community support. In *Community Care in Practice* (eds. A Lavender and F Holloway). John Wiley, Chichester.

Holloway F (1989). Psychiatric day care: the users' perspective. *International Journal of Social Psychiatry*, **35**, 252–264.

Holloway F (1990). Caring for people, a critical review of British government policy for the mentally ill, *Psychiatric Bulletin*, **14**, 641–645.

Holloway F (1991*a*). Day care in an inner city. II, Quality of services. *British Journal of Psychiatry*, **158**, 810–816.

Holloway F (1991*b*). Case management for the mentally ill: looking at the evidence. *International Journal of Social Psychiatry*, **37**, 2–13.

Holloway F (1991*c*). Day care in an inner city. I, Characteristics of attenders. *British Journal of Psychiatry*, **158**, 805–810.

Jahoda M (1981). The impact of unemployment in the 1930s and 1970s. *Bulletin of the British Psychological Society*, **32**, 304–314.

Lavender A and Holloway F (1992). Models of continuing care. In *Innovations in the Psychological Management of Schizophrenia* (eds. M Birchwood and N Tarrier). Wiley, Chichester.

Lee A S and Murray R M (1988). The long-term outcome of Maudsley depressives. *British Journal of Psychiatry*, **153**, 741–751.

Liberman R P (ed.) 1988). *Psychiatric Rehabilitation of Chronic Mental Patients*. American Psychiatric Association Press, Washington.

Linn M W, Caffey E M, Klett C J, Hogarty G E and Lamb H R (1979). Day treatment and psychotropic drugs in the aftercare of schizophrenic patients: a veterans administration cooperative study. *Archives of General Psychiatry*, **36**, 1055–1066.

MacCarthy B, Benson J and Brewin C R (1986). Task motivation and problem appraisal in long-term psychiatric patients. *Psychological Medicine*, **16**, 431–438.

Miles A (1972). The development of interpersonal relationships among longstay patients in two hospital workshops. *British Journal of Medical Psychology*, **45**, 105–114.

Milne D (1984). A comparative evaluation of two psychiatric day hospitals. *British Journal of Psychiatry*, **145**, 533–539.

Milne D (1987). *Evaluating Mental Health Practice: Methods and Applications*. Croom Helm, Beckenham.

Mitchell S and Birley J L T (1983). The use of ward support by psychiatric patients in the community. *British Journal of Psychiatry*, **142**, 9–15.

Mueller D P (1980). Social networks: a promising direction for research on the relationships of the social environment to psychiatric disorder. *Social Science and Medicine*, **14A**, 147–161.

Newby D, Lake B, Sims A C P (1987). Tuke House: initial experience of a new community service for neurotic illness. *Bulletin of the Royal College of Psychiatrists*, **11**, 269–271.

Pilling S (1988). Work and the continuing care client. In *Community Care in Practice* (eds. A Lavender and F Holloway). Wiley, Chichester.

Pilling S (1991). Day and support services. In *Rehabilitation and Community Care* (ed. S Pilling). Routledge, London.

Porter R (1987). *Mind-Forg'd Manacles*. Athlone Press, London.

Pryce I G, Baughan C A, Jenkins T D O and Venkatesan B (1983). A study of long-attending psychiatric day patients and the services provided for them. *Psychological Medicine*, **13**, 875–884.

Ramon S (1988). Towards normalization: polarization and change. In *Psychiatry in Transition: The British and Italian Experiences* (eds. S Ramon and M Giannichedda). Pluto, London.

Shepherd G (1989). The value of work in the 1980s. *Psychiatric Bulletin*, **13**, 231–233.

Shepherd G (1991). Psychiatric rehabilitation for the 1990's. In *Theory and Practice of Psychiatric Rehabilitation* (eds. F N Watts and D H Bennett). Wiley, Chichester.

Shoenfeld D, Halevy J. Hemley-van der velden E and Ruhf L (1986). Long-term outcome of social network therapy. *Hospital and Community Psychiatry*, **37**, 373–376.

Sims A C P, Heard D H, Rowe C E, Gill M M P and Maddock V (1993) 'Neurosis' and the personal social environment. The effects of a time-limited course of intensive day care. *British Journal of Psychiatry*, **162**, 369–374.

Stein L I and Test M A (1980) Alternative to mental hospital treatment. *Archives of General Psychiatry*, **37**, 392–397.

Stevens B C (1973). Evaluation of rehabilitation for psychotic patients in the community. *Acta Psychiatrica Scandinavica*, **49**, 169–180.

Tyrer P J and Remington M (1979). Controlled comparison of day hospital and outpatient treatment for neurotic disorders. *Lancet*, 1014–1016.

Vaughan P J (1983). The disordered development of day care in psychiatry. *Health Trends*, **I5**, 91–93.

Wadsworth W V, Scott R F and Wells B W P (1962). The employability of chronic schizophrenics. *Journal of Mental Science*, **108**, 300–303.

Wainwright T, Holloway F and Brugha T (1988). Day care in an inner city. In *Community Care in Practice* (eds. A Lavender and F Holloway). Wiley, Chichester.

Warner R (1985). *Recovery from Schizophrenia*. Routledge and Kegan Paul, London.

Warr P B and Jackson PR (1985). Factors influencing the psychological impact of prolonged unemployment. *Psychological Medicine*, **15**, 795–807.

Watts F N (1978). A study of work behaviour in a psychiatric rehabilitation unit. *British Journal of Social and Clinical Psychology*, **17**, 85–92.

Watts F N and Bennett D H (1978). Social deviance in a day hospital. *British Journal of Psychiatry*, **132**, 455–462.

Watts F and Bennett D (1983). Neurotic, affective and conduct disorders. In *Theory and Practice of Psychiatric Rehabilitation* (eds. F N Watts and D H Bennett). Wiley, Chichester.

Wilder J F, Levin G and Zwerling I (1966). A two-year follow-up evaluation of acute psychotic patients treated in a day hospital. *American Journal of Psychiatry*, **122**, 1095–1101.

Wing J K and Brown G W (1970). *Institutionalism and Schizophrenia*. Cambridge University Press, Cambridge.

Wing J K and Morris B (eds.) (1981). *Handbook of Psychiatric Rehabilitation Practice*. Oxford University Press, Oxford.

Wolfensberger W (1983). A reconceptualization of normalization as social role valorization. *Canadian Journal of Mental Retardation*, **34**, 22–26.

Wolfensberger W and Thomas S (1983). *PASSING: Program Analysis of Service Systems Implementation of Normalisation Goals*. National Institute on Mental Health, Toronto.

World Health Organization (1980). *International Classification of Impairments, Disabilities and Handicaps*. WHO, Geneva.

Wykes T, Sturt E and Creer C (1985). The assessment of patients' needs for community care. *Social Psychiatry*, **20**, 76–85.

6 Community care, community compulsion and the law

P. Fennell

Community care and the ideology of entitlement

The changing focus of psychiatric care away from hospitals and towards the community has raised new questions about the role of mental health legislation, traditionally geared towards the detention of patients in hospitals. Provisions for community care have always played a somewhat peripheral part. Gostin (1983) argued that patients should be cared for in the least restrictive alternative setting commensurate with their psychiatric care needs, and that access to health and social services should be based on legally enforceable rights, rather than concepts of charity, professional or agency discretion, arguing that that, 'If there is an unreasonable denial of a service, the remedy is, or should be, provided by the law.' He described this notion as part of 'the ideology of entitlement'. Section 117 of the Mental Health Act 1983, included in the legislation after pressure on the government from groups such as MIND, introduced specific duties on health and social services authorities to provide after-care for formerly detained patients. At the time these duties were not seen as adding anything particularly new, but time has proved the contrary and, as we shall see, section 117 has come to occupy a central place in government strategy for delivering after-care services to severely mentally ill people.

Section 117 of the Act applies to those who cease to be detained and leave hospital following detention under the Mental Health Act 1983 for treatment (section 3), under a hospital order (with or without restrictions) made by a criminal court (section 37), or following transfer from prison with or without restrictions (section 47). It puts a joint duty on the local district health authority and the local social services authority to provide, in cooperation with relevant voluntary agencies, after-care services for patients in the above categories until the authorities are satisfied that they no longer need them.

The key case on section 117 is *R* v. *Ealing District Health Authority ex parte Fox* (1993) involving an offender patient detained in Broadmoor under a restriction order. A mental health review tribunal (MHRT) reviewed his detention and directed his conditional discharge but deferred it until it could be satisfied that a number of conditions would be met, including social work support and supervision by a consultant psychiatrist who would act as the patient's responsible medical officer (RMO). All the consultants at the patient's local regional secure unit took the view that he would not be amenable to supervision in the community and declined to supervise him, as did the consultant general psychiatrist for his local area. The health authority therefore refused to supply psychiatric supervision for the applicant, and the MHRT's order for discharge could not take effect until the conditions were met. The applicant sought judicial review. In the health authority's view, the duty under section 117 did not apply because the patient had not yet left hospital.

Fox is important for a number of reasons. First, it shows clearly that the duty under section 117 is to consider the individual needs of each patient to whom the section applies. Otton J rejected the contention that it only came into effect once the patient was discharged from hospital. He considered it to be a continuing duty in respect of any patient who may be discharged and falls within section 117, although the duty to any particular patient was only triggered at the moment of discharge. This is reflected in recent guidance on discharge from the Department of Health emphasizing the need to have a written care plan under the care programme approach in respect of every patient who has a MHRT hearing to determine fitness for discharge, so that the plan can be activated if a decision is taken to discharge (NHS Management Executive 1994*b*).

The judge also concluded that the mere acceptance by the authority of their consultants' opinions was not of itself sufficient to discharge their obligations to proceed with reasonable expedition and diligence and to give effect to the arrangements specified and required by the tribunal. If the health authority's doctors did not agree with the conditions imposed by the tribunal and were disinclined to provide supervision, the authority could not let the matter rest there. They were under a continuing obligation to make further endeavours to provide arrangements within their own resources or to obtain them from other authorities, or, at the very least to make inquiries of other providers of such services. If they still could not make the necessary arrangements they were not entitled to let the matter rest there, but were to refer the matter to the Secretary of State to enable him to exercise his power under section 71 of the 1983 Act to refer the case back to the tribunal.

Although the applicant was entitled to have the health authority's decision quashed, Otton J accepted their contention that it would not be appropriate to make an order compelling them to provide psychiatric supervision in the community. That would, in effect, compel a doctor to supervise a patient against the doctor's will which was based on an honestly held clinical judgment that the treatment was not in the patient's best interests or was not in the best interests of the community in which the supervision would take place. However, he granted a declaration that: (1) the authority had erred in law by not attempting with all reasonable expedition and diligence to make arrangements so as to enable the applicant to comply with the conditions imposed by the tribunal; and (2) a district health authority is under a duty under section 117 to provide after-care services when a patient leaves hospital, and acts unlawfully if it fails to seek to make practical arrangements for after-care prior to that patient's discharge from hospital where such arrangements are required in order to enable the patient to be conditionally discharged from hospital. The ruling entitles patients to expect that the authority will exercise due diligence and act with expedition.

The provision of community care is one of the social services functions of local authorities, and in carrying it out section 7 of the Local Authority Social Services Act 1970 requires them to act under the general guidance of the Secretary of State. According to the Department of Health, guidance documents and circulars are intended to be a statement of good practice, and although not law, 'guidance documents may be quoted or used in court proceedings. They could provide a basis for a legal challenge of an authority's action or inaction' (DoH 1989). Section 7A of the 1970 Act, which was inserted by the National Health Service and Community Care Act 1990, empowers the Secretary of State to issue directions, and requires local authorities to carry out their social services functions in accordance with them. Although directions are obviously intended to be more binding than guidance, unlike orders and regulations, they do not require parliamentary approval.

In 1990 the Department of Health issued a circular to health and social services authorities promoting a care programme approach for mentally ill people who have been referred to specialist mental health services (DoH 1990). From April 1991 health authorities were required to draw up individual written care plans for all in-patients (whether detained or not) who are about to be discharged from mental illness hospitals, as well as for all new patients accepted by the specialist psychiatric services. The needs of each patient for continuing care were to be systematically assessed, and appropriate arrangements made for meeting them. Each patient would be assigned a key worker whose task it would be to keep in touch with patients in the community. Review of patients' needs was to take place at regular intervals. Patients and carers were to be involved in the planning process. Social services authorities were asked to 'collaborate with health authorities in introducing this approach and, as resources allow, to continue to expand social care services to patients being treated in the community'.

Following a number of incidents involving formerly detained patients (discussed below), on 6 February 1995 the Department of Health issued an After Care Form for the Discharge of Psychiatric Patients including those subject to section 117. Its use is not mandatory, but is strongly recommended as good practice, to ensure that details of the patient, his or her key worker and nominated contact are recorded, that the health and local authorities acknowledge in writing their responsibilities for providing after-care, and that responsibility for care can be transferred if the patient moves to another area. (Copies are available from Department of Health, Room 109 Wellington House, 133–155 Waterloo Road, London SE1 8UG.) The form is reproduced at the end of this chapter (p.127–130).

Under section 46 of the National Health Service and Community Care Act 1990, local authorities are required to prepare, publish, keep under review, and periodically modify a plan for the provision of community-care services in their area. In drawing up the plan, they must consult health authorities, family health services authorities housing authorities, and voluntary organizations including those which represent the interests of users and those which provide housing or community-care services.

Section 47 puts a duty on local social services authorities to carry out an assessment of the needs of any person who appears to be in need of community care services and, having regard to the results of the assessment, to decide whether his needs call for the provision by them of any such services. Patients subject to section 117 are expressly entitled to assessment and, if appropriate, provision under section 47, but this also extends more generally to people with problems of mental ill health who have not been detained. The client group covered by the term 'community care services' includes people who 'need such provision because of illness, disability or old age' (National Health Service and Community Care Act 1990, s. 46 (3)). In all three groups mental disorder may be a key factor giving rise to need. This includes people suffering from any form of mental disorder within the meaning of s.1 of the Mental Health Act 1983, National Assistance Act 1948, s. 29.

Once it appears to a local authority that any person for whom they may provide-care services may be in need of such services, section 47 (1) imposes a duty to carry out an assessment. This does not give rise to a right of assessment on demand, but someone who falls clearly within the category of person for whom the authority may provide care services could enforce the duty to assess by way of judicial review. The local authority must assess the person's needs for community care services. Once that has been done, they must then have regard to the results of the assessment and decide whether the person's needs call for the provision by them of any services. (See also Social Services Inspectorate 1992, para. 3.) A refusal to provide services where the assessment clearly indicated that they ought to be provided would be open to challenge by judicial review on grounds of *Wednesbury* irrationality, that it was so unreasonable to refuse the services that no reasonable authority would have done so (*Associated Provincial Picture Houses* v. *Wednesbury Corporation* [1948] 1 KB 223).

Local authorities are required to establish a procedure for considering representations (including complaints) in relation to the discharge of, or any failure to discharge, their social services functions (Local Authority Social Services Act 1970, s. 7B, as inserted by the National Health Service and Community Care Act 1990, s. 50. See Department of Health/Social Services Inspectorate 1993c). They must publicize the procedure, and act in accordance with any directions given by the Secretary of State as regards the consideration of representations and acting in consequence thereof. The Secretary of State has the power under the Local Authority Social Services Act 1970 to establish an inquiry where he considers it advisable to do so in connection with the discharge by any local authority of their social services functions (Local Authority Social Services Act 1970, s. 7C, as inserted by the National Health Service and Community Care Act 1990, s. 50) (except insofar as they relate to persons under eighteen) (separate provision is made for inquiries under the Children Act 1989). Where a local authority fail without reasonable excuse to carry out their social services functions with regard to community care, the Secretary of State may make an order declaring them to be in default, and specifying a time limit for the default to be rectified. The Secretary of State may enforce the order by applying to the High Court for an order of mandamus (Local Authority Social Services Act 1970, s. 7D).

Governments have traditionally shied away from providing patients with express legal entitlements to services, and whilst the common law employs the rhetoric of rights, it is essentially based on providing remedies for individuals who have suffered legal wrongs. Nevertheless, there is an increasing willingness on the part of the legal profession to explore the potential of the complaints procedure and of judicial review to challenge decision-making in relation to community care assessments, as evidenced by Richard Gordon QC's useful guide to such challenges, *Community Care Assessments: A Practical Legal Framework* (Gordon 1993). In this sense we may say that Gostin's 'ideology of entitlement' is reflected in current law because there are legal remedies where services are unreasonably withheld.

Despite growing emphasis on duties to provide community care, as the programme of psychiatric hospital closures has gathered pace in England and Wales, there have been increasing concerns, both about the fate of former in-patients themselves, and the protection of the public from their disturbed and sometimes dangerous behaviour. In some inner city areas it appears that in-patient provision is now so scarce as to be effectively reserved for those who are so ill that they require detention under the Mental Health Act. For many mentally ill clients the reality of community-care has meant a bedsit, a fortnightly visit from a community psychiatric nurse to administer an injection, and perhaps opportunities to visit a day centre or a day hospital. There were also fears that many former psychiatric patients, particularly in London, had, in the words of the Department of Health, 'slipped through the network of care' or become 'lost to care'. By the early 1990s it was clear that hospital accommodation for psychiatric admissions in metropolitan areas was insufficient to cope with demand. The Mental Health Act Commission (MHAC) *Fourth Biennial Report 1989–1991* described squalid conditions in the acute care ward at Hackney Hospital in London and painted a picture of a hospital starved of resources and unable to cope with the demands upon it (Mental Health Act Commission 1991, pp. 18–19). A section in MHAC Fifth Biennial Report entitled 'Crisis in inner city mental health services' sums up the situation in 1993:

> The Commission's concerns have been focused on the high through-put and rapid discharge of detained patients in inner city acute psychiatric wards (40% or more of admissions across inner London are admitted compulsorily ...). On some wards this proportion is 80–90%. The problem of high bed occupancy (sometimes as much as 120%) has become an increasing concern of Commissioners. The result of this overloading is that the patients may be prematurely discharged from hospital on leave, often at a few hours notice and not infrequently to unsupervised accommodation, to make way for more disturbed patients.
>
> (Mental Health Act Commission 1993).

Recording their experiences from 1991 to 1993, the MHAC said that the implementation of section 117 and the care programme approach were 'barely evident' in many inner city acute units. High morbidity levels in inner city populations, lack of alternatives to admission, problems of hopelessness, and poor community service were all contributing factors to the crisis.

As these anxieties have grown, so too has the importance of legal provisions relating to community care become more pronounced. There have been strong arguments for the increase of compulsory powers over mentally ill clients in the community, and at the same time a movement arguing that the necessary quid pro quo of compulsion is increased entitlement for clients to support services in the community. This chapter considers the history of compulsory powers in the community and the changing role of law in compelling patients to accept supervision or treatment in the community, concluding with an analysis of the Department of Health 'ten point plan' and the Mental Health Patients in the Community Bill which is currently before parliament. This Bill is likely to pass with only minor amendments, and, if it does, will come into force in April 1996.

History of compulsory treatment within community settings

Guardianship

The Royal Commission on the Law relating to Mental Illness and Mental Deficiency 1954–7 (the Percy Commission) placed guardianship at the centre of their policy of fostering the reorientation of psychiatric care towards the community, and this was reflected in the Mental Health Act 1959. Mental health guardianship had originated in the Mental Deficiency Act 1913 which provided the guardian of a mental defective with all the powers of a father over a child under 14. Guardianship under the 1913 Act was the equivalent of what is nowadays described as 'extended minority', with the minority being extended potentially indefinitely (Law Commission 1991). The guardian could prevent the patient from giving up work or from leaving home, and had the power to exercise sufficient control to discourage undesirable companionship and anti-social behaviour. The use of guardianship was encouraged by the Board of Control, predecessors of the present day Mental Health Act Commission, and by 1932 there were 2147 cases. Its use increased steadily, reaching a peak in 1947 of 4798. Prior to 1948, guardianship had often been used for financial reasons, because otherwise local authorities had no power to pay for the maintenance of mental defectives in the community. With the arrival of state social security and disability benefit, the incentive disappeared, and guardianship went into steep decline (Fennell 1992).

The 1959 Act brought the treatment of mental illness and mental handicap together under one legal framework, and allowed for the reception of both mentally ill and mentally handicapped people into guardianship. The guardian's powers remained the same – all those of a father over a child under 14. Section 33 of the 1959 Act allowed the local health authority to take on the role of guardian. The Mental Deficiency Act had no express provision to allow this. This marked an important stage in the development of guardianship as a social services function rather than, as the Law Commission puts it 'a means of legitimizing private arrangements' (Law Commission 1991). It was still possible to have a private guardian under the 1959 Act, but where the guardian was not the local health authority, the authority had to approve the appointment.

By the late 1970s there was widespread concern at the failure of guardianship. By then guardianship had become a social services function in every respect, responsibility having been transferred from health to social services authorities. The Department of Health view expressed in the 1981 White Paper on reform of the 1959 Act described the 1959 Act's 'paternalistic approach' as 'out of keeping with modern attitudes to the care of the mentally disordered' (DoH 1981). As well as conferring extensive powers, this paternal role imposed extensive responsibilities for protecting and controlling the behaviour of the person under guardianship. The Department's view was that guardianship powers were needed for 'a very small number' of mentally disordered people who did not need treatment in hospital, but who did require supervision and control in the community. In the government's view, this category included 'people who are able to cope provided they take their medication regularly, but who fail to do so, and those who neglect themselves to the point of seriously endangering their health' (DoH 1981). To achieve this, an 'essential powers' approach was advocated by the government, conferring on the guardian only those powers which are essential to promote the well-being of the patient.

The current powers of a guardian are listed in section 8 of the 1983 Act. Patients may be required to reside at a specified place, to prevent them from living rough or with people who might exploit or mistreat them. If they leave the in place of residence without the guardian's consent, they may be taken into custody and returned there within 28 days. However, there is no power to 'take and convey' patients forcibly to the required place of residence in the first place. Guardians are not empowered to detain patients in the place of residence by locking them in during the daytime.

The guardian is empowered to require the patient to attend at places and times so specified for the purpose of medical treatment, occupation, education, or training. Although the patient may be required to attend for the purposes of medical treatment, the guardian has no power to consent to treatment on the patient's behalf. Furthermore, according to section 56(1), patients subject to guardianship are not subject to the consent to treatment provisions of Part IV of the 1983 Act, and so they cannot be required to accept medical treatment for mental disorder. If a guardianship patient's condition is such that medical treatment is required, and the patient refuses to accept it, a power exists to transfer him or her to hospital (Mental Health (Hospital, Guardianship and Consent to Treatment) Regulations 1983, SI 1983 No. 893).

Guardianship under the 1983 Act is not an option for a learning disabled client unless they are mentally impaired or severely mentally impaired, meaning that their behaviour is abnormally aggressive or seriously irresponsible. This was a factor in the tragic case of Beverley Lewis, a profoundly learning-disabled young woman who died in 1989 having been neglected by her schizophrenic mother. The coroner said that the case highlighted the need for Mental Health Act guardianship to be extended to people like Beverley, who could not have been placed in guardianship because she was neither abnormally aggressive or seriously irresponsible and therefore not 'mentally impaired' within the meaning of the Mental Health Act (Fennell 1989). Others commented that the tragedy could have been averted, had there been some legal mechanism to require the mother to comply with her medication. In fact, there was nothing in law to prevent the care staff, who felt that their hands were tied legally, from applying for a warrant under section 135 of the 1983 Act, and from removing Beverley and her mother to hospital for assessment under section 2 of the 1983 Act, which uses a broad definition of mental disorder and allows for the compulsory admission of mentally handicapped people who are neither aggressive nor irresponsible, if it is necessary for their health or safety or for the protection of others.

Despite the fact that the Mental Health Act Commission has played a similar role to the Board of Control in the promotion of guardianship, the 1983 Act changes failed to prompt any significant increase in its use (Fisher 1988). In 1990–1991 there were 143 patients, and the latest total of patients under guardianship is only 332, compared with 17–20 000 compulsory admissions annually.

Extended leave

Undoubtedly an important reason for the under-use of guardianship has been the availability of a medically controlled power to impose treatment in the community which does not involve the cumbersome decision-making procedures of guardianship. There was a widespread practice under the Mental Health Act 1959, continued under the 1983 Act, of granting leave to detained patients on condition that they continued to take their medication. When the authority to detain the patient was about to lapse, he or she would be recalled to hospital by the psychiatrist in charge of the case (the responsible medical officer (RMO)) to renew the detention. The patient would then be sent out on leave again on condition that he or she continue taking medication. Patients who did not comply could be recalled to hospital. This arrangement came to be referred to by psychiatrists and even by the MHAC as the 'long leash' (MHAC 1985). It could be repeated ad infinitum, and no doubt many patients were subjected to it on a long-term basis until 1986 when it was declared unlawful in *R* v. *Hallstrom ex parte W (No. 2)* and *R* v. *Gardner and another ex parte L*.

Both these cases involved patients with long histories of chronic schizophrenic illness. *Hallstrom* concerned a notional admission for one night, leave of absence being granted the next day, on condition that the patient accepted medication. *Gardner* concerned a patient who had been given leave of absence in February 1985. In May 1985 the RMO renewed the detention for a further six months even though the patient had been living in the community since shortly after her admission. McCullough J ruled that patients may be detained for treatment under section 3 of the 1983 Act only if their mental condition is believed to require a period of in-patient treatment (*Gardner*, p. 316). Whilst it was perfectly lawful to grant leave with a condition of acceptance of treatment, detention could not be renewed while the patient was on leave unless his or her condition at the time warranted actual detention. Under the 1983 Act patients who are liable to be detained under section 3 or 37 are discharged if the period of detention expires while they are on leave or if six months have elapsed and they have not returned to the hospital. Under the Mental Health (Patients in the Community) Bill (discussed below), the six-month maximum period of leave before discharge will be extended to 12 months (Mental Health (Patients in the Community) Bill 1995, cl. 3, which amends s. 17 of the 1983 Act). This can only apply where the patient has already been detained for 12 months; the initial detention and the first renewal only last for a maximum of six months.

Compulsory powers in the community: the ten point plan

The decision in *Hallstrom* led to an outcry on the part of many psychiatrists and both the Royal College of Psychiatrists and the Mental Health Act Commission issued discussion documents which were keenly debated. The Royal College proposed introducing a 'community treatment order', but the preponderance of opinion was against change. The term 'order' is a misnomer since under the 1983 Act only courts can make orders in respect of offender patients. Non-offender patients are admitted under *applications* made to the hospital managers. Michael Cavadino has provided an excellent summary of the earlier proposals of the Royal College and the Mental Health Act Commission as well as a persuasive philosophical argument against compulsory community treatment (Cavadino 1991). The Royal College incurred particular criticism for its description of readmission to hospital as 'the sanction for non-compliance'. Subsequently interest in the subject outside the psychiatric profession died away, and there seemed little prospect that any change would be made in the law. In July 1989 Robert Freeman, then Parliamentary Secretary for Health, said that although the government was prepared to look at it:

> Without prejudicing the discussion, we would need to be very clear both of the benefits, and that they could not be achieved through voluntary means, before seriously asking Parliament to create provision for compulsory treatment in the community.
>
> (Speech delivered at Richmond House)

Within two years a dramatic change came over the fortunes of the lobby for compulsory community powers. Apart from the Royal College of Psychiatrists, it included the National Schizophrenia Fellowship, an organization of sufferers, carers and relatives, and a closely allied organization Schizophrenia – A National Emergency (SANE), founded by the journalist Marjorie Wallace. As well as a help line for sufferers and relatives, SANE ran an aggressive poster campaign in the 1980s arguing that community-care policies were failing and that the public were being put at risk from former psychiatric in-patients who were not receiving adequate care in the community. What was undeniable was the serious shortage of acute psychiatric beds in many areas, necessitating discharge of people who should really be in hospital, and there was a growing perception that the money saved by closing hospitals was not being deployed to provide adequate community care.

The year 1992 was a turning-point in the fortunes of proponents of compulsory community powers. On her appointment as Secretary of State for Health, Virginia Bottomley expressed her concern that vulnerable mentally ill people were 'slipping through the net'. Her views were known to be that the 'pendulum' of mental health law had swung too far in the direction of civil liberties (DoH 1993*a*). In November, the eminent forensic psychiatrist Professor Robert Bluglass, who had spoken against community treatment orders during the debates in the late 1980s, unveiled to a Conference of the Royal College of Psychiatrists in Jersey a set of provisional proposals for 'community supervision orders'. The new name was because they considered that one of the main reasons for the failure of previous proposals had been fear on the part of community psychiatric nurses that they would be required actually to administer treatment to unwilling patients in the community (Royal College of Psychiatrists). The community supervision order would be taken out by the patient's RMO and, if the patient refused treatment, he or she could be returned to hospital, where it could be given forcibly if necessary. The president of the Royal College spoke from the floor, and expressed the view that since opinion was now favourable at the very top of the Department of Health, and the National Schizophrenia Fellowship supported such powers, the time was right for the College to press ahead with its proposals, which had been drafted in conjunction with a working party including the President of the Community Section of the College, Dr (now Professor) Tom Burns, an enthusiastic proponent of compulsory community powers.

On the last day of 1992, Ben Silcock, a young schizophrenic, jumped into the lion's enclosure at London Zoo. Although badly mauled, he survived. The whole affair was captured on amateur video and appeared on network news. It would gradually emerge that, despite providing a powerful image, the case was not ideal proof of the need for compulsory community treatment, first because Ben Silcock had in fact taken his medication, and, what was not revealed at the time, stress due to the fact that he was awaiting trial for assault may well have been the major cause of the tragic episode.

Immediately following the incident, the Secretary of State held meetings with the Royal College and other interested parties. On 12 January the Royal College hurriedly published their proposals, and the next day Mrs Bottomley announced an internal review by Department of Health officials, to consider two questions. First, whether any new legal powers were needed to ensure that mentally ill people in the community receive the care they need; and second, whether the present powers in the Mental Health Act 1983 are being used as effectively as they can be and what action could be taken in advance of any new legislation to ensure that they are (DoH 1993*a*). The signals were obvious. The review team clearly knew at the outset that it was going to have to come up with some kind of compulsory community power or risk the wrath of the Secretary of State.

The review's terms of reference reflected the political importance for the government of identifying the problem in terms of non-compliant patients rather than failures in community care provision or bed shortages following closure of psychiatric hospitals. As the review team began their work, another tragic case came to prominence. In December 1992 Jonathan Zito, a young musician barely three months married, was killed by Christopher Clunis, a paranoid schizophrenic with a long history of violence. Clunis had been released from hospital three months before the attack. He had been supposed to attend Friern Barnet Hospital as a voluntary out-patient but had not turned up. The victim's widow, Jayne Zito, had been a rehabilitation manager for the mentally ill and, following Clunis' conviction, wrote to

Virginia Bottomley deploring the failure of community care in his case, pointing to the crisis in psychiatric services and demanding an inquiry. An inquiry was instituted by the health authorities concerned, which reported in February 1994, identifying a woeful catalogue of failure to provide adequate care for Clunis, that there had been no section 117 after-care plan, and that the authorities had failed to manage or oversee provision of health and social services for him (Ritchie *et al.* 1994).

The Secretary of State announced the outcome of the internal review on 12 August 1993, a 'ten point plan to reinforce the care of mentally ill people in the community'. This included a series of shorter-term measures to make greater use of existing powers. Already amendments to the Mental Health Act Code of Practice had been laid before parliament which encouraged early readmission of patients relapsing following cessation of medication. To prepare the way for supervised discharge, the Department of Health issued two further sets of guidance. The first, on which no consultation was held, introduced supervision registers, a form of 'at risk' register for mentally disordered adults (NHS Management Executive 1994*a*). The second, issued in May 1994, provides guidance on the discharge of mentally disordered people and their continuing care in the community (NHS Management Executive 1994*b*). The legislative changes proposed in the ten point plan included the lengthening to 12 months of the period during which detained patients can remain on conditional leave before they are automatically discharged. The ultimate goal of the ten point plan was the introduction of a new statutory power of 'supervised discharge', for which supervision registers and the guidance on discharge would pave the way. (Compare with the Report of the House of Commons Health Committee, 'Community Supervision Orders' Fifth Report Vol. 1, HC 667–1 (23 June 1993), xxvi.)

Early compulsory admission of patients who are relapsing

The Department of Health's 1993 revision of the *Code of Practice on the Mental Health Act 1983* 'strengthened' the guidance on assessment prior to compulsory admission. This now emphasizes more strongly that a patient may be admitted under sections 2 and 3 of the 1983 Act solely in the interests of his own health, even if there is no risk to his own or other people's safety. Those doing the assessment must consider any evidence that the patient's mental health will deteriorate if he does not receive treatment, including 'the known history of the individual's mental disorder' (DoH 1993*b*). They must also consider the 'reliability of such evidence' – the views of the patient or relatives or friends living with the patient about his possible future deterioration, the impact that any future deterioration would have on those friends and relatives and the patient's ability to cope, and whether there are other methods of dealing with such deterioration. This, in effect, places much greater emphasis than the first version of the Code on the duty of those assessing a patient to consider any evidence suggesting that the patient's mental health will deteriorate if he does not receive treatment.

Supervision registers

A central element of the ten point plan was the introduction of 'supervision registers'. Like the amendment to the Mental Health Act Code, this was achieved without legislation, and this time without even any parliamentary approval, by Health Service Guidance HSG(94)5, issued by the NHS Management Executive. This required the introduction of supervision registers by 1 April 1994. It informs health authorities that they are required, when purchasing mental health care services from NHS trusts or other bodies, to include terms in their contracts ensuring that provider units set up supervision registers which identify and provide information on mentally disordered patients in the community who are at risk. All initial assessments and follow-up reviews of patients under the care programme approach are to consider whether the patient should be registered. All provider units are to be required to 'incorporate the supervision register in the development of mental health information systems to support the full implementation of the Care Programme Approach'. All patients of the specialist psychiatric services fall within the scope of the register.

The decision as to whether a person is to be included rests with the consultant psychiatrist in charge of the patient's care, although it should be made in consultation with the other members of the mental health team involved, including the social worker. The mechanism for making decisions about inclusion on the register is a 'Care Programme review meeting', which will have to consider whether the client is suffering from serious mental illness, and whether he or she is, or is liable to be 'at risk of committing serious violence or suicide, or of serious self neglect' (NHS Management Executive 1994a). The guidance includes among the factors which might trigger such a risk, ceasing to take medication and, treating the adoption of legislation as a foregone conclusion, says that 'patients subject to supervised discharge, when the legislation is passed, will be among those included in the register'. Patients and, where they wish, an advocate, relative, friend or carer, must have an opportunity to state their views and have these taken into account, for example, by attendance at the review meeting or through discussion with the relevant clinician or key worker. Wherever possible the patient's GP is to be involved in the decision.

There will be three categories on the supervision register, and a patient should be assigned to no more than one of them unless there are specific reasons. The categories are: (a) significant risk of suicide; (b) significant risk of serious violence to others; or (c) significant risk of severe self-neglect (para. 9). Where the risk is considered to be contingent on certain specified events (e.g. ceasing to take medication, loss of home or of a supportive relationship) the identified warning signs should be recorded (para. 10). Judgments of risk should always be based on detailed evidence of the patient's psychiatric and social history and current condition, which may include evidence from any criminal justice agencies with which the patient has been involved. The evidence on which these judgments are made must be recorded in writing and should be available for the relevant professionals for the review meeting, although no mention is made in the guidance as to whether patients or their advocates would be entitled to this information, which may contain elements the veracity or accuracy of which the patient wishes to challenge (para. 6).

The guidance advises particular care where patients are being transferred from one type of care to another, or to another area (paras 7 and 8). It says that special hospitals and regional or medium secure units will need to ensure that all relevant information is available on patients discharged from those services into the care of local provider units so that the latter can decide whether the patient should be included on the supervision register. If a patient on a supervision register is transferred to a different provider unit, a copy of their record should, as a matter of urgency, be transferred to that unit. The system manager will be accountable for ensuring that the transfer is rapid, accurate and secure. The patient's inclusion on the receiving unit's supervision register is to be reviewed as part of the care programme drawn up at the new provider unit, which will be responsible for liaising with the new social services department and the GP.

Patients are to be informed orally and in writing of their inclusion on the register, 'broadly' why they are on it, how the information will be used, to whom it may be disclosed, and the 'mechanisms for review'. An exception may be made for clinical reasons, when informing the patient would proba-bly cause serious harm to his physical or mental health, but the guidance makes clear that this is expected to be very unlikely to apply to a patient suitable for care outside hospital. If it does apply, the decision 'should not be taken lightly' and should be agreed by the mental health team including the consultant psychiatrist responsible (para. 12). The patient is to be told as soon as the risk has passed.

Care programme reviews of patients on the register are to take place *every six months*, and these should specifically consider the question of continued inclusion. The patient or, if he or she wishes, a relative, friend, advocate or carer must have a suitable opportunity to state his or her views and to have them considered. Any of the agencies or professionals involved can request a special review meeting to be held to consider withdrawal of 'risk status'. The patient or his chosen advocate have the right to request that the con-sultant remove the patient from the register, but the decision is ultimately a matter for the consultant, who, in conjunction with professional colleagues, is to consider the representations and inform the patient of the outcome and reasons for the decision. The guidance says that withdrawal will be appro-priate in one of three circumstances: (a) where the patient is no longer con-sidered to be at significant risk of serious violence, suicide or severe self-neglect (this decision may only be taken by a review meeting); (b) where the patient's records have been transferred to another provider unit, and here there must be a written transfer agreement with the receiving unit; or (c) where the patient has died. Withdrawal from the register must not auto-matically entail a withdrawal of any services provided for a patient. The guid-ance emphasizes that 'All of the responsibilities set out in the care programme approach will continue to apply to such patients as long as they remain under the care of the specialist psychiatric services' (para. 19).

Patients who remain dissatisfied by a decision to keep them on the regis-ter will have recourse to 'the normal channels of complaint' and the right to a clinical second opinion. Since the decision would be 'taken in consequence of an exercise of clinical judgment' the Health Service Comissioner would have no jurisdiction, unless there was maladministration in carrying the decision out once it had been made, and the normal channels of com-plaint would presumably be through the clinical complaints procedure (DoH 1988).

Where a provider unit has lost contact with the patient the risk status should not be changed but the patient should be designated 'out of contact with the unit'. Providers should make every reasonable effort to re-establish contact. The patient's GP, social worker and other members of the care team are to be urgently notified and asked to advise, and a review meeting is to be convened to which they should be invited.

The register will include the following 'required contents', listed in Appendix A of the guidance:

Part 1. Identification
(i) Patient's full name, including known aliases, home address including post code (or 'no fixed address'), sex and date of birth.

(ii) Patient's current legal status in respect of the Mental Health Act (i.e. whether on leave, under guardianship or subject to supervised discharge when available).

Part 2. Nature of risk
(i) Category of risk and nature of specific warning indicators.

(ii) Evidence of specific episodes of violent or self-destructive behaviour (including *relevant* criminal convictions) or severe self-neglect.

Part 3. Key worker and relevant professionals
(i) Name and contact details for patient's key worker.

(ii) Name and contact details of other professionals involved in the care of the patient including the consultant responsible for the care of the patient.

Part 4. Care programme
(i)   Date of registration.
(ii) Date of last review.
(iii) Date of next programmed review.
(iv) Components of care programme.

The guidance states that the patient's entry on the supervision register will be considered confidential in the same way as any other health record, but information from the register would be rapidly accessible to mental health professionals with a need to know in order to plan or provide care, and this would normally include all members of the care team, any social worker involved, and the patient's GP, who should be given a copy of the care plan. The guidance also states that disclosures from the register to other agencies may be made either if the patient consents or without the patient's consent if disclosure can be justified in the public interest. These agencies might include the social services authorities, private sector institutions and, 'in respect of mentally disordered offenders, probation or other criminal justice agencies'. Where information is to be divulged to criminal justice agencies, whether it should, or even may, be divulged will depend on the nature of the information and the context in which it is sought. In *R* v. *Cardiff Crown Court ex parte Kellam* (1993) it was held that records of patients' movements which were extracted from their medical records were 'excluded material' within the meaning of section 11 of the Police and Criminal Evidence Act 1984, and therefore could not be required to be divulged to the police who were investigating a gruesome murder (see also Zander 1990).

The keeper of the record is the board of an NHS trust or the health authority if it directly manages the unit, and one executive member is to be identified to oversee the process. This means that if information from the register is to be disclosed to a third party, it is not for the RMO to decide, but for the trust or the authority, 'taking full account of the views of the consultant psychiatrist responsible for the care of the patient' (NHS Management Executive 1994*a*). The report on the Clunis case recommends the introduction of a nationally-based register of patients 'subject' to section 117 where 'information which leads to the ready identification of the patient may be stored and which would indicate where confidential information about the patient would be obtained' (Ritchie *et al.* 1994). As a health record, the patient would have rights of access to it, under the Access to Health Records Act 1990 if it is manually stored, or under the Data Protection Act 1984, section 21, as modified by the Data Protection (Subject Access Modification) Health Order 1987 (S1 1987 No. 1903) if it is kept electronically. Under these provisions access may be withheld if disclosure would be likely to cause serious harm to the physical or mental health of the data subject or would be likely to reveal information which, on its own or in conjunction with other information, would enable another person, other than a health professional, to be identified either as a person to whom the information relates, or as the source of the information.

Discharge and continuing care

The purpose of the guidance on discharge is to ensure that psychiatric patients are discharged only when they are ready to leave hospital; that any risk to the public or to patients themselves is minimal and is managed effectively; and that patients who are discharged get the support and supervision they need from the responsible agencies (NHS Management Executive 1994*b*). Referring to the risk of self-harm or harm to others, and the devastating consequences of either eventuality, the guidance particularly emphasizes that those taking individual decisions about discharge, including mental health review tribunals, hospital managers (defined in the Mental Health Act 1983, s 145(1) as amended by the Mental Health (Amendment) Act 1994), and RMOs have 'a fundamental duty to consider both the safety of the patient and the protection of other people. No patient should be discharged from hospital unless and until those taking the decision are satisfied that he or she can live safely in the community, and that proper treatment, supervision, support and care are available' (NHS Management Executive 1994*b*). The guidance points out that certain patients with long-term, more severe disabilities and particularly those with a potential for dangerous or risk-taking behaviour need special consideration at the time of discharge and during follow-up and again stresses that discharge decisions must be fully justified:

> No decision to discharge should be agreed unless those taking the clinical decisions are satisfied that the behaviour can be controlled without serious risk to the patient or to other people. In each case it must be demonstrable that decisions have been taken after full and proper consideration of any evidence about risk that the patient presents.
>
> (NHS Management Executive 1994*b*, para. 23)

Checklist for the After-Care of Psychiatric Patients

Parts 1–6 of the form must be completed by the key worker before the patient is discharged from hospital. Copies of the completed form must be sent to everyone involved in the patient's after-care.

Please complete this form in black ink only

checklist record

Is this the first checklist?

yes ☐   *no* ☐

If no please give number ☐

1 About the patient

(a) the full name of the patient is [   ]

(b) the patient is ☐ *male*   ☐ *female*   [   ] *age in years*

(c) the patient lives at [   ] [   ]

(d) the patient is ☐ *married*   ☐ *single*   ☐ *divorced*   ☐ *separated*

   ☐ *widow*   ☐ *widower*

if yes give preferred language

(f) The patient requires an interpreter ☐ *yes* ☐ *no* [   ]

2 Patient's nominated contact

(a) contact's full name

(b) contact's full address

(c) contact's telephone number

3 Key worker's details

(a) the Key worker's name is

(b) the Key worker's profession is

(c) telephone number

(d) fax number

4 After-care plan

(a) an after-care plan was agreed for the patient on   *give date*   ☐

(b) patient agrees with after-care plan   ☐ *yes* ☐ *no*

(c) the patient is subject to section 117 of MHA 1983   ☐ *yes* ☐ *no*

5 Information to be included in the after-care plan

If any of the following apply to the patient, details must be recorded in the after-care plan

(a) in receipt of local authority care management   ☐ *yes* ☐ *no*

(b) on supervision register   ☐ *yes* ☐ *no*

(c) subject to conditional discharge   ☐ *yes* ☐ *no*

(d) subject to child care legislation   ☐ *yes* ☐ *no*

(e) subject to statutory supervision by probation service   ☐ *yes* ☐ *no*

(f) subject to guardianship   ☐ *yes* ☐ *no*

(g) subject to Criminal Procedure *(Insanity and Unfitness to Plead)* Act 1991   ☐ *yes* ☐ *no*

(h) subject to supervised discharge   ☐ *yes* ☐ *no*

6 Availability of information

Where any of the following information is **not** available a full explanation **must** be recorded in the patient's after-care plan

(a) full contact list of those involved in the patient's care   ☐ *yes* ☐ *no*

(b) patient's health and social needs identified   ☐ *yes* ☐ *no*

(c) patient's health and social needs addressed in the after-care plan   ☐ *yes* ☐ *no*

(d) risk assessment carried out   ☐ *yes* ☐ *no*

Patient's after-care plan contains:

(e) details of signs and symptoms suggesting likely relapse   ☐ *yes* ☐ *no*

(f) steps to be followed in the event of relapse   ☐ *yes* ☐ *no*

(g) steps to be followed if the patient fails to attend for treatment or meet other commitments   ☐ *yes* ☐ *no*

(h) action to be taken if the patient's relative or carer can *no* longer provide assitance and support   ☐ *yes* ☐ *no*

Certificate of agreement to after-care

Signed   Print name

On behalf of the Health Authority   Title

Signed   Print name

On behalf of the Local Authority   Title

A copy of this form with parts 1–6 completed was sent: give date _____

7 Review

If this after-care plan is amended, all those involved in the patient's care *must* be told

Date of next review   yes   no   *If yes, please give*
                                                                      date sent

1. [_____]   care plan amended, copies sent   [ ]   [ ]   [_____]

2. [_____]   care plan amended, copies sent   [ ]   [ ]   [_____]

3. [_____]   care plan amended, copies sent   [ ]   [ ]   [_____]

4. [_____]   care plan amended, copies sent   [ ]   [ ]   [_____]

8 Transfer of responsibility for patient's after-care

This section must be completed if the patient is to be moved to the care of another health or local authority. **Once this section is completed copies of this form must be sent to those involved in the patient's after-care who have a need to know.**

If the information in paragraphs 1–6 has changed, you must complete a new checklist. It should be sent, with this checklist (or any previous one) numbered, to show which is the later version (*in box on front page*).

Responsibility for the patient's after-care **remains** with the current health and local authorities **until** the new authorities have **signed** the certificate of agreement.

(a) Responsibility for the patient's after-care transferred:

from [_____]   Health Authority to [_____]   Health Authority

from [_____]   Local Authority to [_____]   Local Authority

on [_____]

Certificate of agreement to after-care

Signed   Print name

On behalf of the current Health Authority   Title

Signed   Print name

On behalf of the current Local Authority   Title

Signed   Print name

On behalf of the new Health Authority   Title

Signed   Print name

On behalf of the current Local Authority   Title

A copy of this form with parts 1–8 completed was sent: *give date*

9 Discharge from after-care

This section **must** be completed when the patient is discharged from after-care.

Once this section is completed copies of this form must be sent to everyone involved in the patient's after-care.

Certificate of agreement to discharge from after-care

The patient was discharged from after-care on
because (*give reasons*)

Signed   Print name

On behalf of the Health Authority   Title

Signed   Print name

On behalf of the Local Authority   Title

A copy of this form with parts 1–9 completed was sent: *give date*

Extensive information and advice are given in the guidance on the assessment of risk (paras 23–31).

The guidance restates the purpose of the care programme approach as being 'to ensure the support of mentally ill people in the community, thereby minimising the possibility of their losing contact with services and maximising the effect of any therapeutic intervention', and says that it should be applied to all mentally ill people accepted by the specialist psychiatric services, whether or not they have been treated in hospital and whether or not they have been detained under the 1983 Act. In the case of patients who have been detained, the care programme approach is seen as essential to the after-care duty under section 117. Authorities are told that they will need to establish mechanisms to monitor the application of the approach as a whole and to report on progress to authority members (paras 8–9).

The discharge guidance sets out four essential elements of an effective care programme. Those taking discharge decisions are told they must be satisfied that these are met before the patient is discharged. They are:

- *systematic assessment* of health and social care needs (including accommodation), bearing in mind both immediate and longer-term requirements;
- a *care plan* agreed between the relevant professional staff, the patient, and his or her carers and recorded in writing;
- the allocation of a *key worker* whose job (with multidisciplinary managerial and professional support) is:
  – to keep in close contact with the patient
  – to monitor that the agreed programme of care is delivered and
  – to take immediate action if it is not;
- *regular review* of the patient's progress and of his or her health and social-care needs (para. 10).

The guidance also stresses the importance of effective record-keeping and clear arrangements for communication between members of the care team. The patient and others involved (including, as necessary, the carer, health and social services staff, and the patient's GP) should be aware of the plan and have a common understanding of the following matters:

- first review date;
- information relating to any past violence or assessed risk of violence on the part of the patient;
- the name of the key worker (prominently identified in clinical notes, computer records and the care plan);
- how the key worker and other service providers can be contacted if problems arise; and
- what to do if the patient fails to attend for treatment or to meet other requirements or commitments (para. 11).

Where patients have applied for a mental health review tribunal the guidance says that 'it is important that the essential elements of the Care Programme approach have been considered and can be put into operation if the patient is discharged, and that the key worker is made immediately aware of any conditions imposed' (para. 19). The guidance on supervision registers and discharge is intended to pave the way for the central project of the ten point plan, the Mental Health (Patients in the Community) Bill which will introduce a new power of community supervision.

The Mental Health (Patients in the Community) Bill

Medical guardianship?

The new supervision in the community power has been described as a medical form of guardianship, because instead of social services being the lead authority, applications will be made by the responsible medical officer to the health authority (Mental Health (Patients in the Community) Bill, cl 25A(5)–(6)), and patients subject to supervision will be under the clinical authority of a community responsible medical officer (Schedule 1, Para. 4 (4)). However, as the government spokeswoman Baroness Cumberledge put it in the Lords' debates on the Bill, whilst 'the new power is health led [there is] ... a firm commitment for the social services to be fully consulted and involved' (Hansard HL Debs, Vol. 564, No. 86, col. 184, 11 May 1995). She went on to emphasize the links between the new power and section 117:

> Section 117 ... already makes clear that the provision of aftercare is a joint health and local authority responsibility. The imposition of any requirements on the patient in the community is also a joint health and local authority responsibility, as is keeping the aftercare services under review. Those provisions should avoid the risk of a health authority going ahead independently of the local social services authority and we shall also be emphasizing the need for full consultation in our guidance on the operation of the new powers ... The central principle of the Bill is that supervision cannot be separated from the after-care services which it exists to support.   (cols 184 and 189)

Supervision differs from guardianship in that guardianship is a 'free-standing' power which can be used whether or not the person has been detained, whereas supervision is linked to a prior period of detention for treatment. In order to be eligible for this power the patient must be over 16 and liable to be detained in a hospital in pursuance of an application for admission for treatment under section 3 or under a hospital order without restrictions or equivalent (Mental Health (Patients in the Community) Bill, cl. 25A(1)).

Supervisors and community RMOs

Every patient will have a responsible medical officer who applies for the supervised after-care, a community responsible medical officer, who is in charge of medical treatment in the community, and a supervisor, but there is nothing to stop all three being one and the same person (Schedule 1, Para. 4(5)). In the Bill as originally drafted, the community RMO could be any registered medical practitioner, but after initial resistance (Hansard HL Debs, Vol. 563, No. 68, col. 114, 4 April 1995), the government accepted amendments in the Lords which will add a new clause (2A) to section 117 to place a duty on the health authority 'to secure that at all times while a patient is subject to after-care under supervision a person who is approved under section 12 of the 1983 Act as having special expertise in the diagnosis or treatment of mental disorder (a 'section 12 doctor') is in charge of the medical treatment provided for the patient as part of the after-care services provided for him under section 117' (Mental Health (Patients in the Community) Bill, Sched. Para 15(4)).

It is envisaged that the supervisor will be a community psychiatric nurse in most cases, although it could be the community RMO or a social worker. The supervisor will play a 'crucial role' in the success of the new power, 'keeping in touch with the patient, coordinating the care which the patient is to receive, alerting colleagues to any modifications that may be necessary, checking that any requirements laid upon the patient are followed', and if necessary, invoking the controversial power to take and convey the patient to hospital (Baroness Cumberledge, Hansard HL Debs Vol. 563 No. 79, col 1238, 1 May 1995).

At the report stage in the Lords, Baroness Cumberledge was asked whether the legal responsibility for doctors taken on by hospital trusts in cases of litigation will apply to supervisors, or whether they would be responsible for any failings of the social services, hospital services, GP services and others which are needed to provide treatment for the patient. She replied as follows:

> While the supervisor will have professional liabilities and responsibilities along with other professionals in the care team, there will be no additional liability of the kind I think my noble friend has in mind. The supervisor would of course be personally liable in cases involving, for example, serious professional negligence, indiscipline or the abuse of patients. But in general liability would fall on the bodies responsible for providing the section 117 after-care service, not the supervisor personally, just because he or she fulfils that role.

The supervisor and other professionals will be carrying out functions under the Mental Health Act 1983, and therefore will have the defence in section 139 that they cannot be liable in criminal or civil proceedings unless they have acted negligently or in bad faith.

The necessary grounds for supervision

The link between the new power and section 117 is emphasized in the grounds which must be met for a supervision application:

(1) The patient must be suffering from mental disorder in one of the four forms prescribed for admission under section 3:

    (a) mental illness;
    (b) severe mental impairment;
    (c) psychopathic disorder;
    (d) mental impairment;

and

(2) there must be a substantial risk of serious harm to the health or safety of the patient or the safety of other persons, or of the patient being seriously exploited, if he were not to receive the after-care services to be provided for him under section 117 after he leaves hospital;

and

(3) this being subject to after-care under supervision is likely to help to secure that he receives the after-care services to be so provided (Mental Health (Patients in the Community) Bill, cl. 25A(4)).

Although the concerns which have given rise to the Bill relate to mentally ill people, this power will extend to people with mental impairment, severe mental impairment and psychopathic disorder. The inclusion in the risk criterion of risk of serious exploitation was criticized during the committee stage in the Lords as 'being capable of many interpretations'. Baroness Cumberledge refused to remove these words, offering as examples of what the government had in mind the risk of patients being 'lured into prostitution or exposed to the risks of drug abuse (Hansard HL Debs, Vol. 563, No. 68, col. 108, 4 April 1995). The third criterion, that the power is likely to help to secure that the patient receives the after-care is presumably intended to provide a diluted counterpart to the requirement for detention for treatment under section 3 that the treatment cannot be provided unless the patient is detained.

Procedure

The procedure for employing the new power departs radically from civil admission under the 1983 Act. Instead of the applicant being an approved social worker (ASW) and the doctors providing the recommendations, here the RMO applies to the health authority for supervision, with one of the two recommendations coming from an ASW, and the other from a doctor who will be concerned with the patient's medical treatment when he or she leaves hospital. If no doctor other than the RMO will be concerned with the patient's treatment, then the medical recommendation can come from any doctor, not necessarily a section 12 doctor.

The Bill states that before making an application, the RMO must consult the patient, one or more persons who have been professionally concerned with the patient's medical treatment in hospital, one or more persons who will be professionally concerned with the after-care services to be provided under section 117, and any person who the RMO believes will play a substantial part in the care of the patient after he leaves hospital but will not be professionally concerned with any of the after-care services to be provided (hereafter referred to as 'the lay carer'). The RMO must take the views of these people into account (Mental Health (Patients in the Community) Bill, cl. 25B(1)–(2), and, before making the application, must also consider the after-care services to be provided for the patient under section 117 and any requirements to be imposed as part of the after-care under supervision (cl. 25 B(3)). The new statutory application form for supervision will state that the conditions of the application are met and will name the community RMO, the supervisor, and the lay carer. The Department of Health internal review describes the consultation process as designed to produce 'a comprehensive multidisciplinary approach to care'. There would be a named key worker, in practice probably a community psychiatric nurse, a care programme and a clear treatment plan negotiated with the patient. Those drawing up the plan would be responsible for finding out the patient's wishes and ensuring that they were taken into account as far as practicable. The conditions of the patient's supervision would be agreed with the key worker and any other agencies and people (including relatives) involved in the patient's care. The patient's freedom of choice must not be limited 'unnecessarily' (DoH 1993*a*, para. 7.16).

The medical recommendation will state that all the conditions required for a supervision application are met, including that the patient is suffering from one of the four prescribed forms of mental disorder. The social work recommendation will be addressed only to the other two criteria: (1) that there would be substantial risk of serious harm to the health or safety of the patient or the safety of other persons, or of the patient being seriously exploited, if he were not to receive the after-care services; and (2) that after-care under supervision is likely to help to secure that he receives the after-care services to be so provided (Mental Health (Patients in the Community) Bill, cl. 25B(5)–(7)). Accompanying the recommendations there must also be statements from the prospective community RMO accepting that he or she will be in charge of the patient's medical treatment, and from the prospective supervisor that he or she is to supervise the patient, as well as details of the after-care services to be provided and the requirements to be imposed on the patient (cl. 25B(8)).

On making the application, the RMO will be required to inform the patient, the lay carer, and (unless the patient has objected) the nearest relative, that the application is being made, what after-care services will be provided, any requirements to be imposed on the patient, and the names of the community RMO and the supervisor (cl. 25B(9)–(10)). Before accepting a supervision application the health authority will have to consult the local social services authority with the joint duty to provide after-care under s. 117 (cl. 25A(7)–(7)). Although there is no express requirement in the Bill that the health and social services authorities must reach agreement, the government did not think this necessary because, in Baroness Cumberledge's words:

> In practice the statement of services to be provided, which has to be submitted with the supervision application, will need to have been agreed with the local authority's representatives so far as the social services element is concerned (Hansard HL Debs, Vol. 563, No. 68, col. 117, 4 April 1995).

When the health authority accepts an application it must inform the patient, the lay carer, and (unless the patient has objected) the nearest relative (Mental Health (Patients in the Community) Bill, cl. 25A(8)).

Powers of the after-care bodies

Once patients are subject to after-care under supervision, the responsible after-care bodies (the bodies which have the joint duty under s. 117, cl 25D(2)) have power to impose requirements for the purpose of securing that they receive after-care. These include:

(a) that the patient reside at a specified place;
(b) that he or she attend at specified places and times for the purpose of medical treatment, occupation, education or training; and
(c) that access to the patient be given, at any place where he or she is residing, to the supervisor, any doctor or any approved social worker, or to any other person authorised by the supervisor (cl. 25D(3)).

These are modelled on the conditions of guardianship in s. 8(1) of the 1983 Act.

The major difference between guardianship and supervision is that the Bill introduces a power to 'take and convey'. All proponents of compulsory community supervision are agreed that they do not want a power to treat forcibly in the patient's own home – concerns described by Geller (1986) as reflecting ideas of territorial propriety, that any compulsory medication would take place not in 'their community', but in 'our institution'. The Bill provides that:

A patient subject to after-care under supervision may be taken and conveyed by, or by any person authorised by, the supervisor, to any place where the patient is required to reside or to attend for the purpose of medical treatment, occupation, education or training (cl. 25D(4)).

This is, in effect, a power of arrest. Section 137 of the 1983 Act defines 'convey' as including any other expression denoting removal from one place to another, and deems people being taken and conveyed to be in legal custody. The principal reference to the power to take and convey in relation to non-offender patients in the 1983 Act is in section 6(1), which provides that a duly completed application form shall be sufficient authority for the applicant or any person authorized by him/her to take and convey the patient to hospital. The purpose of this is to protect those acting on an application for compulsory admission against an action for wrongful arrest imprisonment. *Winterwerp* v. *The Netherlands* and *X* v. *United Kingdom* set down the criteria for a psychiatric arrest to be lawful under Article 5 of the European Convention on Human Rights. Except in an emergency, before a person can be arrested on grounds of unsoundness of mind, there must be objective expert evidence of mental disorder of a nature or degree warranting detention. A completed application with the accompanying medical recommendations would satisfy those requirements. For a psychiatric arrest to be lawful under the Convention the person must be reliably shown to be of unsound mind of a nature or degree warranting detention, entailing 'the establishment of a true mental disorder before a competent authority on the basis of objective expertise' (see *X* v. *United Kingdom* 1981, para. 40; *Winterwerp* 1979, para. 39, *Luberti* v. *Italy* Series A, No. 75 Judgment of 23 February 1984). The evaluation may come from a general practitioner and need not necessarily come from a psychiatrist (Commission Report *Schuurs* v. *the Netherlands*, Application No. 10518/83, p. 3, para. 5–10, 7 March 1985). However, there is an exception for emergencies. In *X* v. *the United Kingdom* the Court stated that it could not be inferred from the *Winterwerp* judgment that the objective medical expertise must in all conceivable cases be obtained before rather than after confinement of a person on grounds of unsoundness of mind. The Court considered that where a provision of domestic law is designed, amongst other things, to authorize emergency confinement of persons capable of presenting a danger to others, it would clearly be impracticable to require thorough medical examination prior to any arrest or detention. In their view, 'A wide discretion must in the nature of things be enjoyed by the national authority empowered to order such emergency confinements' (*X* v. *the United Kingdom* para. 41 of the judgment) Where there is an emergency involving a risk that the patient will behave in a dangerous manner, the expert evaluation may take place after admission. In such circumstances the interests of the public prevail over the individual's right to liberty to the extent of justifying an emergency confinement in the absence of the usual guarantees implied in Article 5(1)(e) (*X* v. *the United Kingdom*, para. 45). Nevertheless, it must be doubtful whether detention on grounds of the person's own health can be justified without prior medical assessment.

The Bill does not specify the circumstances in which the patient may be taken and conveyed, nor does it attach conditions to the power, beyond that it is exercisable by the supervisor or any other person authorized by him or her, and that whoever is exercising it must, if asked, produce a duly authenticated document showing that he is entitled to take and convey the patient. At the committee stage in the Lords, Baroness Cumberledge said in committee that the power to convey 'would give useful backing to the care team, for example where there is temporary reluctance to cooperate' but would be 'used only in times of emergency' (Hansard HL Debs, Vol. 563, No. 68, cols 154 and 156, 4 April 1995). At the report stage she sent out equally conflicting signals as to the circumstances in which the power would be used, refusing to accept amendments designed to subject the power to limiting criteria and procedures through a 'conveyance application'. Having said that she felt it would be used in only 'fairly rare cases' (Hansard HL Debs, Vol. 563, No. 68, cols 154 and 156, 4 April 1995), but then implied that it might be used other than in emergencies with the following statement:

> If a patient is on supervised discharge, the health authority would have accepted a supervision application at the outset, and ... the authorisation of a power to convey is implicit in that original acceptance. That power would be used only *under limited circumstances. but I understand it may be particularly valuable in emergencies.* (emphasis added) (col. 1254)

The failure to attempt any definition of the circumstances which would justify the exercise of this weighty power leaves open the possibility of arbitrariness in its exercise and raises doubt as to whether an arrest pursuant thereto would be in accordance with a procedure prescribed by law. Quite apart from the problem of arbitrariness, it raises the possibility of the police being enlisted to assist in taking and conveying patients to day centres or hospitals, which poses a threat to the continuing relationship between care professionals and clients. Once the person has been taken and conveyed, there is no statement as to what may happen then and how long they have to remain at the place they are conveyed to. one thing is clear. They may not be forcibly medicated unless compulsorily admitted under section 2 or 3 (Mental Health Act 1983, ss 56 and 58).

Review, modification and transfer of after-care

The after-care bodies have a duty to keep under review the after-care services and the requirements imposed on the patient (Mental Health (Patients in the Community) Bill, cl. 25E(1). Where the patient 'refuses or neglects to receive' any or all of the after-care services provided for him (in most cases this will mean medication), or to comply with any or all of the requirements imposed on him, the responsible after-care bodies must review and (where appropriate) modify the services and the requirements imposed on the patient (cl. 25E(2)–(3)). They must consider whether it might be appropriate for the patient to cease to be subject to after-care under supervision and, if so, must inform the community RMO. They must also consider whether it might be appropriate for the patient to be admitted to hospital for treatment and, if they conclude that it might be, inform an approved social worker. The important aspect here is that under the Bill it would be for the after-care bodies, not the community RMO or the supervisor, to bring in the ASW to consider compulsory admission. The Royal College of Psychiatrists' proposed community supervision order had included a separate power of recall to hospital with less stringent criteria for admission. Under the Bill, as part of the review which would take place in the event of non-compliance, consideration would be given to whether the patient's condition had deteriorated so far as to meet the criteria for compulsory admission under the 1983 Act, as interpreted in the 1993 revision of the Code of Practice (para. 8.14e–f). The Department of Health review expressed concern that a recall power which did not require evidence that the patient was at the time of recall suffering from mental disorder of a nature or degree warranting detention would contravene Article 5 of the European Convention on Human Rights.

Before the after-care bodies modify the services or the requirements of the supervised after-care, they would have to consult the patient, the lay carer and (unless the patient objects) the nearest relative. They would also have to inform the patient, the lay carer, and (unless the patient objects) the nearest relative if they do modify the services or the requirements. The Bill will contain express provisions to deal with the situation where a patient under supervision moves from Scotland (where different arrangements apply) to England or Wales and vice versa. As for transfers within England and Wales, the government considers that section 117 already allows sufficient flexibility, by simply placing a duty on the authorities where the patient is resident, regardless of whether those authorities change because of where the patient resides (Hansard HL Debs, Vol. 563, No. 79, col. 1259, 1 May 1995). The section 117 after-care form provides for the transfer of responsibility between authorities.

Renewal

After-care under supervision will last for six months, renewable for six months and thereafter for a year at a time. The procedure for renewal is that the community RMO examines the patient within the last two months of the current period of supervision and furnishes a report to the responsible after-care bodies if the conditions for after-care under supervision are met. The furnishing of the report has the effect of renewing the supervised after-care. Before furnishing a renewal report, the community RMO must consult the patient, the supervisor, one or more persons (if there is anyone) other than the community RMO who are professionally concerned with the patient's medical treatment, one or more persons professionally concerned with the after-care services provided, and the lay carer. There would be no limit on the number of renewals.

The Community RMO's power of discharge

The Community RMO will have the power of discharge, but before doing so must consult and take into account the views of the patient, the supervisor, one or more persons (if there is anyone) other than the community RMO who are professionally concerned with the patient's medical treatment, one or more persons professionally concerned with the after-care services provided, and the lay carer (cl. 25H(1)–(2)). A patient ceases to be subject to supervised after-care if he or she is admitted to hospital under section 2 or section 3 (but not section 4) of the 1983 Act, or is received into guardianship. When a person ceases to be subject to supervised after-care, the responsible after-care bodies must inform the patient, the lay carer, and (unless the patient otherwise requests) the nearest relative (cl. 25H(4)–(5)). A person who is given a custodial sentence by a court is not required to receive after-care services whilst in custody (cl. 25H(6)).

Safeguards for patients' rights

The mental health review tribunal

The Department of Health review promised adequate safeguards to ensure appropriate use of the power, with rights of appeal at least equivalent to those currently available to detained patients (DoH 1993*a*, para. 7.16). The key role in this will be played by mental health review tribunals (MHRTs). Apart from their role in dealing with appeals against supervision, MHRTs hearing applications by detained patients for their discharge will be able to recommend, but not order, that the RMO apply for supervision in the community. They will have the power to reconvene if their recommendation is not complied with (Mental Health (Patients in the Community) Bill, Sched 1 para. 10(2) which will insert a new s. 72(3A) into the 1983 Act). This power is likely to be widely used.

Turning to their role in safeguarding rights, under the 1983 Act MHRTs deal with the question of whether a patient should be detained or liable to be detained. Although there is a general discretion to discharge non-restricted patients, the burden is on the patient to satisfy the MHRT that the conditions of detention are not met. MHRTs currently come under an obligation to discharge from detention if the patient can satisfy them (a) that he or she is no longer suffering from mental disorder of a nature or degree warranting detention or (b) that detention is no longer necessary in the interests of his or her own health or safety or for the protection of others. The current criteria for discharge mean that a tribunal could in theory continue to detain as long as they are *not satisfied* that the patient is *not suffering* from mental disorder of a nature or degree warranting detention (the infamous 'double negative') even though they are *not satisfied* that the patient is *suffering* from mental disorder of the relevant nature or degree. Although there is no settled law on this, it is doubtful whether this meets the third *Winterwerp* requirement that the validity of continued confinement depends on the persistence of such a mental disorder (see *Winterwerp* (1979), para. 37 of the judgment), which implies that it is for those carrying out and authorizing prolonged detention to satisfy themselves at intervals that the criteria for detention continue to be met.

Article 5 does not apply to supervision because it is not detention. In *L v. Sweden* (Application 10801/84, Decisions and Reports of the European Commission of Human Rights, Vol. 45 pp. 181–189 (Decision of 20 January 1986)), where the applicant had been provisionally discharged by a discharge council, the European Commission on Human Rights held that a decision to release on a provisional basis someone who had been detained in a psychiatric hospital constitutes an interference with his right to respect for private life under Article 8(1) of the Convention. However, the Commission went on to hold that the measure was justified in the interests of the person's health under Article 8(2) because the interference with the right of privacy had been 'in accordance with the law and . . . necessary in a democratic society for . . . the protection of health'. There were reasons to believe that she would stop taking her medication if permanently discharged, and this would lead to a permanent deterioration in her health. The Commission held that the decision not to discharge the applicant permanently was necessary in a democratic society for the protection of her health. In the 1988 case in *W v. Sweden* (Application 12778/87, Decisions and Reports of the European Commission of Human Rights, Vol. 59 pp. 158–161 (Decision of 9 December 1988)) the Commission decided that discharge by a discharge council on condition that the applicant took her medication and presented herself for medical control at the hospital every two weeks did not represent such a severe restriction that the applicant's situation after provisional discharge could be characterized as a deprivation of liberty for the purposes of Article 5.

In the interests of minimum amendment of the 1983 Act, the government has put the burden of proof on supervisees too. The Bill will entitle patients to apply to a MHRT for discharge from supervised after-care once within the first six months, and once in every period for which the supervised after-care is renewed. They will also be able to apply if reclassified as suffering from a different form of mental disorder from that in the application (Mental Health Act 1983, s. 66 as amended by Schedule 1 Para. 7 of the Bill). As with non-restricted detained patients, the tribunals will have a general discretion to discharge patients from supervised after-care in any case. They come under a duty to discharge only if the patient satisfies them that the conditions for an application or renewal of supervised after-care are *not* met (Mental Health (Patients in the Community) Bill, Schedule 1 para. 10(3)). Thus, unless a supervisee can persuade the MHRT to exercise its discretion to discharge, the burden is on him or her to satisfy them:

(a) that he is not suffering from mental disorder being mental illness, severe mental impairment, psychopathic disorder or mental impairment; *or*
(b) that there would not be a substantial risk of serious harm to the health or safety of the patient or the safety of other persons, or of the patient being seriously exploited, if he were not to receive the after-care services provided for him under s. 117 below; *or*
(c) that his being subject to after-care under supervision is not likely help to secure that he receives the after-care services to be so provided (para. 10(3) and cl.s. 25A(4)).

This burden will be hard to discharge. If the medical authorities state that the patient would be at risk if he or she did not continue to accept the after-care services, it will be difficult for the patient to show that there would not be a substantial risk of serious harm to his or her own health or safety or of serious exploitation without the requirement to accept after-care. What the decision will boil down to is whether the MHRT accepts the doctor's assertion that without medication the patient will relapse, or the patient's contention that it can safely be discontinued. It can be confidently predicted that discharges 'as of right' will be few. Whilst decisions about continued detention do present elements of prediction and risk-taking, they do involve a justiciable issue – whether the mental disorder is of a nature or degree warranting detention, i.e. making it necessary. It is hard to see how this is so with supervision (in reality compliance with medication). How will a patient who has remained stable in the community whilst taking medication ever convince a tribunal that this is not because of the medication when the RMO says that it is?

Reviewing medication – second opinions?

MHRTs have no jurisdiction to review treatment, only to discharge from compulsion or not. Although supervised discharge will not authorize forcible administration of treatment in the community, its purpose is to create an obligation to accept treatment. Patients who refuse will be told that they may be taken and conveyed to a place of treatment. Even though they may not be forcibly medicated, the Bill is silent on how long they may be kept there. They will also doubtless be told that if they do not accept medication they will be assessed for readmission. Under these circumstances they are likely to agree to treatment, but this will not be true consent. There is therefore a strong case for extending to supervisees the second opinion procedures under section 58 of the 1983 Act whereby detained patients who are to be given drug treatment without consent are entitled to a second opinion after three months of treatment, and regular reviews under section 61 (Mental Health Act 1983, ss. 58 and 61). Second opinion doctors must currently decide whether the treatment ought to be given 'having regard to the likelihood that it will alleviate or prevent deterioration in the patient's condition', and this would give a patient the opportunity to raise concerns about side effects. The thinking behind not applying the section 58 procedure to supervisees is that supervision is intended to be analogous to the more draconian powers of the Home Office over conditionally discharged offender patients who are subject to restrictions to protect the public from serious harm. Conditionally discharged patients are not entitled to second opinions because in theory they are being treated with consent. They have consented to the conditions of their discharge including submission to the treatment regime ordained by their RMO. In a sense this will be true also of supervised discharge, because it is envisaged that the patient's cooperation and consent to the care plan will be sought. However, the ethical, even if not the legal validity of consent, may be questioned when it is the price of freedom. The aim of the new power is to ensure compliance with medication, and the bulk of patients' complaints will be about the effects of their drugs. Tribunals will only be able to decide whether to discharge or not, and will have no formal powers to negotiate a different drug regimen, so patients will be left with no effective independent review of their medication.

The Mental Health Act Commission

Many, including the Royal College of Psychiatrists, MIND and the Law Society have argued for the extension of the remit of the Mental Health Act Commission to cover supervisees, which would mean that they could visit them and deal with any complaints they might raise about their supervision. The Clunis inquiry proposed that supervised discharge orders should be required to be lodged with and monitored by the Mental Health Act Commission (Ritchie *et al.* 1994). Earl Haig sought to move an amendment in Committee to extend the Commission's jurisdiction under section 120 of the 1983 Act to supervisees, to keep a balance between medical needs and civil liberties. Baroness Cumberledge for the government rejected this on the grounds that there were already sufficient safeguards built into the Bill, and that the Commission would have jurisdiction over the patients while they were detained, and thereby could oversee how the powers were being exercised at that stage (Hansard HL Debs, Vol. 563, No. 70, col. 366, 1 May 1995. 48). It appears under section 120(1)(b)(i) as currently drafted that the MHAC already has jurisdiction to hear complaints by supervisees or others in relation to the exercise of powers and duties under the Act. This states that the Commission must investigate any other complaint as to the exercise of the powers or the discharge of duties conferred or imposed by this Act in respect of a person who is or has been so detained. By definition, supervisees have been detained, and complaints under this subsection are not limited to events which occur during detention. As the Bill will be an amendment to the Act, powers and duties under the Bill will be powers and duties under the Act. In addition to these complaints possibilities under s. 120, since section 117 services are community care within the National Health Service and Community Care Act 1990, complaints can be addressed through the local authorities complaints procedures under that Act.

Conclusion

Although the Bill introduces a new and somewhat convoluted system of procedures for supervised after-care, and has serious implications for both human rights and the relationship between care professionals and their

clients, it is difficult to see it as an improvement on the possibilities for intervention under current legislation. If someone is subject to guardianship and
is considered to need compulsory admission, the nominated medical attendant can ask an ASW to assess with a view to implementing a transfer from
guardianship to hospital. Where someone ceases medication and is beginning to relapse, the Mental Health Act Code of Practice makes it clear that
they can be readmitted to hospital (DoH 1993*b*, para. 2.9; Blom Cooper *et
al*. 1995, Chapter 18). The principal form of treatment which will be given
to supervisees will be depot antipsychotic medication. Members of Survivors'
Groups speak persuasively of the dependence forming properties of antipsychotic drugs, and that abrupt withdrawal can trigger a powerful psychotic
episode. Antipsychotic medication also has well-documented side effects.
What will happen to a mentally ill person who for perfectly sound reasons
wishes to be weaned off antipsychotic medication under medical supervision? Despite the welcome statements in guidance about multidisciplinary-
care plans, will the existence of supervision registers and supervised
discharge serve only to reinforce a dependency of psychiatry and its patients
on these powerful drugs, and a culture of defensive medicine? It also risks
creating an atmosphere of undue faith in these medicines, that as long as
patients comply with their medication all will be well. Medicine is only one
component of community care. These drugs do not cure, they merely control symptoms, and some of the incidents where acts of violence and self-
harm have occurred have involved patients who were taking medication at
the time (Ben Silcock and Andrew Robinson; see Blom Cooper *et al*. 1995).
Although the ten point plan may benefit patients, in that it will encourage
health and social service bodies to take seriously their obligations under section 117, no extra resources are being made available to implement it beyond
what is required to finance the increased number of MHRT hearings. The
new powers and the supposed 'safeguards' in the Bill place compulsory
supervision beyond effective review, and the danger is that many who are
subject to these powers will effectively be obliged to take neuroleptic medication for the rest of their lives.

References

Statutes

The Access to Health Records Act 1990
The Children Act 1989
The Data Protection Act 1984
The Mental Health Act 1983
The Local Authority Social Services Act 1970
The National Assistance Act 1948
The National Health Service and Community Care Act 1990

Regulations

The Data Protection (Subject Access Modification) Health Order 1987, SI 1987
    No. 1903
The Mental Health (Hospital, Guardianship and Consent to Treatment) Regulations
    1983, SI 1983 No. 893.

Cases

Associated Provincial Picture Houses v. *Wednesbury Corporation* [1948] 1 KB 223

L v. *Sweden* Application 10801/84, Decisions and Reports of the European Commission of Human Rights, Vol. 45, pp. 181–189 (Decision of 20 January 1986)

Luberti v. *Italy* Series A: Judgments and Decisions of the European Court of Human Rights No. 75 Judgment of 23 February 1984

R v. *Cardiff Crown Court ex parte Kellam* (1993) 16 BMLR 76

R v. *Ealing District Health Authority ex parte Fox* [1993] 1 WLR 373

R v. *Hallstrom ex parte W (No. 2)* and *B* v. *Gardner and another ex parte L* [1986] 2 All ER (QBD) 306

Re C (adult: refusal of medical treatment) [1994] 1 All ER 819

Schuurs v. *the Netherlands*, Application No. 10518/83, Report of the European Commission on Human Rights, 7 March 1985

Tarasoff v. *Regents of the University of California* (1976) 551 P 2d 334

Van der Leer v. *The Netherlands* (1990) 7 BMLR 105, Judgment of 21 February 1990

W v. *Sweden* Application 12778/87, Decisions and Reports of the European Commission of Human Rights, Vol. 59 pp. 158–161 (Decision of 9 December 1988)

Winterwerp v. *the Netherlands* Commission Report, Publications of the European Court of Human Rights, Series B. Pleadings, Oral arguments and documents, Vol. 31

Winterwerp v. *the Netherlands* (1979) 2 EHRR 387, Judgment of 24 October 1979, Series A: Judgments and Decisions of the European Court of Human Rights No. 33

X v. *United Kingdom* (1982) 4 EHRR 188, (1981) 1 BMLR 98, Judgment of 5 November 1981

Other references

Blom Cooper L, Hally E and Murphy E (1995). *The Falling Shadow*. Duckworth, London.

Cavadino M (1991). 'Community control'. *Journal of Social Welfare and Family Law*, 259–268.

Department of Health and Home Office, (1981). *White Paper, Reform of Mental Health Legislation*, Cmnd. 8405, HMSO, London.

Department of Health (1988). *The Clinical Complaints Procedure*. Circular HC(88)37, HMSO, London.

Department of Health (1989). *The Care of Children – Principles and Practice in Regulations and Guidance*. HMSO, 2, London.

Department of Health (1990). *Care Programme Approach for People with a Mental Illness Referred to the Specialist Psychiatric Services*. Health Circular HC(90)23/LASSL(90)11, HMSO, London.

Department of Health/Social Services Inspectorate (1991). *The Right to Complain: Practice Guidance on Complaints Procedures in Social Services Departments*. HMSO, London.

Department of Health (1993*a*). *Report of the Internal Review of Legal Powers on the Care of Mentally Ill People in the Community*. HMSO, London.

Department of Health and the Welsh Office (1993*b*). *The Mental Health Act Code of Practice* (2nd edn). HMSO, London.

Department of Health/Social Services Inspectorate (1993*c*). *Inspection of Complaints Procedures in Local Authority Social Services Departments*. HMSO, London.

Fennell P (1989). Beverley Lewis – Was the Law to Blame? *New Law Journal*, **139**, 1557–1559.

Fennell P (1992). Balancing care and control: guardianship, community treatment orders, and patient safeguards. *International Journal of Law and Psychiatry*, **15**, 205–235.

Fisher M (1988). Guardianship under the mental health legislation: a review. *Journal of Social Welfare Law*, 316–327, 317 and 323–325.

Geller J L (1986). The quandaries of enforced community treatment and unenforceable outpatient commitment statutes. *Journal of Psychiatry and Law*, 149–158.

Gordon R (1993). *Community Care Assessments: A Practical Legal Framework.* Longman, London.

Gostin L O (1983). The ideology of entitlement. In *Mental Illness: Changes and Trends* (ed. P Bean). John Wiley, London, pp. 27–54.

House of Commons Health Committee (1983). *Community Supervision Orders.* Fifth Report, Vol. 1, HC 667–1 (23 June 1993).

Hunter D J and Judge K (1988). *Griffiths and Community Care: Meeting the Challenge.* King's Fund Institute, London.

Law Commission (1991). *Consultation Paper No. 119: Mentally Incapacitated Adults and Decision-making: An Overview.* HMSO, London.

Mental Health Act Commission (1985). *First Biennial Report 1983–1985.* HMSO, London.

Mental Health Act Commission (1991). *Fourth Biennial Report 1989–1991.* HMSO, London.

Mental Health Act Commission (1993). *Fifth Biennial Report 1991–1993.* HMSO, London.

NHS Management Executive (1993). Health Service Guidelines HSG(94)5: *Introduction of Supervision Registers for Mentally Ill People by 1 April.*

NHS Management Executive (1994b). Health Service Guidelines HSG(94)27: *Discharge of Mentally Disordered People and their Continuing Care in the Community.*

Ritchie J H, Dick D and Lingham R (1994). *The Report of the Inquiry into the Care and Treatment of Christopher Clunis.* HMSO, London.

Royal College of Psychiatrists (1993). *Community Supervision Orders: Discussion Document.* RCP, London.

Social Services Inspectorate (1992). *Guidance on Implementing Caring for People: Assessment.*

Zander M (1990). *The Police and Criminal Evidence Act 1984* (second edn.) Sweet and Maxwell, London.

7 The role of the voluntary sector

R. Brown and R. Dixon

Introduction

Recent changes in social policy and legislation on community care are having a radical effect on voluntary organizations. They are altering the position of the voluntary sector in the provision of mental health care in the community. As a result, there is a need for a fresh evaluation of the relationship between the state and the voluntary sector, and of the quality of mental health care being provided by both sectors. In this chapter we will examine some of the central issues, consider the impact of these changes on multiagency and multidisciplinary care in the community, and look at the future role of voluntary organizations. After some introductory comments, we will consider how people come to make use of mental health services and how this can lead them into contact with voluntary organizations. We will then undertake a brief examination of the historical role of voluntary agencies. The central theme of the chapter is the influence of funding arrangements and the impact such arrangements have on the development of voluntary organizations. We will describe traditional methods of funding and the consequences of adopting such methods, some key elements within the current changes in funding arrangements, and developments that might be affecting the roles of voluntary agencies. We will use one positive local case example to illustrate some of the main points. We will discuss users' views on services and, finally, we will consider possible trends in the future. The chapter is not concerned with private profit-making agencies but with non-profit voluntary organizations and their part in community care provision. We have adopted the broadest definition of such organizations and thus include all those charities and other organizations that are supported and run by boards of managers or trustees who do not receive payments for this work and who act in these capacities as volunteers.

The voluntary sector has played a significant role in the development of welfare provision, particularly in the mental health field. In many ways the services originated by voluntary organizations can be viewed as laying the foundations of welfare provision. State services have then built on these foundations and have tried to make services more universally accessible. After the Second World War a pattern emerged whereby agencies within the voluntary sector were seen as stimulating state provision by several methods. For example, they would appear or move into underresourced areas and demonstrate need by the provision of a new service. The voluntary sector has a tradition of becoming involved in areas which are comparatively poorly resourced by the statutory sector and this continues today. For example, in a review of services for those who have left hospital, Patmore (1987) identified a key role for voluntary agency projects involved in housing and employment issues. One of the main areas of voluntary agency involvement has been accommodation. Pilling (1991) has noted the importance of the voluntary sector in responding to homelessness. Homelessness often has a link with mental health problems but there are frequently other factors involved, and statutory services have sometimes failed to respond to areas of need which do not neatly fit their definitions of their own client group or of the service they provide. There are additional problems where there are overlapping responsibilities across different statutory agencies and where no one of them wishes to take the lead (and probably incur the expense) in tackling the problem.

The identification of a need, the development, and finally the provision of a service by a voluntary agency might lead that voluntary agency to suggest that the statutory agencies should take over or expand the service, or possibly that they should develop similar services in other areas. Alternatively, without providing services directly, a voluntary agency might develop a pressure group function whereby it would articulate needs expressed by people with mental health problems or by their carers. Thus a voluntary organization (such as MIND) may call for an improvement in state services to meet these needs. Where the growing body of legislation has made such provision a mandatory duty, the voluntary organization could press for full implementation of the law. Where the powers are permissive they could try to persuade the authority to make the provision available.

Organizations vary as to how much they listen to the views of those suffering with mental health problems or to their families and friends. Some are dominated by professionals or other people concerned with mental health issues. Service users themselves are not always allowed or encouraged to express their views or to hold positions of influence. Despite these limitations, many voluntary organizations have acted effectively as pressure groups and have been prepared to challenge the statutory sector. One theme of this chapter is that this particular function is under threat because of an increasing dependence on state funding. Before making a closer examination of the funding issues it is necessary to look at the current routes into mental health services for the majority of people, how they are defined as suffering from mental health problems, and how then they may be put in contact with voluntary organizations active in the mental health field.

Routes to mental health services

Goldberg and Huxley (1980) have devised a framework for understanding how people become defined as mentally ill and how they make contact with mental health services. They suggest that there are four filters which determine who will pass through to various levels. They have recently revised this work (Goldberg and Huxley 1992) and estimate that between 260 and 315 people in every 1000 will suffer an episode of mental disorder lasting at least two weeks. However, only a small minority will be seen by mental health professionals (23.5 in every 1000). It will be interesting in 1994–95 to compare these estimates with the results of the OPCS survey into the prevalence of mental illness in the community. For our purposes, what is of particular note is that Goldberg and Huxley found that the majority of distressed people consulted their doctor but that they often did so in relation to associated physical symptoms. Many people with mental disorders were not diagnosed as such by their GPs. Doctors identified 101.5 people in every 1000 of the general population as being mentally disordered and referred 23.5 to mental illness services. (5.71 per 1000 were then admitted as psychiatric inpatients.) The crucial part played by general practitioners in this process raises the question of their relationship with the voluntary sector.

It is to be hoped that Goldberg and Huxley's work will lead to training for GPs to improve their capacity to identify mental illness. This call is echoed by users themselves in a survey conducted in 1993 in the Southampton area (Brown 1993). Wilcock (1990) has also advised that to get best value from a GP users and carers should plan their method of consulting in advance. In any event, the GP's role in referring people to mental health services is of great significance. Williams (1985) has argued that the key question is not how primary care services should fit in with specialist mental health services, but the other way round. If this view is supported, we might expect GPs to become more central, almost as the hub of services, and their liaison with voluntary agencies would take on an even greater significance than in the past. Alternatively, if community mental health teams develop, GPs might still be crucial in terms of deciding whether or not to refer to these teams, but may be less involved after that point, leaving the subsequent coordination of services to a CMHT member.

In situations where GPs remain actively involved, both in referrals to other services and in monitoring their patients' progress and needs, they may develop a broader range of options than the traditional referral on to a hospital-based consultant. The demand for brief psychotherapy or counselling has led in some cases to increased links between GPs and voluntary agencies involved as service providers in this area. Toynbee (1993) has described the work of 120 Relate counsellors based in GP surgeries around the country. Jennifer Newton cites more recent examples of practices working closely with a number of voluntary organizations providing counselling services such as Relate and the Family Welfare Association (Newton 1992). The development of counselling services is a user-led demand and has been shown to be effective in reducing the symptoms of stress and preventing the development of serious symptoms in those rated at high risk of becoming depressed.

There is less evidence of GPs working with voluntary groups that are targeting services at people with serious and long-term mental health difficulties. With the development of GP fund-holding it may be possible that GPs will look to arrangements and services provided by the voluntary sector as alternative referral points for this group involving a direct financial relationship. However, given the priority that GPs are able to give to mental health problems, and the need both to enhance their training and to incorporate them into effective multidisciplinary and multiagency teamwork, this does not promise to be a key area for development for the voluntary organizations who may instead be looking at working with health commissions and local authorities.

Historical role of voluntary agencies

The traditional model of mental health care, as reflected in many texts (e.g. Kuipers and Bebbington 1987; Wilcock 1990) emphasizes the central role of professionals employed by the health authority or the local authority. This model sees the voluntary sector as supplying support, filling gaps and catering for relatives. A counter view (Hatfield and Lefley 1987) stresses that the vast bulk of caring is carried out by the families of mentally disordered people. Voluntary agencies should, therefore, respond to the expressed needs of these carers, and the statutory agencies should be filling in the gaps and providing specialist services and help for those without family support. Both of these models tend to understate the campaigning function of voluntary agencies. Indeed, in the case of the National Schizophrenia Fellowship, much of the campaigning energy has come from the families of those suffering from mental health problems. MIND emerged (as the National Association for Mental Health) immediately after the Second World War and quickly became a pressure group seeking improved rights and services.

Whatever emphasis one might place on the different aspects of voluntary organizations' roles, they have usually offered a balance between self-help, direct services (often of an innovative kind), campaigning, following up individual complaints and offering advice. Many local groups (such as the Falkirk District Association for Mental Health) have maintained this balance despite pressures from statutory authorities to concentrate more on service delivery. The initial energy and funding for these activities has come from voluntary donations and individuals' concern and conscience. They have been non-profit-making and based on a variety of essentially charitable motivations. This has determined the balance of their activities and their priorities. However, recent changes in funding and in particular the reforms linked to the National Health Service and Community Care Act 1990 require a reappraisal of this view.

Traditional funding arrangements

The amount of money raised by voluntary agencies from donations varies, but most have a significant amount of funding which comes from statutory agencies. The relationship between statutory authorities and voluntary organizations has been complementary and, as a consequence, complex and interdependent. Historically these relationships have relied on a great deal of trust, and personal contact between individuals representing the respective bodies. The models and methods of funding that exist between the voluntary and statutory sectors reflect the nature of these relationships. Judge (1982) identified a number of types of such funding arrangements that existed in Britain. These included:

- vendor reimbursement. This is for units of client-specific services and includes the purchase of residential care and boarding-out schemes.
- delegated agency. This involves proportional reimbursement of costs where a voluntary agency undertakes total responsibility for a particular service on behalf of a social services department.
- quasi-contracting. This includes major grants where there is usually some expectation of a service but this is not spelt out and the grant is not cost related.
- community development. This involves the giving of minor grants.

Between 1960 and the 1980s the most common form of funding was the provision by local authorities of grants on a block basis which voluntary organizations took the initiative to apply for. These were usually reviewed and/or renewed on an annual basis. Most local authorities have rules built into their standing orders that govern the process of grant giving. Hampshire County Council Social Services Department, for example, has general criteria which require that grant bids should relate to the legislative responsibilities of the social services department and that all grants over £5000 require the approval of the members' committee.

In spite of such guidelines Judge and Smith (1982) argue that until recently there was little evidence of any clear rationale behind the process of grant giving. They considered that there was considerable political partisanship in the context of very local relationships between local authority members and officers, and the local voluntary organizations. Whilst the rationale may not have been evident, there were clear advantages for both sides in adopting this method of funding. Grants were generally given with a broad remit to provide a service with little specified detail or accountability and were frequently given in response to a request from a voluntary organization to provide or develop a service, rather than by the local authority tendering or recruiting a voluntary organization into providing a service it required or saw as necessary.

This process had a number of benefits. Firstly, the availability of grants allowed for the possibility of voluntary organizations funding, or continuing to develop, innovative schemes that may not have been seen as a priority for the local authority. An example of this was the development of refuges for women fleeing from domestic violence. The movement behind the establishment of refuges was rooted in the radical politics of the women's movement of the 1960s and whilst some refuges remained entirely voluntary or user run, many applied for and received local authority grant aid. The demand for the service came from the voluntary organization not from the local authorities and in many cases the issues around funding such a service were not only new but were also challenging to local authorities.

Grant funding also provided a great deal of autonomy and independence for voluntary organizations to develop service flexibility. It allowed space for the development of campaigning and advocacy. Organizations such as Mencap and MIND in a large number of places were in receipt of grant funding which covered not only the provision of direct services, such as day clubs or sitting services, but which also maintained to some degree the campaigning and advocacy side of their work. This system also allowed for a number of grant applications to be made to a range of authorities. Where effective 'joint funding' between agencies operated, alternative sources of funding may have been limited. However there existed the possibility for some voluntary organizations of obtaining funding from not only more than one statutory agency (central government, local authority or the health service) but also from within separate departments of such authorities.

The advantages of this method of funding were not all to the benefit of the voluntary organizations. The major advantage to statutory agencies was that the provision of a grant may not have borne any direct relationship to the real cost of the service being funded. The statutory authority could see its grant as a contribution to the cost of the service, expecting funding to be sought from elsewhere, either from other statutory funds or from the charitable monies of the voluntary organization. In addition, whilst grants were loosely specified, most commonly they were annually reviewed and this maintained a level of uncertainty for the voluntary organization and thus some power for the funders. The disadvantages of this traditional method of funding from the statutory agencies' point of view included: very little monitoring; an emphasis on inputs rather than outputs; a lack of evaluations; very little accountability of the service providers; a general lack of planning; and a tendency towards short-term arrangements.

The new contract culture

Over the last ten years there has been a radical change in the relationship between the voluntary sector and the statutory agencies, and in particular with local authorities. This change has been accelerated by the current implementation of the National Health Service and Community Care Act 1990, but many of the changes had already appeared before the debate about this legislation began.

Major changes in government policy towards local authorities and state-run services from the early 1980s onward led to the notion of local authorities being considered enablers rather than providers of services. This encouraged the expansion of the voluntary sector as providers and also promoted a market system in social welfare. This policy was enacted through a range of new legislation introduced prior to the NHS and Community Care Act and it shaped the relationships between the voluntary and statutory agencies in the UK. Relevant legislation included the Local Government Act 1988, which introduced compulsory competitive tendering for certain defined local authority services. In general these were not the welfare services but the process gave many local authorities large-scale experience of contracting. Similarly, the Housing Act 1988 introduced restrictions on local authorities' direct role in the provision of housing, and encouraged the expansion of housing associations and the private sector. The Education Reform Act of 1988 introduced the local management of schools, again reducing the powers of local authorities and promoting the role of school governors. The NHS and Community Care Act 1990 (the implementation of which was mainly delayed until April 1993) must be seen in the context of this other legislation, and the government's underpinning ideology.

In essence, the NHS and Community Care Act 1990 requires local authorities and health authorities to assess need, decide what services are available, separate out purchaser and provider functions, reduce direct provision and commission services to meet the identified need on an individual and on a strategic level. In the background document to the Act, the Department of Health's White Paper, *Caring for People* (Department of Health 1989), a new relationship between the voluntary sector and the statutory sector was clearly set out:

> Authorities should seek to move towards funding in partnership with the voluntary sector. Voluntary organisations may need to make major changes in their working methods and there is likely to be considerable advantage for both sides of the partnership if the voluntary sector can be involved at an early stage in negotiation over the contents of the contract.

Different models of contracting

Models of contracting for welfare services from the USA were beginning to influence the British debate in the early 1980s. Diana Leat (1983) has examined the relevance to Britain of a North American model which was first postulated by Kramer (1981). This model suggested five types of financial relationships between voluntary organizations and statutory agencies. These were:

- categorical grants
- subsidies
- payments for service
- contracts for purchase of service
- third-party payments for service.

This model was developed in a climate where far more welfare provision was being provided by voluntary organizations and by the private sector than in Britain. In addition, the use of detailed and legally enforceable contracts was the norm, extending back over two decades. The debate about the value of contracts in the United States has tended to suggest that the use of contracts has enhanced the power of voluntary organizations. The argument runs that it has created a real sense of partnership between them and the statutory agencies and has allowed them to maintain their independence and autonomy. More recent commentators have not been so positive about this or about the potential benefits of applying the North American contracting arrangements to the British context. Gutch (1992), for example, suggests that the relationship in North America between voluntary organizations and statutory agencies has become a vast bureaucratic paper chase combining the worst aspects of the UK grant system with the worst fears of the contract culture.

Thompson and Monkcom (1990) have identified four types of funding commonly in operation in Britain in the early 1990s:

- a per capita fee (e.g. the payment of fees of a person who is in a voluntary sector residential home)
- a grant (usually made for a group to carry out certain broad objectives – essentially a gift depending on the good faith of both sides)

- a formal contract (a legal document which would cover in detail the commitment which both sides are making)
- a service agreement (a compromise between grants and contracts).

Whilst there are some similarities between this and Judge's (1982) list cited earlier, there has been a change in the balance between the different methods of funding. In the context of a significant increase in the total amount of statutory agency funding available there has been a shift away from the provision of simple grants. Hampshire County Council Social Services Department, for example, has eliminated discussion of simple grants and has introduced three methods of funding for voluntary organizations:

- letters of agreement. These are used for sums under £2000.
- service agreements. These are legally enforceable but brief agreements. They contain a minimum of specified detail and are based on a close working relationship between the parties.
- contracts. Again these are legally enforceable agreements but they specify in detail a service to be provided and include specific outcome measures to be achieved.

Apart from formal contracts with private sector providers of residential care Hampshire is positively promoting the use of service agreements.

This trend is reflected elsewhere. In her research in three London boroughs Lewis (1993) suggests that the change in funding arrangements in the UK since 1990 has been a formalization of the relationship between agencies, rather than a move towards contracting on the North American model:

> The stated preference of both the voluntary sector and local authorities has been to move towards a redefined partnership rather than price determined competition; the evidence suggests that trust remains an important and valued component in contracting for the human services, that are often provided to vulnerable people.

She goes on to say, however that:

> For the voluntary organisations to become equal partners they need to be involved in all aspects of the changes; in the process of community care planning, which is intended to provide a vehicle for assessing needs and determining which services will be commissioned. (Lewis 1993, p. 185.)

The issue here is: who is setting the agenda? The statutory services are now leading the way, deciding on the service that they wish to see in place and then commissioning and in some cases tendering for them. It is emerging that in this process the voluntary organisations find that there is a stifling of innovation and a move away from their own priorities towards those of the statutory agency. There is concern that the voluntary organisations are not merely replacing the local authorities as providers of services, but that they are becoming managerially, financially and ideologically tied down and incorporated into local statutory networks at the expense of their autonomy.

A positive example

The implications of these new funding relationships and of the new ideology can be examined in relation to a project funded by the local social services department from mental illness specific grant (MISG). The mental illness specific grant probably had a highly significant effect in the realignment of the relationships between the voluntary and statutory agencies in some areas. MISG came with the first phase of the introduction of the NHS and Community Care Act. It was government revenue money that was on offer to local authorities to fund 70 per cent of the development of community mental health services. Whilst there was a high degree of flexibility in its use it came at a time when local authorities were looking to pilot their roles as enabling authorities and were very positive about using this money to pump prime projects in the voluntary sector. It is also true that the voluntary sector was probably able to respond more quickly and flexibly with projects that could ensure the uptake of the funding available, than the statutory agency.

The Community Support Project in Southampton is a new service which is MISG-funded. In essence it involves mainstream work of the social services department being put out to a voluntary housing organisation. There is a high degree of statutory agency input in terms of steering and providing support.

The Community Support Project was established in 1991 to provide flexible domiciliary support services for people with serious mental health problems. The project was developed from scratch in response to a number of stimuli. The first was an examination of how a needs-led service could be provided in the community for people with mental health problems. The second was a piece of research conducted by a local social worker which indicated the need for support workers to befriend and provide practical support to enable people with serious mental health problems to remain living independently in the community. The third was the fact that local authority home care services had been targeted on very vulnerable groups who required a high level of personal care. This created a gap in terms of support for those who required practical support or social contact. There was also a pressing need to be able to provide services for black and Asian people with mental health problems for whom current community provision was failing. Finally there was the availability of the government's mental illness specific grant funding.

The broad outline of a project to meet these needs based on the use of MISG was taken by a social services manager to a local mental health forum of statutory and voluntary organisations and two voluntary organisations expressed an interest in developing the work. The final selection of the host organisation lay with the social services department and was not done on a tendering basis but on criteria related to the management record of the voluntary body, the fact that there had been a long and close working relationship between the agencies, and finally the fact that there had been the experience of a successful delivery of another similar project. A steering group was set up that included social services staff, health service staff, representatives of the host voluntary organisation and representatives of other key voluntary bodies in the field. This group then developed the project and after a period of three months were able to agree an operational policy which became an annex to a service agreement that was signed between the voluntary organisation, the local authority and the health authority. Funding was to be provided by the local authority with a three-year commitment. The health authority was to provide office space and the voluntary organisation would employ staff and manage the project. The steering group became the project's management committee. The project has been very successful in meeting its aims and in developing a flexible needs-led service with high standards of practice.

There have been a number of key issues that have arisen from the development of this project. The first of these is that a voluntary organisation has clearly taken on an agency role on behalf of the social services authority. Whilst the service provided is new and different from the existing services provided by the local authority, it is within the mainstream of the direction that the local authority is developing. The agency issue was clearly reflected in the prolonged debate that took place between the various voluntary organisations and the statutory agencies about how people were to be referred to the project. Both social services and the health authority clearly established control by ensuring that referrals were filtered through social workers or community psychiatric nurses. The rationale for this was to ensure that the project's resources were meeting the target group and that the project workers were not left isolated, but would be able to work in partnership with the social workers and nurses. A second issue has been the success of the project in developing antidiscriminatory practice. Whilst much of the policy and underpinning principles were written in to the original social services agreement, the project has been highly effective in its implementation and has developed a culture that has not yet been achieved in the local statutory authorities. In fact project workers are now influential on this issue and are feeding their experiences back into statutory agency working groups.

In many ways, whilst most of the power and control still lies with the statutory agencies, the challenge of this project has been to those agencies. The development of the project has been positive for the users who are recipients of the service. A survey of users and carers by Brown (1993) found that, among other positive indicators, the Community Support Project was the only service mentioned which consistently proved able to give its users a sense of choice.

Users' views

The shift away from statutory agencies and towards voluntary agency provision would certainly seem, at first sight, to be in accordance with views expressed by the users of mental health services. Rogers, Pilgrim and Lacey (1993) conducted MIND's People First survey. They found that users tended to be more positive about voluntary agencies than they were about statutory ones. Reasons given were: informality, helpfulness, being treated as equals, and the availability of nontraditional forms of intervention such as telephone help lines, drop-in centres, tranquillizer withdrawal groups and self-help groups. Rogers *et al.* considered that some of these services would be difficult to provide within the statutory sector because they run counter to the traditionally dominant treatment philosophy of a heavy reliance on psychotropic drugs. Similarly, the style of delivery was more flexible and could accommodate users in the service delivery process. Structures were less formal and were less influenced by a professional culture. Users expressed greater satisfaction when they had a role in service delivery. Rogers *et al.*'s data was collected in 1989–1990 but the findings were largely repeated in a more recent local study (Brown 1993). For example, there was evidence in both studies of a growing demand for alternative acute services outside the statutory sector. Typically this might involve a 24-hour community-based crisis intervention team with access to crisis houses and to user-run asylum-type facilities. Campbell (1993) has described user-led projects offering alternative places of safety in times of distress in his examination of developments in the provision of crisis services.

However, despite the general tendency of users' views to support a shift towards more voluntary agency provision, some central doubts remain. Once again, these include the potential threat to voluntary agencies' funding if they adopt a critical stance towards their funding authority. Rogers *et al.* (1993, p. 80) give an individual example: 'Approached local MIND re complaining about treatment at local unit. Given very little help – told that they were aware of situation but were afraid to interfere lest they were deprived of their grant from the local authority'. Ramon comments on the more general issue of the traditional campaigning role of the voluntary sector. In her study of psychiatric hospital closure she states:

> Central Government has also attempted to curtail the campaigning role of the non-profit organisations, arguing that their charitable status excludes campaigning. Such an attempt goes against the grain of the long-honoured tradition of the British non-profit sector, as well as against the interests of the people represented by these organisations.
>
> (Ramon 1992 p. 92.)

Some of the larger voluntary organisations may be in a stronger position to retain their campaigning and 'upholder of complaints' function by linking national campaigns to grass-roots support. For example, MIND's 'Stress on Women' campaign (Sayce 1993) has demonstrated how it is possible to both stimulate and draw on a network of local groups with a high degree of user involvement, through a well-coordinated national campaign.

Another area of doubt is that, although current government policy favours a move towards greater involvement of the voluntary sector, this is based on a model which looks at them as replacing existing statutory-run services rather than providing a range of different alternatives which would increase user choice. Finally, and not surprisingly, Langan (1990) identified that there tends to be less voluntary provision in predominantly working-class areas than in more affluent areas. Thus, perversely, users in those areas of greatest need may be denied access to the more flexible, user-orientated services which the voluntary sector may be able to provide elsewhere.

Multi-agency work

An increased role for the voluntary sector in direct provision should lead to a greater diversity of services and more informality in their delivery but there are a number of challenges. Powell and Lovelock (1992) by adopting a case study approach, have examined some of the implications of decentralizing mental health services. In terms of multidisciplinary teamwork they found that it leads to greater individual autonomy for workers, together with a lack of clarity about accountability and leadership.

These aspects will be heightened by increased involvement of the voluntary sector in multi-agency work. Issues of accountability and management will have to be settled project by project. There will also be issues concerning the reassessment of what skills and training are required for particular tasks. Traditional understanding of the role of nurses, social workers and other community-based workers may have to be radically re-evaluated. Other people with the skills, but not the background or training previously considered necessary, may take on key areas of work. Questions will have to be resolved such as: what are appropriate pay levels? who is responsible for health and safety? will voluntary organisations' workers have access to the training opportunities offered by statutory agencies? There will be a need for a broad understanding of these issues on all sides, at management and at worker level. This cooperation will need to be communicated in an effective and understandable way to service users if multi-agency work is to prove successful.

Conclusion

In this chapter we have evaluated the changes that are occurring in the relationship between the statutory and voluntary sectors. The main practice example we have cited is a positive one, but there are many others which could be quoted to illustrate disadvantages as well as advantages arising from these changes. One clear danger is that the voluntary sector's role as a force for change and development may be dissipated as energies are concentrated on winning contracts and delivering services, rather than on acting as pressure groups. We have also noted that not everything has been straightforward in managing changes in the partnership between funding statutory agencies and recipient voluntary organisations. Difficulties and more complex situations seem to have arisen where there have been long-standing grant aid relationships for the provision of services. This is exacerbated where statutory agencies are seeking to change the current service provided, extend the service or to develop additional 'bolt on' services. Voluntary organisations that have not been specialized and aimed to provide holistic health and welfare services are being squeezed. This may particularly affect neighbourhood and black and ethnic minority organisations which are providing a very wide range of support services or which do not recognize the labels and limitations of the statutory services. The challenge will be to concentrate on meeting needs rather than being dominated by structural funding issues. Finally, we have seen how changes in the role of voluntary agencies are likely to alter the nature of multidisciplinary working. Indeed, multi-agency working will probably be of equal importance and there may be significant changes still to come, in terms of relationships between professional mental health workers and with users of these services.

References

Brown R (1993). *Users' and Carers' Views on Mental Health Services in Southampton and South-West Hampshire*. Unpublished.

Campbell P (1993). New paths to caring? *Open Mind*, **63**, 12–13.

Department of Health (1989). *Caring for People: Community Care in the Next Decade and Beyond*. Cmnd 849, HMSO, London.

Goldberg D and Huxley P (1980). *Mental Illness in the Community: The Pathway to Psychiatric Care*. Tavistock, London.

Goldberg D and Huxley P (1992). *Common Mental Disorders: A Bio-social Model*. Routledge, London.

Gutch R (1992). Contracting Lessons from the US. NCVO, London.

Hatfield A and Lefley H (eds.) (1987). *Families of the Mentally Ill*. Cassell, London.

Judge K (1982). *The Public Purchase of Social Care*: British Confirmation of the American Experience. PSSRU Discussion Paper No 230/2, University of Kent, Canterbury.

Judge K and Smith G (1982). *Why Purchase? The Rationale for POSC in the English Social Services*. PSSRU Discussion Paper No. 243, University of Kent, Canterbury.

Kramer R (1981). *Voluntary Agencies in the Welfare State*. University of California Press, Berkeley.

Kuipers E and Bebbington P (1987). *Living with Mental Illness*. Souvenir Press, London.

Langan M (1990). Community care in the 1990s: The Community care white paper 'Caring for People'. *Critical Social Policy*, **29**, 58–70.

Leat D (1983). Working together: statutory–voluntary relationships. In *Collaboration and Conflict: Working with Others* (ed. J Lishman). Department of Social Work, University of Aberdeen People's Press.

Lewis J (1993). 'Developing the mixed economy of care: emerging issues for voluntary organisations'. *Journal of Social Policy*, **22.2**, 173–192.

Newton J (1992). *Preventing Mental Illness in Practice*. Routledge, London.

Patmore C (ed.) (1987). *Living After Mental Illness*. Croom Helm, Beckenham.

Pilling S (1991). *Rehabilitation and Community Care*. Routledge, London.

Powell J and Lovelock R (1992). *Changing Patterns of Mental Health Care*. Avebury, Aldershot.

Ramon S (ed.) (1992). *Psychiatric Hospital Closure*. Chapman and Hall, London.

Rogers A, Pilgrim D and Lacey R (1993). *Experiencing Psychiatry: Users' Views of Services*. MIND, London.

Sayce L (1993). *The Stress on Women Campaign Pack*. MIND, London.

Thompson C and Monkcom C (1990). *Contracting for Care*. Briefing Paper No.1. National Council for Voluntary Organisations, London.

Toynbee P (1993). The counsellor in the doctor's chair. *The Guardian*, 25 July.

Wilcock G (1990). *Living with Alzheimer's Disease*. Penguin, Harmondsworth.

Williams P (1985). Psychiatric disorder in the community and in primary care. In *Responding to Mental Illness* (ed. G Horobin). Kogan Page, Aberdeen.

8 Managing the psychiatric emergency in the community

J. A. Robertson

A psychiatric emergency may be defined as a situation involving mental disorder where prompt action is necessary to avert serious consequences. These consequences may include physical harm to the patient or others, emotional distress and damage, the risk of physical illness, destruction of property, or rapid deterioration of mental state. These situations, of their nature, involve extremes of emotion and behaviour but such extremes are not unique to mental illness: psychiatric emergencies share common ground with other personal and social crises and responsibility often overlaps with that of other agencies such as the police and social services. A high level of anxiety is usual and the management of anxiety is crucial to the resolution of the crisis. There will be occasions when the degree of anxiety does not appear to be objectively justified in terms of imminent physical danger but it is always a problem and a proper appraisal cannot be made until the situation has been fully assessed. Together with anxiety, a pervasive problem in psychiatric emergencies is confusion over responsibility which feeds the anxiety in a vicious circle. The key to resolving a tense situation often lies in the proper allocation of responsibility so that it can be effectively discharged. Management of these problems in community settings means that responsibility is more widely shared, with the possibility of greater confusion but also with the hope of recruiting more allies such as family, friends and neighbours.

Only in rare instances, such as admission to hospital in cases of major mental illness, will responsibility be assumed totally by one agency: even in this example, the operation of the Mental Health Act involves the family and social worker. Usually responsibility is shared and a proportion belongs to the patient himself, even when he is suffering from mental disorder.

Scope and limits of emergency psychiatry

What is seen as the proper territory of mental health professionals varies widely between services and between disciplines. It also varies between what may be called different psychiatric cultures. Some teams confine themselves to mental illness, narrowly defined: others assume a broader responsibility for psychosocial crises. The former are likely to be relatively restricted in their therapeutic goals. The latter may take up the challenge offered to the emergency psychiatrist by Slaby (1989) 'to use the opportunity offered by a crisis, no matter how induced, to facilitate growth and actualization that would not have been possible if the crisis had not occurred'. This aspiration echoes the enthusiasm of such pioneers as Caplan (1964). Extensive claims have been made to the effect that the way in which a crisis is handled affects the whole future career of the patient, and may indeed determine whether he becomes a patient or not. Reports such as that of Langsley *et al.* (1969) inspired the British Association of Social Workers, in the discussions leading up the 1983 Mental Health Act, to propose that a multidisciplinary crisis team attend all mental health emergencies.

The development of crisis intervention theory and practice expanded greatly in the 1970s and was reviewed by Cooper for the World Health Organization (Cooper 1979; Katschnig and Cooper 1991). Its principles have been summarized by Brandon (1970). Though some services such as that in the London suburb of Barnet (Scott 1980) have continued to operate on such principles, most services now take mental illness as their focus and distinguish it from the broader ground of psychosocial crisis.

The proponents of crisis intervention claimed that their methods reduced the need for admission and hence the number of acute beds needed. In recent years the number of admission beds available has gradually declined to a level where many services are coping with levels equivalent to such experimental units a few years ago. (They may or may not be offering adequate alternatives.) Other approaches such as the vigorous use of day care (Creed *et al.* 1991) or employing deliberately shortened periods of in-patient care (Hirsch *et al.* 1979) also appear to be successful in reducing the need for in-patient treatment.

It seems likely that the benefits of Crisis Intervention can be delivered in other ways, provided the priorities are kept in mind, i.e. the availability of rapid response in the patient's normal environment, avoidance of medicalizing non-medical problems, avoidance of hospitalization unless strictly necessary and ready access to the full range of relevant professional help.

It does not seem necessary or economic for a multidisciplinary team to visit every case and there is a risk of patients and families feeling overwhelmed, but there must be adequate opportunity for face-to-face consultation between workers if required. This said, it must be acknowledged that the idea of a crisis intervention team has the virtues of a unifying ideology and working model which can promote *esprit de corps* and cohesion among workers of different disciplines in a demanding field. If it is abandoned, there is a risk of psychiatric emergencies being managed in an ad hoc way by a disparate group of workers who come together in different combinations only at times of crisis (Szmukler *et al.* 1981). The end result is the not uncommon situation in which a patient is seen by a doctor off an emergency rota, a psychiatrist off the 'approved' list and a duty social worker, none of whom will be involved with the patient's subsequent career and all of them strangers to each other.

Availability of services

A comprehensive and effective psychiatric service must have a clear operational policy for dealing with emergencies. This may take the form of a crisis intervention team, an acute home treatment service or the 24-hour availability of community psychiatric nurses (CPNs) supported by medical staff. It should be backed up by facilities for urgent assessment and intervention on a walk-in or rapid referral basis. This can be sited in a mental health resource centre or hospital department of psychiatry (Mindham *et al.* 1973; Lim 1983).

Clear lines of communication must be established whereby a psychiatric opinion can be readily obtained on patients in casualty departments and police stations. It is especially important in the UK to agree local procedures between the psychiatric department and the police for the operation of section 136 which enables the police to remove people whom they deem to be mentally ill from a public place to a place of safety where they can be assessed. Finally, psychiatric emergencies can present on general medical wards and avoidable tragedies have occurred when intervention has been delayed due to confusion or buck-passing: this seems more likely to occur in general hospitals without a psychiatry department. General medical staff must know to whom they can turn for urgent psychiatric assistance and there must be adequate liaison between in-patient teams and home treatment teams.

Role of the GP and the primary health care team

Clearly, the psychiatric secondary care team cannot operate without the consent and cooperation of the primary health care team whose 'filtering' function with respect to mental disorder is now widely recognized (Goldberg and Huxley 1980). Psychiatric emergencies are more likely than routine referrals to bypass the general practitioner and to come via police and social services but for a large number the professional point of first contact will still be the GP. It is particularly important to reach agreement about the issue of medical responsibility, not only in the narrow sense of prescribing drugs and screening for physical disorder, but because a substantial minority of patients presenting as psychiatric emergencies have unsuspected physical illness (Eastwood *et al.* 1970; Hall *et al.* 1981) and there is a risk of it being missed between the GP, community psychiatrist, admitting psychiatrist and in-patient medical team. Responsibility for follow-up also needs to be decided: some GPs are far keener to be involved than others.

British psychiatric services may be entering a state of flux with regard to responsibility for services in the community. It is widely assumed that major mental illness (of the kind which used to be cared for in hospital) will be looked after by secondary care teams deployed in community settings. However, GPs may prefer to pick and choose the professionals they work with e.g. by-passing psychiatrists but using the services of CPNs. At the time of writing, fund-holding GPs have to pay for all treatment and care apart from episodes of hospital admission, an arrangement which is potentially very destructive of the seamless service we aspire to create. In the planning of services it is clearly important to be aware of the needs and priorities of GPs and in the age of the market it cannot be assumed that they will uncritically buy what the specialist team thinks they ought to have. Sensitive negotiation at the planning and contracting stage might go a long way to avoiding difficult confrontations over disturbed patients in the early hours of the morning. Strathdee and co-workers, in a survey of a group of GPs in a London district, found that three innovations in the provision of emergency services were particularly favoured: a crisis intervention outreach team, a parasuicide service and especially a 'rapid section' service for those in need of formal admission to hospital (Strathdee 1990).

Home treatment or admission?

The goals of emergency management, as of psychiatric treatment in general, are the relief of distress and disability and the promotion of normal mental functioning. Several studies have now shown that this can be achieved without hospital admission at all or with very short periods of admission (Stein and Test 1980; Muijen *et al.* 1992; Merson *et al.* 1992; Dean *et al.* 1993). Thus the movement towards de-institutionalization of long-stay patients has been overtaken by a thrust towards 'community' treatment of acute mental illness. Indeed, if the 1970s was the decade of 'crisis intervention' the 80s and 90s seem to be the age of 'acute home treatment'. Here a note of caution needs to be struck. Few, if any, services have been able to cope without hospital beds. The Birmingham service described by Dean *et al.* (1993) operated with about six beds per 25 000 population. The Daily Living Project described by Muijen entailed the admission of patients as the DLP team thought fit and manic in-patients, for example, averaged 18 in-patient days. Too often managers have exploited the enthusiasm of home treatment teams to push bed numbers down to unacceptable levels. The virtual disappearance of designated medium- and long-stay beds has led to a parlous situation in many British wards where acute beds are at an absolute minimum.

The main rationale for avoiding admission is now that patients and their relatives prefer home treatment (Marks 1992). There are reasons to fear that admission may have adverse consequences such as stigma, institutionalization, rejection or too ready expectation by patient or relatives that admission will solve the problem. However, despite the forebodings of crisis intervention theorists (e.g. Scott 1973), there is little empirical evidence that short periods of admission to units of reasonable quality cause lasting damage.

Common sense and clinical experience suggest that at least some episodes of acute mental illness require humane containment and skilled treatment in hospital. At the time of writing English legislation makes no provision for compulsory psychiatric treatment other than in hospital and an attempt to introduce a community treatment order has just been rejected. The inference is that a balanced system must contain an adequate number of staffed beds in addition to 'outreach' teams and other facilities and that the effort to avoid admission at all costs will not deliver a humane or safe service.

There are circumstances where temporary removal of a distressed person from a fraught situation seems indicated, yet it is not warranted to 'medicalize' the crisis by hospital admission. Unfortunately, few facilities yet exist for this kind of intervention, while increasing pressure on a diminishing number of acute psychiatry beds means that they tend to be reserved for 'real mental illness'. Relatively few services include such designated 'crisis beds' yet they should not be expensive to staff compared with conventional acute beds, being geared to 'time out' from overwhelming social pressure rather than the medical treatment of mental disorder. Workers in the field need to be aware of local alternatives to admission; indeed approved social workers are obliged by the Mental Health Act to consider such alternatives, though the scope is often limited. Examples include some local authority mental health hostels and women's refuges. 'Natural' alternatives such as the possibility of lodging with a suitable friend or relative also need to be considered.

Classification of emergencies

Following these general considerations, we can look in detail at the types of emergency that may confront the psychiatric team. These could be classified in more than one way; they might for instance be listed according to a conventional diagnostic scheme. However, it is not a diagnosis which initially confronts the worker but a call for help with a situation characterized by distress, anxiety and the possibility of danger. An attempt at a psychiatric diagnosis must certainly be made, not least because it helps to define areas of responsibility and to shape a plan of intervention; but there are common elements in psychiatric crises which cut across diagnostic boundaries; a homicidal threat, for instance, might be made in the context of a paranoid illness, a severe depression, a state of intoxication or simply in the course of a furious row. Management will differ according to the assessment made but the important common elements are ensuring safety, reducing anxiety, making the assessment, deciding what needs doing and seeing it gets done. The diagnostic process may conclude negatively, by defining the problem out of the orbit of psychiatry, but the mental health specialist has to get involved in order to reach this point. It seems most useful to survey the field in terms of the nature of the presenting problem.

Suicidal behaviour

The possibility of suicide and self-harm is one of the commonest reasons for urgent referral to a psychiatrist. Suicidal behaviour covers a wide range, from threats, through self-harming acts of various degrees of severity, to achieved suicide. Since the work of Stengel and Cook (1958) it has been recognized that 'attempted suicide' is far from synonymous with 'failed suicide' and that non-fatal self-harm carries a variety of meanings and motives of which the determined wish to end one's life is only one. Though one can draw a statistical profile of the typical suicide in contrast to that of the typical 'parasuicide' the two populations overlap, as is clearly shown by the greatly increased incidence of achieved suicide in those who have previously made attempts and in the record of past attempts in those who have died by suicide. The typical suicide is likely to be male, elderly, suffering from a diagnosable psychiatric illness such as depression, often physically ill, and he is likely to have consulted a doctor in recent weeks. Socially, he is likely to be isolated and may recently have suffered a bereavement. 'Successful' suicide is more often associated with violent means such as hanging, shooting, drowning or jumping from a height.

In contrast, the typical attempted suicide (hereafter referred to as parasuicide) is young, female, involved in a troublesome relationship and not suffering from a major mental illness. The vast majority of parasuicides take drug overdoses which are now the commonest reason for emergency medical admission in females and the second commonest in males.

Someone who has harmed themselves is therefore most likely to make first contact with the psychiatric services in a general hospital ward and every acute medical ward needs to have a system, in conjunction with psychiatric personnel, for the adequate assessment and management of such cases. Several models have been described and the guiding principles have been well delineated by Hawton and Catalan (1982). These could also apply to the assessment of parasuicide at home with the important difference that in hospital the patient's medical safety can usually be assumed: clearly this cannot be taken for granted at home and it may be the first priority of a mental health worker, particularly if non-medical, to get an adequate physical assessment, if necessary conveying the patient to hospital. Should the patient refuse to go, compulsory admission must at least be considered, though it is rarely applicable, since very few such patients are psychotic and most should be considered responsible for their actions. A clear-headed decision needs to be made on this point, preferably in consultation with a colleague, and communicated to the patient and relatives. Particularly difficult problems are posed by those who are intoxicated and histrionic but who are genuinely at risk because of overdose. There are no hard and fast rules for their management but one should bear in mind that hospital admission is reversible while death is not, and also that while the Mental Health Act precludes compulsory admission for uncomplicated intoxication, it is quite legitimate to admit someone for a combination of intoxication and mental illness. Otherwise, patience, persuasion and skilled countermanipulation must be the order of the day.

Once physical safety is assured, and provided the patient is alert enough to be interviewed, assessment can proceed along the lines described by Hawton and Catalan. This seeks to answer a number of questions: (1) What is the explanation for the attempt? (2) What was the degree of suicidal intent? (3) Is the patient at risk of suicide or further overdose or self-injury? (4) What problems, acute and chronic, confront the patient? Was there a particular precipitant? (5) Is the patient psychiatrically ill? If so, what is the diagnosis and how is this related to the attempt? (6) What kind of help would be appropriate and is the patient willing to accept it? In the home situation, one must add: can the patient safely be left at home and what safeguards against further self-harm are available there? This entails careful appraisal of the social supports available.

Hawton and Catalan describe an approach to treatment for those able to use it. It is essentially a practical problem-solving approach which starts with the assessment of the overdose itself and the associated problems, proceeding to the provision of psychotherapeutic help which will first help the patient resolve the crisis and then equip her to overcome subsequent crises without resorting to self-harm.

In practice, a relatively small number of parasuicides accept further follow-up. For many, the act itself concludes the episode, either expressively through the discharge of emotion or instrumentally through securing certain goals, e.g. the return of a spouse or lover. Even those who have made a serious attempt on their lives may feel they were 'meant' to survive and thereby feel enabled to continue with their own resources.

Parasuicide and threats of suicide are so common and so familiar to workers in the mental health field that there is a risk of our becoming blasé and forgetting the immense anxiety that these behaviours cause to relatives and others. Such feelings need to be taken seriously. Family, members of the public and other helpers may assume that any possibility of suicide, however remote, warrants the patient's being removed to hospital forthwith or, if already admitted, being transferred to a psychiatric ward. If this is not done and a degree of risk is implicitly accepted, the reasons for not doing so need to be carefully explained.

The converse problem is presented by the patient who appears to the professionals to be a serious risk when this is not obvious to others. Profound depression should always prompt serious enquiry about suicidal ideation; this needs to be tactful but searching. A precise plan of action is always more worrying than vague ruminations and, when rapport has been established, detailed questions should be asked about possible methods. The availability of firearms, drugs, toxic chemicals and other means of self-destruction should be established and the patient denied access to them if possible.

Special difficulties can arise with 'opaque' patients whose withdrawal, vagueness, psychotic thinking or evasiveness makes adequate assessment impossible; some may show the classical picture of the 'smiling depressive'. Full mental state examination is essential, with particular attention to ideas of guilt, pessimism and hypochondriasis, especially if they verge on the delusional. Some patients show paradoxical calm and lightening of mood once they have formed a suicidal plan which seems to offer them a means of escape. These problems entail serious consideration of admission and the only responsible advice must be to err on the side of caution, but it would be a mistake to assume that all suicidal patients must come into hospital. The saving factor is the patient's ambivalence; only a small number are in the grip of a single minded-determination to end their lives and in many cases a 'therapeutic alliance' can be established. Szmukler's (1981) comparison of a series of compulsory admissions with a series of informally admitted emergencies showed a significant excess of suicide threats and attempts among the informal group, confirming that it is possible to negotiate with this type of patient. Given the right resources and sufficient safeguards, it may be possible to negotiate a home treatment programme as an alternative to admission. The availability of effective non-toxic antidepressants has been a notable advance in this direction. An understanding must be established with the patient and his supporters as to what is being offered and what can reasonably be expected, e.g. that the mood-raising action of antidepressants takes about ten days to take effect. Further help should be available promptly on the end of a telephone if the patient's condition deteriorates.

Aggressive and violent behaviour

Only a small proportion of aggressive behaviour is attributable to mental illness and only a small number of people with mental illness become aggressive (Boker and Hafner 1973). Nevertheless, the overlap is significant for the emotions it arouses and the genuine risks it sometimes poses. There is a general impression that British society as a whole is becoming more violent and that groups who have hitherto been 'immune' such as doctors, nurses and firefighters on duty are becoming targets. If people in general are more prone to resort to violence in fraught situations, this might be expected to apply to the mentally ill as well, especially in situations of acute distress and panic. Psychotic violence may be especially feared because it is seemingly incomprehensible, therefore unpredictable and unmanageable. By the same logic, violence which is unexpected and out of character may be assumed too readily to be due to mental illness – 'he must be mad to behave in that way'.

Violence and the threat of violence raise, in a peculiarly acute form, the questions alluded to above regarding the scope and limits of emergency services, particularly that of responsibility. Most people are assumed to be responsible for their actions and if their actions are illegal or unacceptable, they are culpable in law or legally answerable to others. The control of violence normally falls to the police who have a responsibility to keep the peace.

The attribution of mental illness radically alters the situation (*pacé* Thomas Szasz). Violent behaviour is held to require treatment rather than punishment and its control is seen as the responsibility of the professionals who treat the patient. Things might be simpler if such a neat dichotomy could indeed be made, dividing 'bad' behaviour from 'mad' behaviour. The whole concept of 'psychopathy' with its attendant confusions really stems from attempts to map the no man's land between these two domains. The inclusion of psychopathy in the English Mental Health Act has not helped matters and the extension of 'therapeutic' approaches to non-psychotic violence, while it can be regarded as a civilizing enterprise, raises problems about responsibility.

The approach taken here is consistent with conventional practice. In short, issues of psychiatric diagnosis, treatability, responsibility for control and legal liability need to be separately assessed and generally regarded as distinct, with the important proviso that clear evidence of psychosis does shift responsibility into the medical domain, particularly if there is a causal relationship between the illness and the abnormal behaviour.

An important practical caveat is that, even in cases of psychosis, the police may be the best agency to contain aggression, because of their experience, physical presence and the influence of a uniform. As with self-harm, the priority must be safety, and if this can only be assured by taking the patient into police custody, it may have to be done. There are a number of legal routes back into mental health care from the police and penal system, the quickest being a Mental Health Act section after calmer assessment at the local police station.

The involvement of the police entails some difficulties. Some police officers are outstanding for their patience and forbearance even in the face of provocation, insult and physical threat. Others, particularly if angry or frightened, may be stung into retaliation. They are also used to being in charge and may have difficulty sharing authority with doctors, social workers and others. A quick door-step conference between all concerned will help to establish what is to be expected, both of the client and of the professionals.

As with suicidal behaviour, the assessment of aggression comprises an attempt to understand it in psychological terms, a psychiatric diagnosis, assessment of treatability and assessment of risk. Conditions which may be associated with aggressive behaviour include organic psychosis, especially acute confusional states, acute schizophrenic excitement, mania, paranoid states and psychotic depression. The latter may occasionally lead to the tragedy of homicide followed by suicide. Violent situations are very commonly associated with substance abuse and the most widely implicated is undoubtedly alcohol, either through excessive intake or the effects of sudden withdrawal; paranoid states associated with amphetamine abuse also need to be considered.

Psychiatric investigations should include inquiry into previous personality: violent behaviour which is out of character is suggestive, though not conclusive evidence of illness, psychiatric or neuro-psychiatric. Outbursts of violence are characteristic of undercontrolled personalities such as the explosive or anti-social varieties of personality disorder but simply applying such a label should not be a substitute for attempting to understand the individual and the situation. One also needs to be aware of the possibility of a psychotic 'break' in such brittle personalities.

Epilepsy has probably been overemphasized in the past as a cause of violence, which is uncommon as the direct manifestation of a seizure but can sometimes arise from post-epileptic confusion. There is a relationship between epilepsy and personality disorder and anti-epileptic drugs can sometimes cause irritability and explosive behaviour.

Mental illness can give rise to aggression in a number of ways, some of them psychologically understandable, some more obscure. Sometimes the patient can be 'talked down', sometimes he is so inaccessible that the only safe option is firm control, with or without the aid of drugs. By no means all psychotic violence is directly motivated by delusions; it may spring from diffuse fear, excitement or disinhibition and is often a direct reaction to the professionals' interference. This is different from the planned and purposive violence that may be perpetrated by the paranoid patient who is seriously deluded but otherwise well organized.

Dangerousness is notoriously difficult to predict (Scott 1977). The most robust predictor is generally agreed to be previous behaviour, and a record of violence, whether or not associated with previous mental illness, must be taken seriously. It is much harder, in the absence of such a record, to decide whether threats will escalate to actions or trivial destructive behaviour to serious violence against the person. The possession of a weapon, particularly a firearm, multiplies the patient's capacity for violence many times and every effort should be made to check whether this is the case; amateurs in the field should then stay clear till police experts have taken control.

As in other emergencies, a relatively limited choice of strategies confronts the mental health team; treatment at home, voluntary admission, compulsory admission or treatment on a day or out-patient basis. Other solutions are in the hands of the police.. Unlike other situations, one cannot simply walk away from the scene if one decides the problem is beyond the responsibility or capability of the team. Options include clear warnings to victims and their removal to safety, or the removal of the aggressor to custody as described above. In the case of women, direction to a refuge may be appropriate. The safety of children may need to be ensured through the operation of the Children's Act (1989) by seeking an emergency protection order.

In dealing with actual or threatened violence, safety is best ensured by having a clear superiority of forces which will either deter aggression or ensure that it can be subdued without damage. It is wise not to challenge or confront the patient until the situation is clearly in the professionals' favour from a physical point of view. Often the patient accepts compulsory admission after at most a token show of resistance. Sedation is rarely indicated at the scene since the amount of force necessary to administer it is the same as that needed to get the patient into the ambulance and little is gained by the delivery of a comatose patient to hospital. If the physical safety of the patient or others can only be ensured by rapid sedation, the intravenous route is preferred: an intramuscular injection may simply result in an enraged patient who still takes several long minutes to lose consciousness and can do much damage in the meantime. Intravenous diazepam, 10–20 mg, will give rapid control and can be followed through the same cannula by intravenous haloperidol 10–15 mg to give a long period of sleep. If it is impossible to give medication intravenously, intramuscular lorazepam can be useful.

Acute alteration of mental state

Sudden alteration of mental state and behaviour, the expression of bizarre beliefs, incongruous emotions or fantastic perceptions are of themselves deeply disturbing to those close to the patient, whether or not they have any reason to fear for their safety. Equally, anxiety can be raised in public places by some flagrant breach of accepted social boundaries and taboos, such as going naked. Mental health workers have to judge how seriously to take such situations. In an age when more people with active mental illness are at large in the community, odd behaviour will be more common and the public need to be educated to expect and tolerate it to some extent.

However, more extreme instances of deviant conduct, such as the example above, are, prima facie, strongly suggestive of mental illness which needs intervention. Some may object that if someone is doing no obvious harm and has made no request for help they should simply be left alone. This is to ignore the possibility that seemingly innocuous behaviour change may be the first sign of a deteriorating mental illness that may have more serious consequences. It may rarely be a sign of organic brain disease. Furthermore, patients may look back with embarrassment at such an episode and regret that they were not brought under control at the time. An episode of mania may have dire social consequences such as debt or promiscuity due to disinhibition.

Management of these problems needs a great deal of tact and diplomacy on the part of the team who must balance the needs and rights of the patient against those of others who insist that something must be done. Even harder is balancing the individual's right to liberty and autonomy against his right to be controlled against his will, in his own interest, when his judgment is impaired (Bloch and Chodoff 1991). Happily, effective intervention in such circumstances need not entail compulsory measures, especially if helpers have time to establish rapport, negotiate with the patient and agree a mutually satisfactory plan. Hoult (1986) has described how this approach led to a striking decrease in hospital admissions in Sydney. Szmukler (1981) has shown that compulsory admission is often the end result of a process whereby people with persistent psychotic illness lose touch with helpers, abandon medication, become socially dislocated and finally come to attention through behavioural disturbance: the moral is that assertive follow-up and persuasion to remain in treatment programmes could prevent many such emergencies arising.

Acute emotional distress and non-psychotic disturbance

People can, of course, become intensely emotionally upset without suffering from a major diagnosable syndrome or psychotic process. Whether they are to be regarded as mentally ill is partly a matter of semantics. The DSM 111 definition of mental illness excludes 'expected reactions to events' which would exclude normal grief but Parkes (1965) explicitly accepts grief, with its characteristic patterns of distress and disability, morbidity and mortality, as a mental disorder. What seems certain is that many such situations will continue to be referred to doctors and other professionals who are likely to seek the help of mental health teams.

Some neurotic crises will present as medical emergencies, the converse of acute medical conditions presenting as behavioural disturbance. Acute panic with tachycardia and overbreathing is a notorious example. On the other hand, a wide range of medical conditions can mimic or actually produce panic attacks. Breadth of vision in the emergency team is essential, as is access to an adequate range of emergency medical investigations. Once medical disorder is excluded beyond *reasonable* doubt(and one cannot do better) authoritative reassurance becomes possible. At this point it is important to decline further bids for investigation on the part of the patient or relatives. The sooner the emotional nature of the problem is accepted, the sooner it can be dealt with in psychological terms. The well-known physiological effects of overbreathing can be alleviated by re-breathing into a paper bag.

While the labels 'hysteria' and 'hysterical' have disappeared recently from conventional diagnostic schemes they retain some usefulness to describe conditions in which the unconscious simulation of disorder, mental or physical, dominates the picture. Such conditions may affect individuals or groups. Acute conversion hysteria, the production of physical symptoms, is not common in developed countries, though it occurs occasionally. Dissociated states such as trances and fugues are also relative rarities. Factitious psychosis is a related phenomenon which will present like the acute psychotic episodes discussed above, though its emotional precipitants and imitative nature may be evident. The increasing popularity of charismatic religious sects may have increased the incidence of 'possession' both as an hysterical phenomenon and as the content of psychosis.

There are two important diagnostic traps. The lesser, at least in an emergency context, is to mistake a hysterical condition for true psychosis. It is more important not to miss a psychotic or organic state masquerading as hysteria. It is also important to realize that hysterical mechanisms can be facilitated by major alterations of mood from which they distract attention, particularly if behaviour is florid and histrionic when it may be dismissed as attention seeking. It is wisest not to accept hysteria or any of its modern analogues as the primary diagnosis until other underlying possibilities have been explored.

If the team is satisfied that the emotional state and behaviour are explicable in psychological and social terms, they may be in a position to manage the problem in its natural setting. This is a situation where the crisis intervention model is very pertinent, since socially induced behaviour is susceptible to social re-enforcement and the earlier a pseudo-medical situation can be 'de-medicalized' the sooner things can be resolved. One should, however, bear in mind the paradox that it often takes a medical expert to de-medicalize things and the patient may not be able to abandon psychogenic symptoms without loss of face unless doctors take him seriously.

Management of disasters

Lindemann's (1944) classic work on acute grief, the stimulus for much subsequent work on crisis management, originated with a disastrous fire at the Coconut Grove night club. The last few years in the UK have seen a series of mass tragedies and efforts by health and social services to deploy speedy and effective help, not only to survivors and the bereaved but to rescuers and witnesses who have been emotionally traumatized. This has been paralleled by increasing interest in post-traumatic stress disorder, both in a military and civil context, and improving emergency assistance around the time of the original trauma has clearly been driven by the hope of avoiding sequelae in the form of PTSD and some suggestive evidence that this can be done (Parkes 1991).

While public and professional interest invariably returns to this area in the aftermath of a major public tragedy, it is important to recall the continual stream of private disasters and tragedies which mar the lives of individuals. It would not be appropriate to treat all these as psychological emergencies but one needs to be aware of events which might have long-term damaging effects and of individuals who are especially vulnerable, as well as being prepared to render psychological first aid for reasons of ordinary compassion.

It is clear that a relatively small part of such work will be done by specialist professionals. The specialist team needs to establish communications which will come into action either on a large or small scale; planning for the former should be linked with local plans for dealing with major disaster which are the responsibility of the director of social services; the latter entails making links with local police, rescue and victim support services, to be called into action as required.

Hodgkinson and Stewart (1993) describe a cognitive model and a method of crisis intervention in disaster called 'psychological de-briefing' which can be applied to individuals and small or large groups as required. They emphasize the importance of timing and suggest that de-briefing should take place around 48–72 hours after the event, since those involved will pass through a period of little reaction in the early stages. A balance must be struck between availability and intrusion, allowing normal social supports to become effective but rendering specialist help when they are insufficient.

Vagrancy, destitution and neglect

These are problems of gradual onset which may present as emergencies when crisis point has been reached, through physical illness, accident, fire or because someone has suddenly called attention to the person's plight. Such people are also vulnerable to violence, robbery or exploitation. Tragedies occur when patients have 'slipped through the net' or when the onset of their condition has been so insidious that they have not come to attention in time. Examples occur among the homeless mentally ill and in isolated individuals who allow their homes to decay into chaos and squalor. It is a particular problem of the demented elderly.

As with other emergencies, the first priority is assuring physical safety, then making an assessment, diagnosis and decision about responsibility. The latter can be particularly difficult and hard decisions may have to be made as to whether to allow someone 'the dignity of risk' (Perske 1972) or to take compulsory measures. The differentiation between eccentricity, paranoid personality disorder and mental illness, for example, is often far from easy. It may be argued that the patient has chosen to live like that, but what is the validity of 'choice' if thinking is disordered and judgment clouded by delusions? This is the kind of issue which can split the team along professional lines, with social workers emphasizing the right to choice and doctors the right to treatment (but individuals do not always follow professional stereotypes).

The more one can establish and maintain physical and emotional contact with the patient, the more opportunity there is of extending help on a voluntary basis and of avoiding compulsory admission. Admission on a voluntary basis may be appropriate while accommodation problems are solved or the place cleaned up. Patients may be willing to accept practical, social or financial help while declining treatment and of course this should be made available where practical. Once such a bridge has been built, specific treatment may become acceptable. The problem of the homeless mentally ill in cities is becoming desperate, numerically as well as individually. Contrary to popular opinion, they do not seem to be the long-term residents of traditional mental hospitals decanted on to the street; they tend to have had multiple short admissions but to have lapsed from follow-up and never to have engaged with services. This group presents a major challenge to community psychiatry. Unless 'assertive outreach' is kept up, their clinical and social gains are rapidly lost (Marks 1992) and they become revolving door patients, presenting as recurrent emergencies. While care plans and key workers may clarify decision-making and responsibility, they are unlikely to be sufficient without increased staffing levels, resources for day care, provision for occupation and accommodation, help back to employment and a number of beds that provide more than a first aid service.

In our present crisis, this group warrants a specialized team to cover night shelters, lodging houses and the street, at least in the inner city. They could also cover casualty departments. More favoured districts should consider integrating their emergency services with day-to-day provision for the sake of continuity.

A multidisciplinary parasuicide team in a district general hospital

The Parasuicide Counselling Group (PCG) at Kidderminster General Hospital provides an example of interdisciplinary work with psychiatric emergencies. All cases of deliberate self-harm admitted to the hospital are seen by a member of the PCG. Cases are initially assessed by counsellors drawn from a variety of disciplines – trained nurses, social workers, psychologists, psychiatrists in training and others. Basic instruction in the assessment of parasuicidal acts and the examination of mental state is given and thereafter the counsellors are expected to attend regular monthly training sessions in addition to the weekly clinical meeting. As soon as they have seen a case they are required to seek support from a senior mental health worker, usually a consultant psychiatrist or senior psychologist. They are expected to seek a psychiatric opinion if there are the least grounds to suspect serious disorder and to have a low threshold of suspicion for such disorder. All cases are then discussed at the weekly meeting of the team at which senior psychiatrists are present but which is not chaired by a psychiatrist.

Patients are nearly always seen initially on 'foreign ground' where the authority of physicians or surgeons holds sway; clearly it is essential for the team to have credibility with these authorities and prompt clearing of their beds has been a major asset in this regard. No attempt is made by the team to encroach on their area of decision-making and it is made clear that the final decision to discharge still rests with the medical firm concerned. The credibility of the PCG is now such that they exert considerable influence on the decision but we do not feel it is right to burden the non-medical workers with what is normally seen as the medical prerogative of discharge.

Decisions about future management are made partly in discussion with the support worker, in collaboration with the duty psychiatrist if one is involved, and finalized at the weekly review. Cases are discussed in an egalitarian way but the principle of expertise applies. In other words, the psychiatrists carry most authority with cases where there is clear evidence of mental illness, the social workers where there are prominent family difficulties or children at risk and so forth. In practice, the shared area where skills and interests overlap is much larger than these specialist enclaves of knowledge. In the relatively rare event of transfer to the psychiatric ward, negotiated between psychiatrists and physicians, clinical responsibility passes to the former as they take the patient into their own territory.

The group has now established sufficient cohesion to weather the difficulties inherent in such work: disagreement is more often friendly and creative than unpleasantly abrasive. In the early stages, psychiatric registrars found it difficult to be called to account for decisions to admit that were considered inappropriate by other disciplines.

Difficulties occasionally arise at interfaces, often coinciding with the arrival of new junior medical staff, but on the whole regular medical and nursing staff have cooperated well with the system. Attempts are sometimes made to by-pass the system by GPs who know their patients well and feel they would be better handled in a different way. Most trouble is caused by people who only partly use the system without understanding its principles or procedure.

The PCG illustrates a number of points relevant to clinical responsibility and primacy, decision-making, boundaries and interfaces. The solutions depend on a commitment to cooperation despite the professional discomfort involved. It has also required the blessing of the consultant psychiatrists and a willingness on their part to accept 'umbrella' responsibility for the service without pedantically controlling every detail of it. It provides, in microcosm, an example of both the problems and opportunities inherent in multidisciplinary work. Figures show that the rate of completed suicide in the District is the same as the national rate, implying that the system is as safe as any other. Disappointingly, the rate of repeated attempts does not seem to be influenced by the PCG but few, if any services have yet succeeded in reducing attempted suicide.

References

Bloch S and Chodoff P (1991). *Psychiatric Ethics*. Oxford University Press.

Boker W and Hafner H (1973). *Crimes of Violence by Mentally Disordered Offenders in Germany: A Study in Psychiatric Epidemiology*. Springer–Verlag, Berlin.

Brandon S (1970). Crisis theory and possibilities of intervention. *British Journal of Psychiatry*, **117**, 627–633.

Caplan G (1964). *Principles of Preventive Psychiatry*. Basic Books, New York.

Cooper J E (1979). *Crisis Admission Units and Emergency Psychiatric Services*. Public Health in Europe 11, Regional Office for Europe, World Health Organization, Copenhagen.

Creed F, Black D, Anthony P, Osborn M, Thomas P and Tormenson B (1991). Randomized control trial of day patients' vs. in-patients' psychiatric treatment. *British Medical Journal*, **300**, 1033–1037.

Dean C, Phillips J, Gadd E M, Joseph M and England S (1993). Comparison of community based service with hospital based service for people with acute severe psychiatric illness. *British Medical Journal*, **308**, 473–476.

Eastwood M R, Mindham R H S and Tennent T G (1970). The physical status of psychiatric emergencies. *British Journal of Psychiatry*, **116**, 545–550

Goldberg D and Huxley P (1980). *Mental Illness in the Community: Pathways to Psychiatric Care*. Tavistock, London.

Hall R C V, Gardner E R, Poplin H K, Lecann A F and Stikney S R (1981). Unrecognized physical illness prompting psychiatric admission: A prospective study. *American Journal of Psychiatry*, **138** (5), 629–635.

Hawton K and Catalan J (1982). *Attempted Suicide*. Oxford University Press.

Hirsch S R, Platt S, Knight A and Weiman A (1979). Shortening hospital stay for psychiatric care: effects on patients and relatives. *British Medical Journal*, **1**, 442–446.

Hodgkinson P E and Stewart M (1993). Trauma crisis intervention and psychological debriefing. *Industrial and Environmental Crisis Quarterly*, **7** (2).

Hoult J (1986). Community care of the acutely mentally ill. *British Journal of Psychiatry*, **149**, 137–144.

Katschnig H and Cooper J E (1991). Psychiatric emergency and crisis intervention services. In *Community Psychiatry* (eds. D H Bennett and H L Freeman). Churchill Livingstone, Edinburgh.

Langsley D G, Flomenhaft R and Machotka P (1969). Follow up studies of family crisis therapy. *American Journal of Orthopsychiatry*, **39** (5),753.

Leff J P, Kuipers L, Berkowitz R, Eberlein-Fries R and Sturgeon D (1982). A controlled study of intervention in the families of schizophrenic patients. *British Journal of Psychiatry*, **141**, 121–134.

Lid N (1983). A psychiatric emergency clinic: a study of attendance over six months. *British Journal of Psychiatry*, **143**, 460–466.

Lindemann E (1944). Symptomatology and management of acute grief. *American Journal of Psychiatry*, **101**, 141–148.

Marks I (1992). Innovations in mental health care delivery. *British Journal of Psychiatry,* **160**, 589–597.

Merson S, Tyrer P, Onyett S, Lack S *et al.* (1992). Early intervention in psychiatric emergencies: a controlled clinical trial. *Lancet,* **339**, 1311–1314.

Mindham R H S, Kelleher N J, Birley J L T (1973). A psychiatric casualty department. *Lancet,* **ii**, 1169–1171.

Muijen M, Marks I, Conolly J and Audini B. (1992). Home based and standard hospital care for patients with severe mental illness: a randomized control trial. *British Medical Journal,* **304**, 749–754.

Parkes C M (1965). Bereavement and mental illness Pt I. A clinical study of the grief of bereaved psychiatric patients. *British Journal of Medical Psychology*, **38**, 1–12.

Parkes C M (1991). Psychiatric aspects of disaster. Planning for the aftermath. *Journal of the Royal Society of Medicine*, **84**, 22–25.

Perske R (1972). The dignity of risk and the mentally retarded. *Mental Retardation*, Feb., 24.

Scott P D (1977). Assessing dangerousness in criminals. *British Journal of Psychiatry,* **131**, 127–142.

Scott R D (1973). The treatment barrier. *British Journal of Medical Psychology*, **48**, 45.

Scott R D (1980). A family orientated treatment service to the London borough of Barnet. *HMSO Health Trends*, **12**, 65–66.

Slaby A E (1989). Emergency psychiatry. In *Comprehensive Textbook of Psychiatry* (eds. H I Kaplan and E J Sadock). Williams and Wilkins, Baltimore.

Stein L J and Test M A (1980). Alternative to mental hospital treatment I: Conceptual model, treatment programme and clinical evaluation. *Archives of General Psychiatry*, **37**, 392–397.

Stengel E and Cook N (1958). *Attempted Suicide: Its Social Significance and Effects.* Maudsley Monographs, No 4. Chapman and Hall, London. *Journal of the Royal Society of Medicine*, **83**, 222–225.

Szmukler G I (1981). Compulsory admissions in a London borough: II Circumstances surrounding admission. *Psychological Medicine*, **11** (4), 825–838.

Szmukler G I, Bird A S and Button E J (1981). Compulsory admissions in a London borough: I Social and clinical features and a follow-up. *Psychological Medicine*, **11** (3), 617–636.

9 Interventions with long–term clients

J. Carson and F. Holloway

Introduction

> Schizophrenia remains the most perplexing of psychiatric disorders. Its cause is poorly understood, its course variable and highly unpredictable, and its management exceedingly difficult. (Falloon *et al.* 1987, p. 394)

This chapter focuses on psychological approaches to the treatment of people with a diagnosis of schizophrenia and is written from our perspective as workers within a psychiatric rehabilitation service. Schizophrenia is the commonest diagnosis amongst patients or clients in contact with long-term, high-intensity mental health services (Clifford *et al.* 1991; Holloway, 1991*a*). We assume that readers are familiar with the characteristic problems that people with a diagnosis of schizophrenia experience, notably the 'positive' symptoms of psychosis (delusions, hallucinations, thought disorder) and the very handicapping and less clinically obvious 'negative' symptoms (e.g. social withdrawal, lack of drive and initiative, underactivity, poverty of speech). Community teams will also have to provide long-term support to people with a range of other psychiatric problems notably chronic affective illness (depression and mania), severe anxiety disorders and obsessive-compulsive disorder, eating disorders, severe personality disorders (particularly those with a borderline personality disorder) and a small but demanding group of patients who present their mental health problems in terms of multiple somatic symptoms. Hawton *et al.* (1989) provide a useful introduction to the psychological management of this whole range of psychiatric problems from the perspective of the cognitive behaviour therapist. Increasingly drug and alcohol problems, which also tend to be chronic and relapsing in course, are managed by specialist teams.

Despite an enormous mass of research into schizophrenia since its initial description by Kraeplin at the turn of the century under the name dementia praecox, we still understand relatively little about the underlying causes of the condition (Birchwood *et al.* 1988). Indeed some authorities dispute its very existence, despite the reliability with which the diagnosis can now be made if standardized techniques of assessment are used and the mass of evidence that has accumulated about the hereditability of the condition (Owen and McGuffin 1992), the existence of structural and functional abnormalities in the brains of people with schizophrenia (Pilowsky 1992) and evidence of neuro-psychological deficits in patients with first episode illnesses who have never received antipsychotic drugs (Saykin *et al.* 1994).

Kraeplin initially defined schizophrenia by its poor prognosis, conceiving it as an illness of early onset with an inevitable downward course. We now know that this is not the case: some patients with a diagnosis of schizophrenia will have a single episode of illness; the majority will have a relapsing and remitting course, often with residual disability between episodes; and some patients will have an unremitting illness, which in the past would inevitably have led to prolonged hospital stay (Johnstone 1993). Even for those who are initially very severely affected by the illness, very long-term follow-up indicates that improvement is the norm (Harding *et al.* 1987; Harding *et al.* 1992).

Our interests as rehabilitation specialists are with the majority of patients with a schizophrenic illness who either have repeated episodes of illness or fail to return to their previous level of functioning after their first illness, as they are the most likely to come into contact with our services. The difficulty in predicting outcome for people with schizophrenia is at once a great challenge for rehabilitation workers, and at the same time probably one of the greatest frustrations. Ekdawi and Conning (1994) describe it thus: 'One of the challenges of working in psychiatric rehabilitation is that there is rarely a "right" answer, a prescribed way of intervening in a particular situation, with a guaranteed degree of success' (p. 16).

Other chapters in this book (our own on day care, Elizabeth Kuipers' on family interventions, Malcolm Peete's on long-term medication and Debra Hall's chapter on daily living skills) address areas that we would also consider to be crucial in the delivery of comprehensive care to people with a mental illness (Huxley *et al.* 1993).

Our starting-point is to present the reader with the conceptual model which guides our clinical work. After this we discuss the historical development of psychological interventions in rehabilitation. We then consider the practice of social skills training. Psychological treatments that seek to control schizophrenic symptoms are discussed. The possibility of early intervention and the detection of early warning signs of relapse are outlined. We next look at the issues of depression, self-identity, coping and grief in schizophrenia. Finally we discuss case management and the role that such systems may play in the delivery of comprehensive psychiatric care.

Biosychosocial model

Many rehabilitation workers utilize a biopsychosocial model which guides their work with people with schizophrenia and other major mental disorders (Birchwood *et al.* 1988). One of the first authors to describe such a model was the American psychologist Paul Meehl.

This neural integrative defect which I shall christen schizotaxia, is all that can properly be spoken of as inherited. The imposition of a social learning history upon schizotaxic individuals results in a personality organiza-

tion which I shall call following Rado, the schizotype .... Only a subset
of schizophrenic personalities decompensate into clinical schizophrenia. It
seems likely that the most important causal influence pushing the schizotype toward schizophrenic decompensation is the schizophrenogenic
mother.   (Meehl 1962, p. 828)

Meehl's model, sometimes referred to as a diathesis-stress model, was the
first of what later came to be known as vulnerability-stress models (Zubin
and Spring 1977; Nuechterlein and Dawson 1984; Birchwood et al. 1988).
Such models hypothesize, rather as Meehl did, that the person with schizophrenia has an underlying weakness or vulnerability. This might be at the
neuro-chemical level, (Snyder 1982), the neuro-anatomical level,
(Weinberger et al. 1982) or the neuro-physiological level (Turpin and
Clements 1992). While the individual is posited to have an inherited
or acquired weakness in the structure or functioning of their brain, it is the
experience of stress that will determine whether or when the person breaks
down.

The role of life stresses in causing or precipitating mental illnesses has
been the subject of intensive study (Creed 1993). There is abundant evidence
that patients who develop schizophrenia and other mental illnesses, or
relapse after a previous episode of illness, have experienced increased psychosocial stress prior to the onset of symptoms (Creed 1993). Whilst it has
been demonstrated fairly convincingly that adverse life events, notably losses,
can act as a cause of a depressive illness this is less clear in the case of schizophrenia. Bebbington and Kuipers (1992) in a review of the literature on life
events and schizophrenia concluded that 'social influences probably have an
effect on the first emergence of the condition, at least in its timing' (p. 139).
The evidence for relapse (i.e. re-emergence of positive psychotic symptoms
in someone who has recovered from an acute episode) is that life events
(both favourable and unfavourable) act as a precipitant rather than a cause
of relapse, bringing forward in time a relapse that would have occurred at
some stage (Creed 1993).

One important source of both stress and support for all of us is the family. During the 1960s the family was often seen as the cause of schizophrenia in the identified patient (Meehl 1962; Lidz et al. 1965; Laing and Esterson
1964), as in the case of Meehl's schizophrenogenic mother described above.
More recently careful empirical studies have begun to tease out the role of
the family in influencing the course of schizophrenia, particularly whether
or not the patient will experience a florid relapse of positive psychotic symptomatology (Vaughn and Leff 1976; Leff et al. 1982). A reliable link has been
demonstrated between the level of 'expressed emotion' (hostility, critical
comments and overinvolvement) in a family and the likelihood of later
relapse (Kavanagh 1992a). The cynic might wonder whether the family is
any better off moving from a position as being seen as 'schizophrenogenic'
to 'relapsogenic'! More positively there is now growing experience in the
value of family interventions in the management of schizophrenia. These are
aimed at reducing tensions within the family liable to increase the risk of
relapse, increasing the understanding of family members about the disorder
and improving the abilities of the sufferer and carers to cope with the effects
of the illness (see Liz Kuipers' chapter in this book).

Wing (1978) has proposed an alternative biopsychosocial model which has proved popular with British workers. It provides a model of psychiatric disability on three levels. The first level is that of *primary or intrinsic impairments*. These arise as a direct result of the illness and encompass both positive and negative psychotic symptoms. (We could also call these biological factors.) *Secondary handicaps* arise from the responses of other people in the patient's environment to the illness (for example the stigma of receiving a diagnosis of mental illness) and the individual's views about him- or herself. The reactions of the patient and the family to the experience of illness are crucial here and will largely determine the individual's self-confidence, motivation and self-esteem. Caring staff can also exert a significant effect, either by a positive attitude to the patient that fosters adaptive coping behaviours or by a negative and rejecting attitude that engenders hopelessness in the patient and informal carers. (These are psychological factors.) Finally, *tertiary or extrinsic handicaps* are disadvantages that may be independent of the illness itself, but which may have played some part in its etiology. This includes factors such as social isolation, poverty and unemployment. (These are clearly social factors.) The actual level of disability experienced by the patient will be a result of the interaction between the degree of primary impairment and secondary and tertiary handicaps.

Biopsychosocial or stress-vulnerability models are important as they force rehabilitation workers to adopt a broad approach to tackling schizophrenia. Intervening at one level on its own is not likely to be particularly effective. Changing a person's medication may reduce their positive psychotic symptoms, but will not provide them with a valued social role or address the patient's low self-esteem. Equally, providing a treatment programme for people with schizophrenia that does not incorporate pharmacological intervention is likely not only to be unsuccessful but, given the benefits of antipsychotics in controlling positive symptoms and preventing relapse, unethical. It is vital that a holistic approach to the needs of sufferers and carers is adopted that provides help with their real-life everyday problems rather than focusing exclusively on symptoms or deficits in functioning (Holloway 1994).

A further refinement of the biopsychosocial model into one that takes account of the coping strategies of the patient and carers allows us to begin to look at how we can enable the sufferer to cope with the disorder and its effects on their life (Liberman 1988). Patients and carers make active adaptations to the illness in an attempt to minimize its effect on their lives: these adaptations may be more or less successful. This stress-vulnerability-coping model allows us to see the ways in which sufferers are active participants in their recovery from psychosis: outcome is the result of complex interactions between the person, their illness and their environment (Harding *et al.* 1992).

Early psychological interventions

A significant feature of rehabilitation in the last few decades has been the tendency to import approaches from America. Inevitably such approaches have to be tailored for British consumption. In the mid to late 1960s in America the token economy was 'king'. This approach revolutionized rehabilitation efforts towards the treatment of people with the most chronic illnesses (Ayllon and Azrin 1968; Atthowe and Krasner 1968). This development had been largely inspired by the work of Skinner (1953) and it represented one of the first attempts to apply principles of 'learning theory' derived from animal experimentation to work with the long-term mentally ill.

The token economy built on individual case studies in which behavioural psychologists utilized strategies of 'operant conditioning' to 'reinforce' desired behaviour and 'extinguish' inappropriate behaviours in chronically institutionalized patients with a diagnosis of schizophrenia (Rachlin 1969). The approach meant that ward staff, working on a unit specifically dedicated to the purpose, rewarded patients for performance of prespecified target behaviours with plastic tokens. These tokens could later be exchanged for a variety of back-up reinforcers in the ward shop. Psychologists eager to apply this new behavioural technology were probably able to do so as few other mental health professionals were concerned with the people on the 'backwards'. They found ready allies in nursing staff who effectively ran the ward token economies with psychology back-up. Encouraging early pilot programmes gave way to a number of controlled outcome studies of which the classic American study was that of Paul and Lentz (1977). British researchers adopted the token economy somewhat later but were not slow in launching their own series of evaluative studies (Presly *et al.* 1976; Hall *et al.* 1977; Elliott *et al.* 1979; Stoffelmayr *et al.* 1979). These studies demonstrated the success of token economy programmes, even when compared with established control treatments such as milieu therapy.

Despite the impressive research findings, the token economy fell from grace almost as rapidly as it had emerged. Today it has largely been relegated to a small group of private hospitals such as St Andrew's, Northampton. The demise of the token economy has gone virtually unreported, though problems in its operation were apparent from its earliest days (Hall and Baker 1973; Gripp and Magaro 1974). One of the early pioneers of the approach in Britain, Roger Baker (personal communication) suggested that its demise may have been hastened by the greater acceptance of other models of care or philosophy such as normalization (Wolfensberger 1970; Ramon 1991). Some of the more punitive aspects of early token economies, such as time-out, response cost and giving 'Complan' as a meal substitute, were also counter to moves to improve conditions for patients in our mental hospitals (Martin 1984). Equally the notion that patients were being treated in the same way as animals in a Skinner box was no doubt a great concern to many. From a more scientific perspective a major problem with these early behaviouristic approaches to treatment is their lack of a plausible underlying theory about the nature of the problems that the therapy was trying to address. We are only now just beginning to understand the extraordinarily complex interactions between brain structure and function, basic neuro-psychological functioning (e.g. attention, information processing, memory) and higher psychological functioning (e.g. response to social cues, social learning) that go to produce the impairments and handicaps typical of schizophrenia. In retrospect it is now apparent that much of the positive effect of the token economy wards was due to the social reinforcement staff gave to patients (Shepherd 1991) rather than the material rewards that patients received for 'appropriate' behaviour.

For all their problems, token economies proved popular with many nursing staff. Observational studies of nurse–patient interaction on ordinary psychiatric wards (Sanson-Fisher *et al*. 1979; Rezin *et al*. 1983) demonstrated the low frequency of interactions and equally the maladaptive nature of many of those that did occur. Ward staff (and other carers) often reinforce negative behaviour (for example by only beginning to pay attention to someone when they act in a disturbed fashion). Token economies ensured high frequency of staff–client interactions. They also showed how staff behaviour could be shaped to focus on more positive aspects of patient behaviour. Perhaps most importantly the token economy gave staff a clear model to guide their work with patients, and established a clear language of communication – the token exchange.

Contemporary with the token economy research, and in the long-term far more influential, were the careful studies of Wing and Brown (1970), on the effects of ward environment and rehabilitation efforts on the functioning and attitudes of patients with schizophrenia. Wing and Brown (1970), showed that impoverished ward environments (where patients, for example, lacked personal possessions and spent much time doing nothing) were associated with the development of the 'negative' symptoms of schizophrenia, whilst prolonged length of stay in hospital resulted in patients becoming increasingly institutionalized in their attitudes towards discharge. They identified aspects of a care environment that were conducive to active rehabilitation, emphasizing the importance of a motivated staff group that had positive but realistic expectations of their patients and made demands on the patients to function as normally as possible.

Social skills training

On average people with schizophrenia have markedly smaller social networks than average and show significant deficits in the basic skills of social interaction (for example responding to questions or engaging others in conversation). One obvious treatment intervention is therefore to try and teach patients the social skills that they lack, with the long-term aim of allowing them to develop larger and more appropriately structured social networks.

Unlike the token economy, which clearly had its roots in American psychology, social skills training could be described as much as being a British development as an American one. Hollin and Trower (1986) claim that social skills training arose from three main influence: second, from research into pre-morbid social competence and the outcome from major psychiatric illness (Strauss *et al*. 1977); and third, from social psychological research conducted into verbal and non-verbal communication (Argyle *et al*. 1971). Much of this research was conducted in Britain by Michael Argyle and his colleagues (see Argyle 1967 for a review of this early work). Along with Peter Trower and Bridget Bryant they began to seek clinical applications for this research (Trower *et al*. 1978). As many psychiatric patients have deficits in social skills (Lindsay 1982), and as social skills training was a method purposely developed to improve social skills, it seemed only logical to assume that social skills training could be applied to help people with schizophrenia overcome their interpersonal difficulties. From the mid-1970s to the early 1980s there was a massive expansion in the social skills literature, and a number of textbooks described how to apply social skills training to people with major mental disorders (Goldstein *et al.* 1976; Bellack and Hersen 1979; Wilkinson and Canter 1982; Curran and Monti 1982; Spence and Shepherd 1983; L'Abate and Milan 1985).

Unfortunately the early optimism for this new psychological approach was not matched by its success in routine clinical practice. As with many behavioural approaches, generalization of skills to non-treatment environments proved problematic even in early research studies (Shepherd 1977, 1978). American workers continue to feel that the approach has much to offer the long-term client and have developed elaborate packages for training patients in a variety of social and instrumental skills as part of a comprehensive psychosocial rehabilitation intervention (Liberman 1988; Liberman *et al.* 1989). However, it is significant that two new textbooks on schizophrenia (Kavanagh 1992*b*; Birchwood and Tarrier 1992) have not been able to find British workers to describe social skills training in practice.

Why did such optimism about the potential of social skills training dissipate, at least amongst British rehabilitation workers? Perhaps the greatest problem was that the early motor skills model of social skills was too simplistic to cover the complexities of social behaviour. Argyle's original model (Trower *et al.* 1978) was soon reformulated by Trower and other workers to include a more pronounced cognitive component (Trower 1984). However few models developed by social skills theorists encompassed the myriad of factors that contribute to whether a person is perceived as socially competent or not. Even if we focus on basic social skills, in addition to the often studied verbal and non-verbal behaviour, skills such as reciprocity, rewardingness, self-disclosure, empathy and learning from experience are critical, (Argyle 1980; Argyle and Henderson 1985). Individual attitudes and factors such as persistence and motivation are no doubt important. Similarly, parental influences and upbringing are critical in the development of self-esteem and self-confidence. Sociocultural factors were often neglected by early workers in the field. Additionally a range of other factors such as finance, opportunities, physical attractiveness, previous success and failure, and even luck play a role. The inclusion of such factors would broaden out the training curriculum from the narrower focus given to it by many social skills practitioners. Again the model of a person that social skills training presented (Bannister 1983) was that of an expert (the trainer) knowing the skills the trainee was deficient in and then instructing the trainee until they became proficient in them. The individual was therefore seen as being both passive and inexpert. Moreover some 'abnormal' aspects of the social behaviour of people with schizophrenia may actually be adaptive: for example, some patients find intimate social contact highly stressful to the point that their positive psychotic symptoms worsen if they spend too much time with others. Social withdrawal may, for these people, serve to reduce unpleasant symptoms. For such patients environmental manipulation that offers them the opportunity of 'company without intimacy' (for example the availability of an unstructured drop-in facility) may be of great value.

Social skills training with the long-term population also failed on Meehl's (1954) distinction between statistically significant and clinically significant change. While there are a host of outcome studies which demonstrate statistical changes following social skills training (e.g. Liberman *et al*. 1984; Foxx *et al*. 1985; Wallace and Liberman 1985), there are fewer studies that can demonstrate that the training had a major impact on the patients' lives. Patients' conversation skills may have improved after training, they may have done better at role-play tests, but did they make any more friends as a result of the training? The answer unfortunately is no. A clinical vignette will outline a typical problem in social skills training.

Case study

John was a 48-year-old man with a long history of psychiatric problems. He was admitted to the rehabilitation ward for help with developing a more independent lifestyle. Prior to his most recent breakdown he had been living at home with his elderly parents. As part of his rehabilitation programme, he participated in the ward social skills training group. In the first phase of this group, he had 12 sessions on the ward, held twice weekly for an hour. In the second phase six sessions were conducted in the community in 'in vivo' settings. On one of these real-life assignments his social skills task was to ask to join a local library. The psychologist accompanying him on this trip stood about eight feet away to watch how he performed the task. Unfortunately the librarian must have had a counselling qualification, as, noting our trainee's hesitant skills, she asked 'You don't really seem very certain about wanting to join?' At this our trainee exclaimed 'I'm not! I'm only doing it because the psychologist over there asked me to!'

Many workers would immediately wonder at the ineptitude of getting patients to perform skills they did not necessarily want to become proficient in. Unfortunately this was the way a great deal of social skills training was conducted, in violation of the most basic tenets of rehabilitation (MacCarthy *et al*. 1986).

Despite these comments on the practical limitations of social skills training with the long-term mentally ill, these groups are often very popular with both staff and patients. Again the most likely reason for this is probably that such groups are very clearly structured and both staff and patients have a clear idea of what is expected of them, as with the token economies. This contrasts markedly with the views that staff and patients have towards unstructured ward groups (Carson and Sharma 1994).

Is there then no role for social skills training with the long-term client? Given the severe and handicapping deficits in interpersonal skills experienced by many people with a long-term mental illness the answer must be 'no' However, different strategies need to be adopted than the traditional social skills group held weekly in the day hospital. Services should be structured to encourage the exercise of appropriate social skills among users, with staff utilizing behavioural therapy skills such as modelling and feedback in their day-to-day interactions with clients. One important practical point is that staff should be working with the client rather than doing things to or for him or her: in the days of the back-ward patients lost very basic instrumental skills because it was quicker, for example, for the nurse to shave the patient than encourage the patient to shave himself. The generalization problem can be overcome by working with clients in their environment of need. Importantly, services should be aiming at early intervention with psychotic patients prior to the development of fixed patterns of abnormal behaviour and the loss of the patient's ordinary social network.

Psychological interventions for delusions and hallucinations

Somewhat surprisingly, given the negative findings of some of the early research in this area, there is now a resurgence of interest in psychological interventions with schizophrenic symptoms (Birchwood and Shepherd 1992). Although antipsychotic medication currently has a central role in the management of psychotic symptoms, these drugs have unpleasant and potentially damaging side effects, are unacceptable to some patients, and are ineffective in a proportion of cases. Therefore, despite the massive investment by drug firms in antipsychotic medication, psychologically-based treatments could play an important role.

The earliest interventions were not only inconclusive in outcome but also rather crude in manner. For instance a study by Bucher and Fabricatore (1970) used patient-administered electric shock to suppress hallucinations. Similarly a number of early attempts to reduce the amount of delusional speech used social reinforcement to shape more normal speech (Ayllon and Haughton 1964). Both approaches were empirically rather than theoretically based, and again neither were successful in reducing symptoms once contingencies were removed.

A number of psychologists have tried to modify delusional beliefs using cognitive belief modification procedures. Early studies by Watts *et al.* (1973) and Milton *et al.* (1978) were not followed up properly until a study by Chadwick and Lowe (1991). In a series of case studies, they described how they challenged patients' delusional beliefs in three stages. First; they pointed out any irregularities within patients' belief symptoms. Second, they showed patients that there was a viable alternative explanation for what was happening to them. Third, they showed patients that the evidence available to them supported the alternative explanations, and not their own beliefs. Using this approach systematically they were able to demonstrate significant weakening in patients' delusional beliefs. While Chadwick and Lowe's results are encouraging, they require replication in other centres before we can be certain that this approach represents a major step forward in modifying delusional beliefs.

Research into the modification of hallucinations has also continued apace. Again, a number of the approaches adopted here have not been very sophisticated whatever their underlying rationale. For instance, Birchwood (1986), described an approach to reducing the frequency of hallucinations using monaural auditory occlusion – since renamed 'ear-plug therapy' by some workers in the field. This approach was said to be based on a neuro-psychological model of symptoms linked to hemispheric asymmetries of function. Hallucinations were said to reflect nondominant hemisphere verbalizations which interfered with dominant hemisphere speech (Green,

Glass and O'Callaghan 1979). According to the model, the decision which ear the ear-plug went into needed to be determined by a dichotic listening task. Dutch colleagues have discovered that it does not seem to matter which ear is selected (Van der Gaag personal communication). Nelson *et al.* (1991) found that teaching long-term hallucinating patients to use a Walkman was another effective technique.

In a comprehensive review of studies, Slade and Bentall (1988) suggested that methods could be categorized into three main groups. The first consisted of anxiety-reduction techniques such as systematic desensitization (Slade 1973). Patients will often spontaneously withdraw to their room when assailed by abnormal experiences; and withdrawal may serve to reduce the sufferer's level of arousal. The second method consisted of distraction techniques (Erickson and Gustafason 1968): this is a commonly adopted natural coping mechanism whereby patients try to engage their attention on alternative stimuli. The third consisted of focusing methods (Fowler and Morley 1989). Haddock *et al.* (1993) describe an approach to treating hallucinations using focusing. They describe it thus:

> the patient is encouraged to explore the content and meaning of the voices within a therapeutic relationship. It was hoped that by gradually exposing the patient to his voices, this would allow him to identify their true origin and to resolve any difficulties reflected in their context. (p. 337)

Unfortunately, the approach was successful in only one of the two cases presented.

This last study highlights the major problem of psychological interventions to control psychotic symptoms. It is that the successful studies conducted to date have tended to be single case studies, or studies with a small series of patients. The results of two major ongoing randomized control trials of cognitive behavioural therapy for psychosis from both the Liverpool and the Maudsley research groups are eagerly awaited. An additional difficulty arises from the fact that neither of these approaches have been tried in the absence of patients receiving antipsychotic medication. Unlike cognitive therapy for depression (Rush *et al.* 1977; Shaw 1977), which has been shown to be as effective as drug treatment, and which has a synergistic effect when used in combination with drugs, the same cannot be said for existing psychological modification of schizophrenic symptoms. Such work would seem to have a long way to go before we can be certain of its efficacy.

Psychological interventions to arrest relapse

A number of studies demonstrate that there are signs of an impending relapse in patients, often several weeks before such relapses actually occur (Herz and Melville 1980; Birchwood *et al.* 1989). The symptoms most frequently reported by patients themselves or by their family members are dysphoric in nature. In the Birchwood study, problems of anxiety and agitation were most common, followed by problems of depression and withdrawal. Birchwood (1992) suggests that each patient will probably have their own unique prodrome which can be called a 'personalized relapse signature'.

Identifying what this unique signature is, however, can only take place retrospectively after relapses have occurred. In Birmingham, Birchwood and his colleagues (Smith and Birchwood 1990) have established an Early Intervention Research Group to monitor early warning signs and to attempt to forestall psychotic relapses. Such an approach depends on close liaison between the patient, their carer and mental health professionals.

It may then be possible for patients to avoid relapses with close monitoring of their prodromal signs by both themselves and their relative by taking appropriate action prior to the onset of florid symptomatology. (At present this means restarting or increasing the dose of antipsychotic medication, although in principle psychological or social manipulation may be useful.) Early signs monitoring is generally carried out with low-dose antipsychotic treatment regimens or in patients who are medication-free. Birchwood (1992) notes that this approach may be of limited value for patients who are already on high maintenance doses of medication, for those with drug-resistant psychotic symptoms and for those lacking in insight. As yet few services have attempted to include such strategies in their delivery of care, with the exception of studies such as the Buckingham Project (Falloon *et al.* 1990) and Birchwood's own work. It may be possible to incorporate some of this work into the functioning of case management services (Shepherd 1990) so that early signs monitoring is conducted in a more systematic way.

Depression, coping and grief

Birchwood and Shepherd (1992), commenting on the high incidence of depression in people with schizophrenia, suggest that it might be 'a psychological response to a chronic and apparently uncontrollable illness' (p. 327). A number of other research workers have looked at depression in schizophrenia as being a form of unresolved grief (Appelo *et al.* 1994). Looking at Wing's primary impairments, Appelo and his colleagues argue that it is hardly surprising that the problems in information processing, difficulties in social functioning, lack of energy, emotional blunting, etc., depress sufferers with schizophrenia. Following Strauss *et al.* (1989) they argue that these primary impairments result in additional psychological difficulties such as the loss of hope and self-esteem. They argue that these secondary handicaps 'can be understood as grief reactions to loss' (p. 56). Their own rehabilitation programme places great emphasis on helping patients adjust to the losses that have occurred in their own lives, and towards acceptance and resolution of these losses. Interestingly Miller *et al.* (1990) found a similar pattern occurring in relatives, and they suggest that families may undergo a delayed grief response. Rehabilitation workers need to be sensitive to such responses in both relatives and patients with schizophrenia.

A sense of loss is one of the many psychodynamic issues raised by the experience of long-term mental illness. Although there is no evidence that psychodynamic therapy has any general value in the treatment of schizophrenia (Mueser and Berenbaum 1990) psychodynamic concepts may be of value in helping patients cope with the human issues raised by having a chronic illness and deal with everyday life difficulties. Supportive psychotherapy has a significant role to play in the long-term management of schizophrenia.

A number of studies (Strauss 1989; Taylor and Perkins 1991) have focused on the issue of self-identity and how this might be involved in helping patients cope with long-term psychiatric problems. Societal images of mental illness may actually interfere with patients' attempts to create a more positive self-image for themselves. Notions of violence, the need for segregation, patients being a danger to small children, etc., all help convey a negative image of mental illness which hinders self-acceptance. Where patients do accept their illness this seems to be associated with more positive outcomes (Warner *et al.* 1989). Birchwood and Shepherd (1992) argue that workers need to 'encourage blame-free acceptance of the illness and [the development of] a sense of mastery over it through education and inculcating strategies for self-control' (p. 329).

Normalization principles (Wolfensberger 1983) suggest that we should focus on issues of image and competency enhancement. This remains problematic. Szivos and Travers (1988) have used consciousness raising as an approach with people with learning difficulties to try and enhance their self-image. It would be interesting to see if this approach could be applied systematically to people with long-term mental health problems. Certainly people involved in the 'survivor' movement, who view themselves as having survived the mental health system, gain much sense of support from being engaged in active self-help rather than remaining passive recipients of care.

It is important to consider what we can learn from patients themselves. Increasingly service providers are having to listen to the concerns of users (Lieper and Field 1993). Users are in a unique position to inform practitioners of what approaches have been of help to them, and indeed a number of workers have already incorporated such perspectives into their own interventions (Falloon and Talbot 1981; Tarrier *et al.* 1990). While some users accounts can be extremely critical of service interventions, often on the lack of a caring intervention (Campbell 1992), others are more positive. Describing his own breakdown, Chadwick (1993) stated:

> For me the disease model in action, with its inference of hardware disorder, although of questionable validity in isolating necessary causal factors thus far has, in the general sense, nonetheless been protective and practically helpful rather than condemnatory and confusing. (p. 249)

The developing mental health consumer movement may further encourage diminished stigma and according to Warner *et al.* (1989) 'may reduce the disability associated with mental illness even more effectively than do professional psychosocial interventions' (p. 408).

Increasingly clinicians are learning to build on patients' natural coping strategies (for example the Walkman that shuts out the voices) and to develop a collaborative relationship with the patient and their carers. At the heart of effective collaboration is the provision of information about what is known about the illness (and what is not known!) and its treatment (Corrigan *et al.* 1990). In clinical practice most psychotic relapses occur after the patient has made the decision to stop taking medication. Such a decision often occurs when the patient is free of psychotic symptoms and reflects a judgment about the balance between risk and benefit. Patients may be unconvinced that medication will stave off a psychotic relapse and consequent readmission to hospital (the benefit side of the equation), but all too aware of the unacceptable side effects that they are experiencing from the medication (the risk side of taking treatment). Clinicians have to help patients and carers come to an informed decision about the treatment that they receive.

Case management

Helping long-term clients involves a judicious mixture of specific therapeutic interventions (both biological and psychological) and environmental manipulation. People with long-term disabilities require care environments that both make positive demands for social functioning and minimize stress (Wing and Brown 1970). Any system of long-term care will require a range of resources including day care, sheltered work facilities, residential provision and systems for income maintenance.

However, as Shepherd (1991) has noted:

> Rehabilitation is not therefore just about systems of facilities. It is not even really about resources. Fundamentally it is about people and how they behave towards one another and about the attitude society takes towards them.   (p. xli)

The new community-based services are highly fragmented and often appear impenetrable to the sufferer and carers. With the transition from institutional to community care the relationship between long-term clients and their key workers assumes an added importance. It has been suggested that the key worker, adopting the role of the 'case manager' can function as the 'glue' that will hold the new community-based service together, serving to guide the client through its complexities (Intagliata 1982).

While there are numerous definitions of case management and of its constituent components (Holloway 1991b; Thornicroft 1991), in this chapter we will focus on 'clinical case management' (Kanter 1989). Surber (1994) argues that it is through the relationship with the case manager that long-term clients change, develop and attain goals. He suggests that there are a number of key service principles that need to be addressed in the delivery of effective case management services:

- *Comprehensiveness*
  This includes mental health treatment, the provision of basic support for health and social problems, and help to achieve goals.
- *Continuity*
  Care must be available over time and for as long as it is needed.
- *Individualization*
  Services should be designed to respond to the unique needs of each client. Implementation of the plan should also be tailored to each individual's circumstances. One case manager is responsible for each client.

- *Flexibility*
  Services should be provided that are acceptable to clients. Workers should be prepared to see clients whenever they come to the office. Staff should have the ability to be flexible in their interventions.
- *Capability*
  Caseloads should be within manageable limits. Staff mobility needs to be backed up by administrative resources.
- *Meaningfulness*
  A major purpose for case management services is that they must facilitate clients working towards goals and ambitions as specified by the clients.
- *Willingness and acceptance*
  Clients should not be excluded from care on the grounds of their problematic behaviours. Staff, as far as possible, should try to understand and accept clients.
- *Cultural competence*
  Services should conduct assessments that are sensitive to clients' cultural backgrounds. Competence means understanding the clients' cultural values and norms, understanding one's own cultural values and norms, and trying to utilize the clients' culture as a support to enhance treatment.
- *Resourcefulness*
  Team members need to try and utilize all the resources of a local community to help carry out treatment plans.
- *Participation*
  Active client participation is crucial to the issues of any case management endeavour, especially in developing and carrying out service plans.
- *Accessibility*
  Case management services need to be situated where clients can access them.

Surber concludes that there are a number of key skills that case managers must possess to be effective:

- an understanding of human behaviour and how to influence it
- an understanding of culture and how to support it
- an understanding of families and how to involve them
- an understanding of community resources and how to use them.

Case management is clearly seen as one of the main contemporary innovations in intervention for the long-term client. In a recent review of the outcome literature (Holloway *et al.* 1995) we were unable to be as positive in our conclusions as many of the advocates of case management (Stein and Test 1980; Muijen *et al.* 1992). Few outcome studies have used randomized control designs. Similarly few studies specify in detail what experimental or control conditions consisted of. It becomes difficult to assess, therefore, what case managers actually did. Our own East Lambeth Continuing Care Research Project and other current studies will hopefully enable us to make a more informed appraisal of the efficacy of case management. However it is clear that the humanistic principles outlined by Surber do have relevance to the day-to-day practice of staff working with long-term severely handicapped clients.

Conclusions

This review of interventions for long-term clients has concentrated on the needs of people with schizophrenia. We have purposely avoided discussion of the crucial role of antipsychotic medication, the importance of family interventions and the teaching of daily living skills. All of these interventions are crucial to any comprehensive service system and are discussed elsewhere in this book. The components of an effective rehabilitation service have been clearly articulated by a number of workers and do not require further rehearsal here (Anthony *et al.* 1982; Pilling 1991; Ekdawi and Conning 1994). Instead we have chosen to focus our attention on psychological interventions. The early promise and optimism of the token economy in rehabilitation has not yet been fulfilled. The generalization problem, and a major shift in how we perceived our patients accounted for its demise. Equally social skills training has with the fullness of time also failed to live up to its early promise with a rehabilitation clientele. Interventions to control psychotic symptoms and to monitor early signs of relapse appear promising, but require much further evaluation before their general adoption can be advocated.

These more recent developments, along with case management and our increased understanding of the experience of illness and how people overcome their disabilities, suggest that rehabilitation workers need to utilize a more collaborative approach than they may have followed in the past. We need to enhance our understanding of how patients cope with their illnesses. We need to listen more clearly to how patients perceive our supposedly rehabilitative services. We also have to try and ensure that we create more valued social roles for our patients. While it is sometimes assumed that social role valorization was a concern addressed only by workers operating from a normalization perspective, it has always been seen as crucial by traditional rehabilitation workers (Wing and Brown 1970; Parry 1991).

We have argued that the stress-vulnerability-coping model provides the best framework for interventions with long-term clients. It is important that the help people receive covers the whole range of psychosocial needs and is not merely focused on symptoms and deficits. Such approaches will always be delivered best by a team with a range of skills to offer clients (Onyett 1992; Øvretveit 1993).

References

Anthony W, Cohen M and Farkas M (1982). 'A psychiatric rehabilitation treatment program. Can I recognize one if I see one?' *Community Mental Health Journal*, **18**, 83–96.

Appelo M, Sloof C, Woonings F, Carson J and Louwerens J (1994). Grief: its significance for rehabilitation in schizophrenia. *Clinical Psychology and Psychotherapy*, **1** (1), 53–59.

Argyle M (1967). *The Psychology of Interpersonal Behaviour*. Harmondsworth.

Argyle M (1969). *Social Interaction*, Methuen, London.

Argyle M (1980). Interaction skills and social competence. In *Psychological Problems: The Social Context* (eds. P Feldman and J Orford). Wiley, Chichester.

Argyle M and Henderson M (1985). *The Anatomy of Relationships*. Penguin, Harmondsworth.

Argyle M, Alkema F and Gilmour R (1971). The communication of friendly and hostile attitudes. *British Journal of Social and Clinical Psychology*, **10**, 386–401.

Atthowe J and Krasner L (1968). Preliminary report on the application of reinforcement principles (token economy) on a chronic psychiatric ward. *Journal of Abnormal Psychology*, **73**, 37–43.

Ayllon T and Azrin N (1968). *The Token Economy: A Motivational System for Therapy and Rehabilitation.* Appleton Century Crofts, New York.

Ayllon T and Haughton E (1964). Modification of symptomatic verbal behaviour of mental patients. *Behaviour Research and Therapy*, **2**, 87–97.

Bannister, D (1983). The internal politics of psychotherapy. In *Psychology and Psychotherapy – Current Trends and Issues* (ed. D Pilgrim). Routledge, London.

Bebbington P and Kuipers L (1992). Life events and social factors. In *Schizophrenia: An Overview and Practical Handbook* (ed. D Kavanagh). Chapman and Hall, London.

Bellack A and Hersen M (eds.) (1979). *Research and Practice in Social Skills Training.* Plenum, New York.

Birchwood M (1986). 'Control of auditory hallucinations through occlusion of monaural auditory input. *British Journal of Psychiatry*, **149**, 104–107.

Birchwood M (1992). Early intervention in schizophrenia: Theoretical background and clinical strategies. *British Journal of Clinical Psychology*, **31** (3), 257–278.

Birchwood M and Shepherd G (1992). Controversies and growing points in cognitive behavioural interventions for people with schizophrenia. *Behavioural Psychotherapy*, **20** (4), 305–342.

Birchwood M and Tarrier N (eds.) (1992). *Innovations in the Psychological Management of Schizophrenia.* Wiley, Chichester.

Birchwood M, Hallett S and Preston M (1988). *Schizophrenia: An Integrated Approach to Research and Treatment.* Longman, London.

Birchwood M, Smith J, Macmillan F, Hogg B, Prasad R, Harvey C and Bering S (1989). Predicting relapse in schizophrenia: The development and implementation of an early signs monitoring system using patients and families as observers. *Psychological Medicine*, **19**, 649–656.

Bucher B and Fabricatore J (1970). Use of patient administered shock to suppress hallucinations. *Behaviour Therapy*, **1**, 382–385.

Campbell P (1992). A survivor's view of community psychiatry'. *Journal of Mental Health*, **1** (2), 117–122.

Carson J and Sharma T (1994). In–patient psychiatric care – What helps? Staff and patient perspectives. *Journal of Mental Health*, **3**, 99–104.

Chadwick P (1993). The step-ladder to the impossible: a first hand phenomenological account of a schizoaffective psychiatric crisis. *Journal of Mental Health*, **2** (3), 239–250.

Chadwick P and Lowe F (1991). The measurement and modification of delusional beliefs. *Journal of Consulting and Clinical Psychology*, **58**, 225–232.

Clifford P, Charman A, Webb Y and Best S (1991). Planning for community care. *British Journal of Psychiatry*, **158**, 190–196.

Corrigan P W, Liberman R P and Engel K D (1990). From non–compliance to collaboration in the treatment of schizophrenia. *Hospital and Community Psychiatry*, **41**, 1203–1211.

Creed F (1993). Life events. In *Principles of Social Psychiatry* (eds. D Bhugra and J Leff). Blackwell, London.

Curran J and Monti P (eds.) (1982). *Social Skills Training.* Guildford, New York.

Ekdawi, M and Conning A (1994). *Psychiatric Rehabilitation: A Practical Guide.* Chapman and Hall, London.

Elliott P, Barlow F, Hooper A and Kingerlee P (1979). Maintaining patients' improvements in a token economy. *Behaviour Research and Therapy*, **17**, 355–367.

Erickson G and Gustafson G (1968). Controlling auditory hallucinations. *Hospital and Community Psychiatry*, **19**, 327–329.

Falloon I and Talbot R (1981). Persistent auditory hallucinations: coping mechanisms and implications for management. *Psychological Medicine*, **11**, 329–339.

Falloon I, Boyd J and McGill C (1987). *Family Care of Schizophrenia*. Guildford, New York.

Falloon I, Krekorian H, Shanahan W, Laporta M and McLees S (1990). The Buckingham Project: a comprehensive mental health service based on behavioural psychotherapy. *Behavioural Change*, **7**, 51–57.

Fowler D and Morley S (1989). The cognitive behavioural treatment of hallucinations and delusions: a preliminary study. *Behavioural Psychotherapy*, **17**, 267–282.

Foxx R, McMorrow M, Bittle R and Fenlon S (1985). Teaching social skills to psychiatric in-patients. *Behaviour Research and Therapy*, **23**, 531–537.

Goldstein A, Sprafkin R and Gershaw N (1976). *Skill Training for Community Living: Applying Structured Learning Therapy*. Pergamon, New York.

Green P, Glass A and O'Callaghan M (1979). Some implications of abnormal inter-hemispheric interaction in schizophrenia. In *Hemispheric Asymmetries of Function and Psychopathology* (eds. J Gruzelier and P Flor-Henry). Elsevier, Amsterdam.

Gripp R and Magaro P (1974). The token economy programme in the psychiatric hospital: a review and analysis. *Behaviour Research and Therapy*, **12**, 205–228.

Haddock G, Bentall R and Slade P (1993). Psychological treatment of chronic auditory hallucinations: two case studies. *Behavioural Psychotherapy*, **21** (4), 335–346.

Hall J and Baker R (1973). Token economy systems: breakdown and control. *Behaviour Research and Therapy*, **11**, 253–263.

Hall J, Baker R and Hutchinson K (1977). A controlled evaluation of token economy procedures with chronic schizophrenic patients. *Behaviour Research and Therapy*, **15**, 261–283.

Harding C M, Brooks G W, Ashikaga T *et al.* (1987). The Vermont longitudinal study: II. Long term outcome of subjects who retrospectively met DSM–III criteria for schizophrenia. *American Journal of Psychiatry*, **144**, 727–753.

Harding C M, Zubin J and Strauss J S (1992). Chronicity in schizophrenia: revisited. *British Journal of Psychiatry*, **161** (suppl. 18), 27–37.

Hawton K, Salkovskis P M, Kirk J and Clark D M (1989). *Cognitive Behaviour Therapy for Psychiatric Problems*. Oxford Medical Publications, Oxford.

Herz M and Melville C (1980). Relapse in schizophrenia. *American Journal of Psychiatry*, **137**, 801–812.

Hollin C and Trower P (eds.) (1986). *Handbook of Social Skills Training*, Volume 2. Pergamon, Oxford.

Holloway F (1991*a*). Day care in an inner city. *British Journal of Psychiatry*, **158**, 805–810.

Holloway F (1991*b*). Case management for the mentally ill: looking at the evidence. *International Journal of Social Psychiatry*, **37** (1), 2–13.

Holloway F (1994). Need in community psychiatry: a consensus is required. *Psychiatric Bulletin*, **18**, 321–323.

Holloway F, Oliver N, Collins E and Carson J (1995). Case management: a critical review of the outcome literature. *European Psychiatry*, **10**, 113–128.

Huxley P, Hagan T, Hennelly R and Hunt J (1993). *Effective Community Mental Health Services*. Avebury, Aldershot.

Intagliata J (1982). Improving the quality of community care for the chronically mentally disabled: the role of case management. *Schizophrenia Bulletin*, **8**, 655–674.

Johnstone E (1993). A concept of schizophrenia. *Journal of Mental Health*, **2** (3), 195–207.

Kanter J (1989). Clinical case management: Definition, principles, components *Hospital and Community Psychiatry*, **40**, 361–368.

Kavanagh D (1992*a*). Recent developments in expressed emotion and schizophrenia. *British Journal of Psychiatry*, **160**, 601–620.

Kavanagh D (ed.) (1992*b*). *Schizophrenia: An Overview and Practical Handbook.* Chapman and Hall, London.

L'Abate L and Milan M (eds.) (1985). *Handbook of Social Skills Training and Research.* Wiley, New York.

Laing R and Esterson A (1964). *Sanity, Madness and the Family.* Tavistock, London.

Leff J, Kuipers L, Berkowitz R, Eberlein-Vries R and Sturgeon D (1982). A controlled trial of social intervention in the families of schizophrenic patients. *British Journal of Psychiatry*, **141**, 121–134.

Liberman R P (1988). *Psychiatric Rehabilitation of Chronic Mental Patients.* American Psychiatric Press, Washington DC.

Liberman R, Lillie F, Falloon I, Harpin E, Hutchinson W and Stouts B (1984). Social skills training for relapsing schizophrenics: An experimental analysis. *Behaviour Modification*, **8**, 155–179.

Liberman R, De Risi W and Mueser K (1989). *Social Skills Training for Psychiatric Patients.* Pergamon, New York.

Lidz T, Cornelison A, Singer M, Schafer S and Fleck S (1965). The mothers of schizophrenic patients. In *Schizophrenia and the Family* (eds. T Lidz, S Fleck and A Cornelison). International Universities Press, New York.

Lieper R and Field V (eds.) (1993). *Counting for Something in Mental Health Services.* Avebury, Aldershot.

Lindsay W (1982). Some normative goals for conversation training. *Behaviour Psychotherapy*, **10**, 253–272.

MacCarthy B, Benson J and Brewin C R (1986). Task motivation and problem appraisal in long–term psychiatric patients. *Psychological Medicine*, **16**, 431–438.

Martin J (1984). *Hospitals in Trouble.* Basil Blackwell, London.

Meehl P (1954). *Clinical Versus Statistical Prediction.* University of Minnesota Press, Minneapolis.

Meehl P (1962). Schizotaxia, schizotypy, schizophrenia. *American Psychologist*, **17**, 827–831.

Miller F, Dworkin J, Ward M and Barone D (1990). A preliminary study of unresolved grief in families of seriously mentally ill patients. *Hospital and Community Psychiatry*, **41** (12), 1321–1325.

Milton F, Patwa V and Hafner J (1978). Confrontation versus belief modification in persistently deluded patients. *British Journal of Medical Psychology*, **51**, 127–130.

Mueser K T and Berenbaum H (1990). Psychodynamic treatment of schizophrenia: is there a future? *Psychological Medicine*, **20**, 253–262.

Muijen M, Marks I and Connolly J (1992). The Daily Living Program: preliminary comparison of community versus hospital based treatment for the severely mentally ill facing emergency admission. *British Journal of Psychiatry*, **160**, 379–384.

Nelson H, Thrasher S and Barnes T (1991). Practical ways of alleviating auditory hallucinations. *British Medical Journal*, **302**, 307.

Nuechterlein K and Dawson M (1984). A heuristic vulnerability stress model of schizophrenic episodes. *Schizophrenia Bulletin*, **10**, 300–312.

Onyett S (1992). *Case Management in Mental Health.* Chapman and Hall, London.

Øvretveit J (1993). *Co-ordinating Community Care: Multidisciplinary Teams and Care Management.* Open University Press, Buckingham.

Owen M and McGuffin P (1992). The molecular genetics of schizophrenia. *British Medical Journal*, **305**, 664–665.

Parry G (1991). Domestic roles. In *Theory and Practice of Psychiatric Rehabilitation* (eds. F Watts and D Bennett). Wiley, Chichester.

Paul G and Lentz R (1977). *Psychosocial Treatment of Chronic Mental Patients: Milieu versus Social Learning Programs.* Harvard University Press, Cambridge, Mass.

Pilling S (1991). *Rehabilitation and Community Care.* Routledge, London.

Pilowsky L S (1992). 'Understanding schizophrenia. *British Medical Journal*, **305**, 327–328.

Presly A, Black D, Gray A, Hartic A and Seymour E (1976). The token economy in the National Health Service: possibilities and limitations. *Acta Psychiatrica Scandinavica*, **53**, 258–270.

Rachlin R (1969). *Introduction to Modern Behaviourism.* Freeman, San Francisco, Ca.

Ramon S (1991). Principles and conceptual knowledge. In *Beyond Community Care: Normalization and Integration Work* (ed. S Ramon). Macmillan, London.

Rezin V, Elliott P and Paschallis P (1983). Nurse–patient interaction in a token economy. *Behaviour Psychotherapy*, **11**, 225–234.

Rush A, Beck A, Kovacs M and Hollon S (1977). Comparative efficacy of cognitive therapy and imipramine in the treatment of depressed out-patients. *Cognitive Therapy and Research*, **1**, 17–37.

Sanson-Fisher R, Poole A and Thomas V (1979). Behaviour patterns within a general hospital psychiatric unit: an observational study. *Behaviour Research and Therapy*, **17**, 317–332.

Saykin A J, Shtasel D L, Gur R E *et al.* (1994). Neuropsychological deficits in neuroleptic naive patients with first-episode schizophrenia. *Archives of General Psychiatry*, **51**, 124–131.

Shaw B (1977). Comparison of cognitive therapy and behaviour therapy in the treatment of depression. *Journal of Consulting and Clinical Psychology*, **45**, 543–551.

Shepherd G (1977). Social skills training: the generalization problem. *Behaviour Therapy*, **8**, 1008–1009.

Shepherd G (1978). Social skills training: the generalization problem, Some further data. *Behaviour Research and Therapy*, **16**, 287–288.

Shepherd G (1990). Case management. *Health Trend* 1990s. Foreword in *Theory and Practice of Psychiatric Rehabilitation* (eds. F Watts and D Bennett). Wiley, Chichester.

Skinner B (1953). *Science and Human Behaviour.* Macmillan, New York.

Slade P (1973). The psychological investigation and treatment of auditory hallucinations: a second case report. *British Journal of Medical Psychology*, **46**, 293–296.

Slade P and Bentall R (1988). *Sensory Deception: A Scientific Analysis of Hallucinations.* Croom Helm, London.

Smith J and Birchwood M (1990). Relatives and patients as partners in the management of schizophrenia. *British Journal of Psychiatry*, **156**, 654–660.

Snyder S (1982). Neurotransmitters and CNS disease in schizophrenia. *Lancet*, **ii**, 970–974.

Spence S and Shepherd G (eds.) (1983). *Developments in Social Skills Training.* Academic Press, London.

Stein L and Test M (1980). Alternative to mental hospital treatment. 1. Conceptual model, treatment programme and clinical evaluations., *Archives of General Psychiatry*, **37**, 392–397.

Stoffelmayr B, Faulkner G and Mitchell W (1979). The comparison of token economy and social therapy in the treatment of hard core schizophrenic patients. *Behavioural Analysis and Modification*, **3**, 3–17.

Strauss J (1989). Subjective experiences of schizophrenia: towards a new dynamic. *Schizophrenia Bulletin*, **15**, 179–188.

Strauss J, Klorman R and Kokes R (1977). Premorbid adjustment in schizophrenia: Part V. The implications of findings for understanding research and applications. *Schizophrenia Bulletin*, **3**, 240–244.

Strauss J, Rakfeld J, Harding C and Liberman R (1989). Psychological and social aspects of negative symptoms. *British Journal of Psychiatry*, **155**, 128–132.

Surber R (ed.) (1994). *Clinical Case Management: A Guide to Comprehensive Treatment of Serious Mental Illness*. Sage, California.

Szivos S and Travers E (1988). Consciousness raising among mentally handicapped people: a critique of the implications of normalization. *Human Relations*, **41**, 641–653.

Tarrier N, Harwood S, Yusopoff L, Beckett R and Baker A (1990). Coping strategy enhancement (CNE): a method of treating residual schizophrenic symptoms. *Behavioural Psychotherapy*, **18**, 283–293.

Taylor K and Perkins R (1991). Identity and coping with mental illness in long stay rehabilitation. *British Journal of Clinical Psychology*, **30**, 73–85.

Thornicroft G (1991). Case management in long–term mental illness. *International Review of Psychiatry*, **3**, 125–132.

Trower P (ed.) (1984). *Radical Approaches to Social Skills Training*. Croom Helm, London.

Trower P, Bryant B and Argyle M (1978). *Social Skills and Mental Health*. Methuen, London.

Turpin K and Clements K (1992). Psychophysiological contributions to clinical assessment and treatment. In *Schizophrenia: An Overview and Practical Handbook* (ed. D Kavanagh). Chapman and Hall, London.

Vaughn C and Leff J (1976). The influence of family and social factors on the course of psychiatric illness: a comparison of schizophrenic and depressed neurotic patients. *British Journal of Psychiatry*, **129**, 125–137.

Wallace C and Liberman R (1985). Social skills training for people with schizophrenia: a controlled clinical trial. *Psychiatry Research*, **14**, 239–247.

Warner R, Taylor D, Powers M and Hyman J (1989). Acceptance of the mental illness label by psychotic patients: effects on functioning. *American Journal of Orthopsychiatry*, **59**(3), 398–409.

Watts F, Powell G and Austin S (1973). The modification of abnormal beliefs. *British Journal of Medical Psychology*, **46**, 359–363.

Weinberger D, DeLisi L, Penman G, Torgum S and Wyatt R (1982). Computed tomography in schizophreniform disorder and other acute psychiatric disorders. *Archives of General Psychiatry*, **39**, 778–783.

Wilkinson J and Canter S (1982). *Social Skills Training Manual*, Wiley, Chichester.

Wing J (1978). Clinical concepts of schizophrenia. In *Schizophrenia: Towards a New Synthesis* (ed. J Wing). Academic Press, London.

Wing JK and Brown GW (1970). *Institutionalise and Schizophrenia*. Cambridge University Press, Cambridge.

Wolfensberger W (1970). The principle of normalization and its implication for psychiatric services. *American Journal of Psychiatry*, **127** (3), 291–297.

Wolfensberger W (1983). Social role valorisation: a proposed new term for the principle of normalisation. *Mental Retardation*, **21** (6), 234–239.

Wolpe J and Lazarus A (1966). *Behaviour Therapy Techniques*. Pergamon, New York.

Zubin J and Spring B (1977). Vulnerability: a new view of schizophrenia. *Journal of Abnormal Psychology*, **86**, 260–266.

10 Coping with drug and alcohol misuse

P. Groves and M. Farrell

Introduction

The use of psychoactive substances appears to be universal throughout history and through most communities. Whereas the use of some substances, notably alcohol in Western societies, is sanctioned and to some extent regulated by social mores, the use of other drugs such as heroin is taboo and its users stigmatized. For the latter, any use of the substance is generally viewed as misuse. The increase in use of illicit drugs over the last two decades has led to considerable public concern. By contrast the rise in alcohol use has been complacently noted, yet it affects much larger numbers and the overall damage caused by alcohol is much greater than that caused by, for example, heroin because the extent of use of the former is greater.

Extent of the problem

General population surveys suggest about 23 per cent of men and 6 per cent of women in England report drinking more than the recommended weekly limit (Benzeval *et al.* 1992). A further 7 per cent of men and 2 per cent of women are likely to have experienced complications as a result of their drinking and of these 5 per cent of men and 2 per cent of women may be alcohol dependent. The heaviest drinking occurs in men under the age of 30. Self-reporting surveys are likely to be an underestimation, but nevertheless may give a general indication of the extent of use. The quantity of alcohol consumed by the UK population doubled between 1950 and the mid 1980s (Royal College of General Practitioners 1986), and has remained at about the same level since then (Cox *et al.* 1993).

About 2.5 per cent of men and 5 per cent of women are taking benzodiazepines on a daily basis (Ashton and Golding 1989), although these figures are probably falling. The number of prescriptions issued for benzodiazepines almost halved from about 30 million in 1979 to 16 million in 1992.

Prevalence rates for the misuse of illicit drugs are more difficult to ascertain. The Home Office Addicts Index gives information on those who have presented to doctors for treatment. In 1992 24 703 drug addicts were notified to the Home Office (Home Office Statistical Bulletin 1993*a*). This included 16 964 for heroin, 10 011 for methadone, and 1951 for cocaine (an individual may be notified for more than one drug). These figures probably represent only a fifth or less of the opiate and cocaine misusers in the UK (Hartnoll *et al.* 1985). Nevertheless this can give useful indications of trends over time. There is marked geographical variation, with the highest prevalences in London, Glasgow, Edinburgh and the north-west of England. Useful prevalence estimates may be obtained from local community surveys which attempt to include those not in contact with treatment services. In an inner city area it is likely that about 20 per cent of young people will have used drugs or volatile substances at least once, and in the worst areas up to 10 per cent will have tried or be using heroin (Swadi 1988; Parker *et al.* 1987). The prevalence of drug misuse appears to have steadily increased since the late 1960s, with a doubling in the Home Office notifications between 1988 and 1992. Cocaine seizures increased from 635 (103 kg) in 1986 to 2365 (2248 kg) in 1992 and amphetamine seizures increased from 3047 (116 kg) to 10 570 (569 kg) over the same period (Home Office Statistical Bulletin 1993*b*). Despite this increase in stimulant use, cocaine does not yet appear to have reached the epidemic proportions seen in the United States during the 1980s (Strang *et al.* 1993).

Problems associated with drug and alcohol misuse

The problems caused by drugs and alcohol are pervasive, affecting physical, psychological and social domains. Among alcohol misusers physical problems such as liver disease, gastritis and pancreatitis may not appear until the early forties as a direct toxic effect of the alcohol. Other physical disorders associated with alcohol include hypertension, cardiomyopathy and cancer of the mouth, larynx and oesophagus. At an earlier age the effects of intoxication may produce major problems such as accidents, marital disharmony domestic violence, loss of job or arrest. An estimated 800 people were killed in drink/driving accidents in 1990, about a sixth of all road deaths (HMSO 1992). Approximately 8 million working days are lost each year through drink-related absenteeism (HMSO 1992). In 1989 over 90 000 people were convicted of or cautioned for drunkenness offences (HMSO 1992). Much alcohol-related crime consists of petty offences. Alcohol is also associated with some crimes of violence. Psychological problems result both from the direct toxic effects of alcohol and indirectly from the social and physical problems. These include depression, anxiety, suicide and acute and chronic brain damage. An individual who continues to drink heavily is likely to die about 15 years earlier than the general population, the main causes being heart disease, cancer, accidents and suicide (Schuckitt 1989).

Heroin and other opiates, in particular methadone, cause respiratory depression which can be fatal in overdose. This may occur after a period of abstinence when tolerance has been lost, with a drug of unexpectedly high purity, or in association with other drug use. The route of administration is associated with physical complications. Injecting of any illicit drug may lead to abscesses, septicaemia and endocarditis. Sharing injecting equipment is associated with HIV and hepatitis B and C. Drug inhalation may be associated with asthma, pneumonia and tuberculosis. Financing illegal drugs is associated with crime particularly property offences. Between one-third and two-thirds of opiate addicts admit to such offences (Johnson *et al.* 1985).

Use of amphetamine or cocaine can lead to a psychosis with paranoid delusions and auditory, visual and tactile hallucinations. This usually subsides after a few days once the drug has been cleared from the system. Depression, sometimes with suicidal ideation, and fatigue may follow in the wake of stimulant use. Other problems are associated with route of administration as described above for heroin. Amphetamine may be injected or taken by mouth. Cocaine powder may be snorted or injected. 'Crack' or 'freebase' is cocaine in a form which can be smoked and has a similar rapidity of action to injecting. Cocaine use may be associated with increased HIV risk behaviour (Chaisson *et al.* 1989; Magura *et al.* 1993).

The principal problem with benzodiazepines is dependence. Symptoms of the withdrawal syndrome include shakiness, dizziness, insomnia, impaired concentration and heightened sensory perception. Occasionally fits and confusion can occur. Among those who misuse other drugs, benzodiazepines are sometimes injected with its attendant risks. High doses may also be associated with increased HIV risk behaviour (Klee *et al.* 1990), which may be due in part to disinhibition and amnesia.

Assessment

Owing to the multidimensional nature of the problems of substance misuse, assessment needs to encompass the different aspects of the client's life. A client may present asking for help, but frequently the problem may go unrecognized unless alcohol or drugs are specifically asked about. Any of the possible complications described above should alert the clinician to the possibility of such a problem. For alcohol, screening questionnaires may be helpful. These include the MAST (Michigan Alcohol Screening Test) and the CAGE. The former has 25 items with two subsets consisting of objective alcohol-related events and consequences, and of self-perception of drinking habits (Selzer 1971). The CAGE comprises just four questions, with each letter of CAGE standing for one of the questions. The questions are:

- Have you ever thought you ought to **C**ut down on your drinking?
- Have people **A**nnoyed you by criticizing your drinking?
- Have you ever felt **G**uilty about your drinking?
- Have you ever had a drink first thing in the morning (**E**ye-opener) to steady your nerves or get rid of a hangover?

The cut-off point is a positive answer to at least two of these questions (Mayfield *et al.* 1974).

Once a problem is identified, a detailed history should be taken of the substance use. This should include quantity and pattern of use. For drug users route of administration and current and past HIV risk behaviours should be assessed. Periods of not using and reasons for restarting should be explored. Psychological and physical complications should be elicited. Useful laboratory investigations include full blood count, liver function tests including gamma GT (for alcohol), and hepatitis B and C (for drugs). The effects of the substance use on the client's social functioning including friends and family, work and involvement with crime should be elucidated. It is helpful to involve family members who may be able to give a fuller picture of the client's substance use and lifestyle. The family is a major determinant in the success or otherwise of a client's attempt to change his or her substance use and so involvement at an early stage is highly desirable.

ICD10 classification distinguishes between dependence on a psychoactive drug (including alcohol) and harmful or hazardous use. Dependence implies a strong desire to take the substance plus a withdrawal syndrome, which is a set of symptoms which occur when the substance is stopped or the amount is reduced. Tolerance, which is the need for increasing amounts of the substance to produce the same effect, may also be present. The other key feature is narrowing of lifestyle and drug using repertoire. Hazardous use refers to consumption which carries a high risk of future damage to physical or mental health. Harmful use refers to damage having already occurred. Such damage may occur even if an individual is not dependent on the substance. For this reason it is helpful to describe a client on separate dimensions in terms of dependence, which will have implications for treatment if the individual stops using the substance, and in terms of substance-related problems or damage.

Longitudinal studies

Like major mental illnesses, drug and alcohol misuse have high rates of relapse. Nevertheless over time a considerable proportion will become abstinent. The course of substance misuse over time may be considered as the natural history which reflects the likely biological changes due to toxic effects of the substance or as a career which refers to the individual's sequential behaviour within a substance-using role (Edwards 1984; Raistrick 1991). Both aspects are important to understand an individual's substance use with interacting biological, psychological and social influences.

A 10-year follow-up of 99 men with drinking problems found that 18 had died (Edwards *et al.* 1983). Of the 68 who could be traced 25 per cent had been in a state of continuous troubled drinking and 12 per cent had been continuously abstinent. Apart from one man who was continuously a light social drinker, the remaining 60 per cent moved between problem drinking and abstinence with a few having periods of social drinking (Taylor *et al.* 1985).

A 12-year follow-up of 100 alcoholics by Vaillant (1988) found 37 per cent dead, 25 per cent stably abstinent, 17 per cent alcohol dependent and 21 per cent status unknown or institutionalized.

Vaillant (1973) in a 20-year follow-up of 100 heroin addicts reported 23 per cent dead, 35 per cent stable and abstinent, 25 per cent continuing to use opiates and 17 per cent could not be traced. A 24-year follow-up of California narcotic addicts reported that most of them had started drugs before the age of 20 years. In the first 10 years 13 per cent of the sample had died and 28 per cent had tested negative for opiates. In the second

10-year phase 27 per cent had died and 25 per cent had tested negative for opiates. Of those who continued to test positive for opiates there was a high level of criminal involvement among the sample in their late forties. At any point in time less than 10 per cent of the sample participated in community based treatment programmes such as methadone maintenance. Disability, long periods of heavy alcohol use, heavy criminal involvement and tobacco use were among the strongest predictors of mortality (Hser *et al.* 1993).

Winick (1962) has described the term 'maturing out', reporting 73 per cent of narcotic addicts having stopped using by 37 years and 95 per cent by 57. However a 12-year follow-up of 405 opioid addicts found that continued use or stopping was not related to age (Simpson *et al.* 1986). Furthermore, with regard to individuals who misuse alcohol, a study by Temple and Leino (1989) suggested that while heavier drinkers tend to die prematurely, those over 50 were likely to drink as much or more heavily than 20 years ago.

Factors associated with remission of substance misuse include physical complications, interventions by family or friends including finding a new partner, geographical relocation, spiritual conversion or religious involvement including Alcoholics Anonymous (AA), and financial or legal problems including community compulsory supervision (Robins *et al.* 1974; Saunders and Kershaw 1979; Tuchfield 1981; Vaillant 1983, 1988; and Ludwig 1985). In addition to these predominantly external factors, how people cope with adverse life circumstances appears to be important. Approach coping such as positive reappraisal, seeking support and problem solving are more likely to assist remission of substance misuse, whereas avoidance coping such as trying not to think about a problem may be less effective (Moos 1994).

Over an individual's substance-using career, an episode of treatment may form but a small part and many of the factors given above leading to remission of substance misuse may not be brought about by formal treatment. Nevertheless, treatment may still have a significant effect on a variety of outcome measures such as health cost benefits (Holder and Blose 1992), crime rates (Maddux and Desmond 1979) and alcoholic cirrhosis (Mann *et al.* 1988; Holder and Parker 1992). In addition, favourable social circumstances and helpful coping strategies may enable individuals to engage better in treatment and so gain more from it (Moos 1994). For example, Edwards *et al.* (1987, 1988) found that those who started with a high dependence score, and who obtained a good outcome, attributed their improvement to an 'active' coping style with a positive personal commitment to change. Both AA and formal treatment seemed to be helpful. Those with an initial low dependence score and a good outcome attributed their success to a 'responsive' style of coping with drinking problems which reflected a reaction to threatened or perceived consequences of drinking. Involvement in AA for these people seemed to be counterproductive.

Approaches to treatment

Goals of treatment

In recent years there has been a move away from abstinence as the only goal of treatment. Considerable benefits may be gained by encouraging safer substance use. In particular with the advent of HIV, there has been much focus on harm reduction among opiate misusers. This leads to a hierarchy of goals such as moving from sharing injecting equipment to cleaning equipment or preferably to using sterile equipment, and from there moving to stopping injecting and taking an oral opiate, before eventually perhaps becoming drug-free. Intermediate goals for problem drinkers might include not driving after a drinking episode or reducing the quantity of alcohol consumed. Where an individual is not dependent on alcohol, is younger and has not incurred alcohol-related physical damage, controlled drinking may be appropriate (Ritson 1982). At a population level, reducing the consumption of the larger numbers who drink too much alcohol but are not dependent may lead to greater overall reduction in harm than that which could be obtained by treating the minority with more severe drinking problems. Other important goals include attempting to alleviate concomitant social and psychological problems where this is possible since this may facilitate a change in problem substance use.

Readiness to change behaviour varies over time and this needs to be taken into account when attempting to set goals. Prochaska and DiClemente (1986) have described a stages-of-change model which is represented in Fig. 10.1.

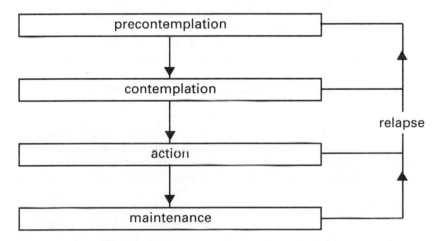

Figure 10.1 Stages of change (in boxes). Relapse may occur from one stage to any of the previous stages.

An individual in the stage of precontemplation has not even considered trying to change and may not feel that they have a problem. Treatment strategies include giving information about the substance and the consequences of its use. This needs to be done in an empathic and non-judgmental way in order not to alienate the individual. Attention may also be given to limiting the harm to the individual, for example giving thiamine to dependent heavy drinkers to prevent Wernicke's encephalopathy, syringe exchange schemes for injecting drug users, and helping third parties, such as assisting the spouse with coping strategies (Tober 1991).

At the stage of contemplation an individual is thinking about changing, but is ambivalent. Advice given on how to change is likely to be counterproductive, unless the ambivalence is first acknowledged and addressed. Probably only a third of heavy drinkers are ready to change, the rest being in the contemplation or precontemplation stages (Rollnick *et al*. 1992). Change may be facilitated by motivational interviewing (Miller and Rollnick 1991) in which the therapist takes a non-confrontational stance while seeking to develop discrepancy between the client's current behaviour and important goals. The aim is to lead the client to give reasons for wanting to change their behaviour, thereby increasing motivation to change. This is then fostered by supporting self-efficacy, that is, confidence that the individual can change. This may be achieved by conveying a message of personal responsibility to the client for changing and offering a selection of treatment choices.

By the stage of action an individual is ready to attempt change and it is at this point that conventional forms of treatment are appropriate. Goals should be set jointly with the client again to increase self-efficacy which predicts good outcome (Solomon and Annis 1990; Wilkinson and LeBreton 1986). Where spouse or other family members are supportive they too may usefully join in the setting of goals.

Once an individual has effected a change, different strategies may be needed to maintain the change. For example Prochaska (1983) found self-liberation, helping relationships, reinforcement management, counter-conditioning and stimulus control were all used in the action stage by smokers, but only the latter two were used in the maintenance stage. Treatment at this stage may include follow-up appointments for support and encouragement, self-help groups, 'dry' houses and residential rehabilitation.

An individual may be at different stages with different behaviours. For example an injecting drug user may be at the action stage with regard to sharing (using sterile equipment), contemplating with regard to stopping injecting (thinking of seeking treatment in the form of a methadone prescription), and at the precontemplation stage with regard to abstinence (no intention of stopping using opiates). Thus one can conceptualize a cascade of stages of change as an individual moves through a hierarchy of goals (Strang 1990).

At any stage an individual may relapse back to any of the earlier stages. Prochaska and DiClement's original work was done with smokers where they found smokers tended to move through the stages between three and seven times (with an average of four) before quitting for good. Thus earlier attempts at changing, rather than viewed with despondency, may be seen as dry runs which may teach lessons for later success. In addition the likelihood of relapse may be anticipated. Relapse prevention work (Marlatt and Gordon 1985) looks at high-risk situations where the client will be tempted to use. The main three high-risk situations are intrapersonal mental states such as anxiety or boredom, interpersonal conflicts such as arguments with the spouse, and social ones such as peer pressure and availability. A distinction is made between a lapse which is a slip or one-off use of the substance and relapse which is a return to the previous level of problem use. A lapse does not necessarily lead to relapse and can provide useful information to learn from. The treatment emphasis is on acquiring coping skills to deal with the high-risk situations and seeking to promote a more balanced and overall rewarding lifestyle.

Treatment of problem drinking

Excessive drinking may be successfully reduced with brief interventions (Bien *et al.* 1993). Key components include giving advice about the hazards of alcohol and ways to cut down or stop, giving reading materials on alcohol, and personalizing the health effects by, for example, linking symptoms of gastritis or the results of a blood test (such as liver function) to alcohol consumption. Such interventions may be carried out effectively in primary care or by generic community mental health workers. The majority of problem drinkers do not come into contact with specialist alcohol treatment services and so brief interventions by non-specialists may be a useful way of reaching a larger population of problem drinkers.

Individuals who are dependent on alcohol may require additional help. Detoxification can be done in an in-patient setting if available, although the majority occur in out-patients which may be more acceptable to some clients. Completion rates are enhanced if the individual has social support and the medication can be supervised (Stockwell *et al.* 1990). Alcohol withdrawal symptoms are covered by a benzodiazepine such as diazepam or chlordiazepoxide, or by chlormethiazole over a period of not more than ten days, and B vitamin supplements, particularly thiamine, are often given. Following detoxification, strategies to maintain abstinence focus on psychosocial support. In addition, alcohol sensitizing agents such as disulfiram, which causes unpleasant symptoms if taken with alcohol, can be effective in maintaining abstinence where support such as a spouse is available. Behaviour therapy and cognitive-behavioural therapy in the form of behavioural self-control training (Miller and Hester 1986), community reinforcement (Azrin *et al.* 1982), cue exposure (Drummond and Glautier 1994), relapse prevention (Annis and Peachey 1992), social skills training and marital therapy (Miller 1990) have been shown to be useful. Some individuals find self-help groups such as Alcoholics Anonymous (AA) to be helpful, and similar support for spouses may be obtained through Al-Anon. Drinkers with major social problems such as homelessness need a comprehensive social and health care management plan to achieve sustainable changes.

Treatment of opiate dependency

Brief detoxification over a period of up to three weeks can be conducted in an in-patient or out-patient setting. Symptomatic relief may be given with, for example, thioridazine plus diphenoxylate and atropine or with a substitute opiate, usually methadone, or with α adrenergic agonists such as clonidine or lofexidine. As an out-patient, slower detoxification with methadone is usually carried out in about three months. Longer term methadone prescribing is useful to allow individuals to attain a more stable lifestyle with improved physical and social well-being, in which criminal activity is reduced (Bell *et al.* 1992). Methadone maintenance has also been shown to be useful in helping reduce HIV risk behaviour (Ward *et al.* 1992). An important component of treatment with opiate misusers is counselling to reduce injecting and sexual risk-taking behaviours, together with the provision of sterile injecting equipment and condoms. Providing hepatitis B vaccination is also an important measure.

Some opiate misusers have additional psychopathology, particularly depression and anxiety, and these individuals may benefit from additional psychotherapy, such as supportive-expressive or cognitive-behavioural, while receiving methadone (Woody *et al*. 1987). More intensive psychotherapy with a relapse prevention focus in the context of a specialized in-patient setting has been shown to be more effective than routine care on a general psychiatric ward (Dawe *et al*. 1993). Such high-quality in-patient care may lead to abstinence in almost half of the treatment group at six months (Gossop *et al*. 1989). Residential rehabilitation projects provide shorter- or longer-term rehabilitation.

Similar to AA, Narcotics Anonymous (NA) provides peer support. Longer-term drug-free rehabilitation, sometimes with similar philosophies to NA, may be provided by therapeutic communities.

Treatment of benzodiazepine dependence

Broadly there are two main groups of individuals who are dependent on benzodiazepines. The larger are those who are legally prescribed them, usually as hypnotics or anxiolytics, although sometimes for depression. A minority use mainly illicit benzodiazepines, often chaotically in large doses in a binge fashion and with other illicit drugs.

Although only about a third of long-term benzodiazepine users will experience withdrawal symptoms, it is impossible to predict who will, and since such symptoms are potentially dangerous withdrawal should be slow, over at least six to eight weeks for the former group. It is usually best to convert the benzodiazepine to a long-acting one such as diazepam. In addition individuals may require psychological help for the disorder for which the medication was originally given. The latter group may need substitute prescribing and slow withdrawal, plus assistance with other illicit drugs or alcohol which are being misused. Temazepam is best avoided owing to its risk of being injected (Ruben and Morrison 1992; Strang *et al*. 1994).

Treatment of stimulant misuse

Individuals misusing stimulants such as amphetamine or cocaine can be advised to stop the drug use abruptly. Substitute prescribing in a manner similar to opiates is advocated by some practitioners but to date there is no good evidence of the benefits of such prescribing. There is some evidence that antidepressants such as desimpramine may help abstinence through reducing craving and anhedonia (Gawin and Ellinwood 1990). Useful forms of psychotherapy include relapse prevention and cognitive-behavioural therapy (Carroll *et al*. 1991). Cocaine Anonymous (CA), again similar to AA, has recently appeared as a self-help group.

Services for drug and alcohol misusers

There are two main levels of services for drug and alcohol users: those with a special interest in drugs or alcohol problems and other agencies without a special responsibility for these problems. The former include statutory and non-statutory residential and community-based services as well as self-help groups such as AA and NA. Drug and alcohol misusers, although coming into contact with a wide variety of agencies, may not make contact with specialist treatment services, particularly where individuals are in the precontemplation or contemplation stages of change. Obtaining money for illicit drug use often brings these individuals into contact with the police, prison or probation services. Many have housing or financial problems and may come into contact with the housing department or social services. A drug user may not have a GP, so may frequent the casualty department. A problem alcohol user may visit his or her GP for a gastric upset but not mention the alcohol use.

All these contacts are opportunities for intervention to nudge the individual's drug or alcohol career in a more beneficial direction. This may include the brief interventions described above, helping the individual to realize there is a problem, or suggesting a referral to a more specialist agency. However, this requires the workers at the non-specialist agencies to be able to identify drug and alcohol problems and to have the confidence and willingness to be able to intervene. The latter 'therapeutic commitment' for working with problem drinkers has been shown to depend on having knowledge of alcoholism and how to counsel problem drinkers, feeling supported to work with problem drinkers, and having experience of working with problem drinkers (Shaw *et al.* 1978; Clement 1986). Moreover, although many individuals working in agencies may not have therapeutic commitment, training may help to develop it (Shaw *et al.* 1978; Cartwright and Gorman 1993).

Some generic agencies have among their team individual social workers or probation officers with a special interest in drug or alcohol problems. They may act to enhance interagency cooperation and support others in their own agency to work with drug and alcohol misusers.

Community drug and alcohol teams

Community alcohol teams began to appear in the 1970s, followed a decade later by community drug teams. More recently combined teams have appeared who work with both drug and alcohol misusers. Their philosophy has been to facilitate the care of drug and alcohol misusers by generic workers by providing both training and support. They aim to stand at the interface between generalist care providers (such as general practitioners and generic social workers) and secondary specialist care (such as regional drug dependency units and residential therapeutic communities) and so in addition to be able to act as conduit to the latter specialist services.

Most of these teams provide information and advice (in person or by telephone) and offer counselling to drug and alcohol misusers. Support for generic workers may be provided in the form of consultation or shared care. The latter has sometimes been shown to be effective in involving general practitioners in the care of drug users (Greenwood 1992), although elsewhere this has been less successful (Strang *et al.* 1992). Providing a consultation service, despite being an aim of community drug teams at their inception, appears to be much harder to achieve. Thus community drug teams, rather than facilitating involvement by generic workers, may end up just providing a local specialist service (Strang *et al.* 1992). The same tension appears to operate in community alcohol teams, with a pressure from busy generic workers to refer on their problem drinkers rather than manage them themselves with assistance. A critical component to the success of a community alcohol team to support generic workers seems to be how much backing the generic workers have from their own management or expectation from colleagues from other professions to work with problem drinkers (Clement 1987). In effect not only must the individual have therapeutic commitment to working with drug and alcohol misusers, but so also must the agency within which the individual works have therapeutic commitment. The latter may be beyond the ability of a community drug or alcohol team alone, and may require political will in the form of a higher priority given to working with drug and alcohol misusers by generic agencies and the resources to be able to do this.

Concomitant with community teams increasingly providing direct care, additional services emerging include outreach or detached street work, physical primary health care and needle exchanges. There is evidence that needle exchanges may have helped to reduce sharing equipment among injecting drug users (Donoghoe *et al.* 1992; Keene *et al.* 1993). The outreach work has aimed to contact groups who may find it difficult to access existing services and who may be at high risk of misusing substances or have special needs. This may include the young, women, ethnic minorities, and stimulant users. Such outreach services manage to contact users who are not in contact with services, but in many settings the volume of activity and the cost per contact may call into question the overall utility of such services (Department of Health 1993; Rhodes 1993).

Targeting treatment for particular groups

Young

The young are of particular concern, since most adults with drug and alcohol problems start the substance use before adulthood, although 90 per cent of adolescent drug abusers will not go on to have drug problems as adults. Over the last two decades there has been a steady increase in prevalence of drug and alcohol use among the young, with a threefold increase in the prevalence of alcohol use. There has also been a fall in the age of induction into drug and alcohol use with initiation into drug use decreasing from 18–20 years to 13–15 years for drugs. Alcohol is about two years earlier. The main substance regularly used is alcohol, plus experimentation with cannabis and solvents, although there is also increasing use of 'Ecstasy' and 'crack' cocaine. (Zeithlin and Swaidi 1991).

Parental attitudes appear to affect whether a young person takes drugs or not. Peers seem to influence the pattern of drug use. Drug use in adolescence is likely to lead not only to continued drug use, but also to a high rate of aggression, anti-social behaviour, and legal, occupational and marital problems. Some of these difficulties may predate the onset of drug use, although drug use may also be a causal or aggressive factor.

Treatment of this group is difficult since they are hard to access. Wherever possible it is generally helpful to involve the parents and generic youth services have a key role to play. To date there are very few specialist services for the young user. Prevention is probably best targeted at children before they have been introduced to drugs with the aims of altering attitudes and preventing or at least delaying initiation. So far, prevention programmes have tended to be targeted at an older age group and have not been well evaluated (Zeitlin and Swadi 1991).

Women

Although the onset of problem drinking occurs at a later age in women than in men, women are more vulnerable to brain and liver damage. Heavy drinking during pregnancy is associated with the fetal alcohol syndrome which can include reduced growth, mental retardation and various other physical abnormalities. Opiate abuse during pregnancy may be less directly toxic, mainly leading to low birth weight. The lack of antenatal care plus poor nutrition and general health care may lead to premature delivery and obstetric complications. Pregnant drug and alcohol users may be afraid to present to antenatal care owing to fears of staff attitudes and of their baby being taken into care. There is the risk of transmission of HIV and babies born to opiate-dependent women may show signs of withdrawal (Gerada and Farrell 1990).

It is important to attempt to attract pregnant drug and alcohol users into antenatal care as early as possible and to liaise with all agencies involved to attempt to improve health and antenatal care and ameliorate the drug or alcohol problem.

Elderly

The main problem substances among the elderly are alcohol and tranquilizers, especially benzodiazepines. The elderly are more sensitive to the adverse effects of these drugs, yet their misuse may be easily missed (McInnes and Powell 1994). Elderly people may find it difficult to fit into services designed predominantly for younger adults so their treatment may be best delivered through existing services for the elderly (Dunne 1994).

Prostitutes

A high proportion of prostitutes may also be injecting drug users (Green *et al.* 1993) and so are at health risks from both sexual activity and drug use. Only a minority of drug-using prostitutes may be in contact with community drug teams and a half may be without a general practitioner. They may fail to make appropriate use of health care services because of the covert nature of most prostitution, the fear of admitting to illegal drug use, a chaotic lifestyle centred around procuring drugs and the fear of losing care and custody of their children (Faugier *et al.* 1992). In addition they may have practical, social and legal problems which may seem more pressing than their own health. Male prostitutes are at particular risk.

Ethnic minorities

The needs of different ethnic minority communities should be considered as part of general service needs assessment. There is generally a lack of good data on the prevalence of drug dependence and problems among differing groups and it may be difficult to ascertain whether the needs are being properly served by simply counting past service contacts. Often services will be perceived as being difficult to access and there is a need to target information and tailor services in a culturally sensitive manner to ensure maximum access for all members of the community. Outreach services in particular may be specifically targeted at ethnic groups and may involve the mobilization of ethnic peer group projects. It is as important not to assume the presence of problems in one ethnic group by extrapolating from the general community, as it is to be able to identify and respond to unique probems.

Conclusion

Alcohol and drug misuse presents a great challenge to the community. It leads to a substantial morbidity and mortality as well as legal and other social problems. Typically it has been an area where intervention has been viewed with pessimism or seen as best left to specialist services. However, the extent of the problem makes it impossible for specialist services alone to deal with it and many substance misusers never make contact with such services. Over time individuals do change their substance misusing behaviour and this may be facilitated by workers who are therapeutically committed to working with these clients. To be successful this requires cooperation by workers from all disciplines who may contact substance misusing individuals. By taking a long-term perspective, they may assist clients with drug or alcohol problems to move towards a healthier way of life.

References

Annis H M and Peachey J E (1992). The use of calcium carbide in relapse prevention counselling: results of a randomized controlled trial. *British Journal of Addiction*, **87**, 63–72.

Ashton H and Golding J F (1989). Tranquillisers: prevalence, predictors and possible consequences. Data from a large United Kingdom survey. *British Journal of Addiction*, **84**, 541–546.

Azrin N H, Sisson R W, Meyers R and Godley M (1982). Alcoholism treatment by disulfiram and community reinforcement therapy. *Journal of Behavior Therapy and Experimental Psychiatry*, **13**, 105–112.

Bell J, Hall W and Byth K (1992). Changes in criminal activity after entering methadone maintenance. *British Journal of Addiction*, **87**, 251–258.

Benzeval M, Judge K and Solomon M (1992). *The Health Status of Londoners: A Comparative Perspective*. King's Fund, London.

Bien, T H, Miller, W R and Tonigen J S (1993). Brief interventions for alcohol problems; a review. *Addiction*, **88**, 315–336.

Carroll K M, Rounsaville B J and Gawin F H (1991). A comparative trial of psychotherapies for the treatment of cocaine abuse. *American Journal of Drug and Alcohol Abuse*, **17**, 229–247.

Cartwright A K J and Gorman D M (1993). Processes involved in changing the therapeutic attitudes of clinicians toward working with drinking clients. *Psychotherapy Research*, **3**(2), 95–104.

Chaisson R E, Bacchetti P, Osmond D, Brodie B, Sande M A and Moss A R (1989). Cocaine use and HIV infection in intravenous drug users in San Francisco. *Journal of the American Medical Association*, **261**, 561–565.

Clement S (1986) The identification of alcohol-related problems by general practitioners. *British Journal of Addiction*, **81**, 257–264

Clement S (1987). The Salford experiment: an account of the community alcohol team approach. In *Helping the Problem Drinker: New Initiatives in Community Care* (eds. T Stockwell and S Clement). Croom Helm, London.

Cox B D, Huppert F A and Whichelow B (eds.)(1993). *The Health and Lifestyle Survey: Seven Years On*. Dartmoor Publishing Company Limited, Aldershot.

Dawe S, Powell J, Richards D, Gossop M, Marks I, Strang J and Gray J A (1993). Does post-withdrawal cue exposure improve outcome in opiate addiction? A controlled trial. *Addiction*, **88**, 1233–1245.

Department of Health, Scottish Office Home and Health Department, Welsh Office (1991). *Drug Misuse and Dependence. Guidelines on Clinical Management*. HMSO, London.

Department of Health (1993). *AIDS and Drug Misuse Update*. Report by the Advisory Council on the Misuse of Drugs. HMSO, London.

Donoghoe M C, Dolan K A and Stimson G (1992). Life-style factors and social circumstances of syringe sharing in injecting drug users. *British Journal of Addiction*, **87**, 993–1003.

Drummond D C and Glautier S (1994). A controlled trial of cue exposure treatment in alcohol dependence. *Journal of Consulting and Clinical Psychology*, **62**(4), 809–817.

Dunne F (1994). Misuse of drugs or alcohol by elderly people. *British Medical Journal*, **308**, 608–609.

Edwards G, (1984). Drinking in longitudinal perspective: career and natural history. *British Journal of Addiction*, **79**, 175–183.

Edwards G. Duckitt A, Oppenheimer E, Sheehan M and Taylor C (1983). What happens to alcoholics? *Lancet* **ii**, 269–271.

Edwards G, Brown D, Duckitt A, Oppenheimer E, Sheehan M and Taylor C (1987). Outcome of alcoholism: the structure of patient attributions as to what causes change. *British Journal of Addiction*, **82**, 533–545.

Edwards G, Brown D, Oppenheimer E, Sheehan M, Taylor C and Duckitt A (1988). Long term outcome for patients with drinking problems: the search for predictors. *British Journal of Addiction*, **83**, 917–927.

Faugier J, Hayes C and Butterworth C A (1992). *Drug Using Prostitutes, Their Health Care Needs, and Their Clients*. University of Manchester.

Gawin F and Ellinwood E H (1990). Cocaine abuse treatment: open pilot trial with desipramine and lithium carbonate. *Archives of General Psychiatry*, **41**, 903–909.

Gerada C and Farrell M (1990). Management of the pregnant opiate user. *British Journal of Hospital Medicine*, **43**, 138–141.

Gossop M, Green L, Philips G and Bradley B (1989). Lapse, relapse and survival among opiate addicts. *British Journal of Psychiatry*, **154**, 348–353.

Green S T, Goldberg D J, Christie P R, Frischer M, Thomson A, Carr A T and Taylor A (1993). Female streetworkers – prostitutes in Glasgow: a descriptive study of their lifestyle. *AIDS Care*, **5**(3), 321–335.

Greenwood J (1992). Persuading general practitioners to prescribe – good husbandry or a recipe for chaos? *British Journal of Addiction*, **87**, 567–575.

Hartnoll R L, Mitcheson M C, Lewis R and Bryer S (1985). Estimating the prevalence of opioid dependence. *Lancet*, **i**, 203–205.

HMSO (1992). *Lord President's Report on Action Against Alcohol Misuse*. HMSO, London.

Holder H and Blose J O (1992). The reduction of health care costs associated with alcoholism treatment: a 14 year longitudinal study. *Journal of Studies on Alcohol*, **53**, 293–302.

Holder H and Parker R N (1992). Effects of alcoholism treatment on cirrhosis mortality: a 20-year multivariate time series analysis. *British Journal of Addiction*, **87**, 1263–1274.

Home Office (1993*a*). *Statistics of the Misuse of Drugs: Addicts Notified to the Home Office, United Kingdom 1992*. Home Office, London.

Home Office (1993*b*). *Statistics of Drug Seizures and Offenders Dealt with, United Kingdom 1992*. Home Office, London.

Hser Y, Anglin D and Powers K (1993). A 24-year follow-up of California narcotics addicts. *Archives of General Psychiatry*, **50**, 577–584.

Johnson B D, Goldstein P J, Preble E, Schmeidler J, Lipton D S, Sprunt B and Miller T (1985). *Taking Care of Business: The Economics of Crime by Heroin Abusers*. Lexington Books, Lexington, Mass.

Keene J, Stimson G V, Jones S and Parry-Langdon N (1993). Evaluation of syringe-exchange for HIV prevention among injecting drug users in rural and urban areas of Wales. *Addiction*, **88**, 1063–1070.

Klee H, Faugier J, Hayes C, Boulton T and Morris T (1990). AIDS-related risk behaviour, polydrug use and temazepam. *British Journal of Addiction*, **85**, 1125–1132.

Ludwig A M (1985). Cognitive processes associated with 'spontaneous' recovery from alcoholism. *Journal of Studies on Alcohol*, **46**, 53–58.

Maddux J F and Desmond D P (1979). Crime and drug abuse behaviour: an area analysis. *Criminology*, **19**, 281–302.

Magura S, Kang S Y, Shapiro J and O'Day J (1993). HIV risk among women injecting drug users who are in jail. *Addiction*, **88**, 1351–1360.

Mann R E, Smart R G, Anglin L *et al.* (1988). Are decreases in liver cirrhosis rates a result of increased treatment for alcoholism? *British Journal of Addiction*, **83**, 683–688.

Marlatt G A and Gordon J R (1985). *Relapse Prevention: Maintenance Strategies in the Treatment of Addictive Behaviors*. Guilford, New York.

Mayfield D, MacLeod G and Hall P (1974). The CAGE questionnaire: validation of a new alcoholism screening instrument. *American Journal of Psychiatry*, **131**, 1121–1123.

McInnes E and Powell J (1994). Drug and alcohol referrals: are elderly substance abuse diagnoses and referrals being missed? *British Medical Journal*, **308**, 444–446.

Miller W R (1990). Alcohol treatment alternatives: what works? In *Treatment Choices for Alcohol and Substance Abuse (*eds. H B Milkman and L I Sederer). Lexington Books/D C Heath, Lexington, Mass.

Miller W R and Hester R (1986). Inpatient alcoholism treatment: who benefits? *American Psychologist*, **41**, 794–805.

Miller W R and Rollnick S (1991). *Motivational Interviewing. Preparing People to Change Addictive Behavior*. Guilford, New York.

Moos R H (1994). Why do some people recover from alcohol dependence, whereas others continue to drink and become worse over time? *Addiction*, **89**, 31–34.

OPCS (1988). *General Household Survey*, HMSO, London.

Parker H, Newcombe R and Bakx K (1987). The new heroin users: prevalence and characteristics in Wirral, Merseyside. *British Journal of Addiction*, **82**, 147–157.

Prochaska J O and DiClemente C C (1983). Stages and processes of self-change of smoking: towards an integrative model of change. *Journal of Consulting and Clinical Psychology*, **51**, 390–395.

Prochaska, J O and DiClemente C C (1986). Toward a comprehensive model of change. In *Treating Addictive Behaviours. Processes of Change* (eds. W R Miller, and N Heather). Plenum Press, New York, pp. 3–26.

Raistrick, D. (1991). Career and natural history. In *The International Handbook of*

Addiction Behaviour (ed. I B Glass). Routledge, London.

Rhodes T (1993). Time for community change: what has outreach to offer? *Addiction*, **88**, 1317–1320.

Ritson B (1982). Helping the problem drinker. *British Medical Journal*, **284**, 327–329.

Robins L N, Davis D H and Goodwin D W (1974). Drug use by the US army enlisted men in Vietnam: a follow-up on their return home. *American Journal of Epidemiology*, **99**, 235–249.

Rollnick S, Heather N, Gold R and Hall W (1992). Development of a short 'readiness to change' questionnaire for use in brief, opportunistic interventions among excessive drinkers. *British Journal of Addiction*, **87**, 743–754.

Royal College of General Practitioners (1986). *Alcohol – A Balanced View*. RCGP, London.

Ruben S M and Morrison C L (1992). Temazepam misuse in a group of injecting drug users. *British Journal of Addiction*, **87**, 1387–1392.

Saunders W M and Kershaw P W (1979). Spontaneous remission from alcoholism – a community study. *British Journal of Addiction*, **74**, 251–265.

Schuckitt M A (1989). *Drug and Alcohol Abuse: a Clinical Guide to Diagnosis and Treatment*, 3rd edn. Plenum Press, New York.

Selzer M C (1971). The Michigan alcoholism screening test: the quest for a new diagnostic instrument. *American Journal of Psychiatry*, **127**, 1653–1658.

Shaw S, Cartwright A, Spratley T and Harwin J (1978). *Responding to Drinking Problems*. Croom Helm. London.

Simpson D D, Joe G W, Lehman W E K and Sells S B (1986). Addiction careers: etiology, treatment, and 12-year follow-up outcomes. *The Journal of Drug Issues*, **16** (1), 107–121.

Solomon K E and Annis H M (1990). Outcome and efficacy expectancy in the prediction of post-treatment drinking behaviour. *British Journal of Addiction*, **85**, 659–665.

Stockwell T, Bolt L, Milner I, Hugh P and Young I (1990). Home detoxification for problem drinkers: acceptability to clients, relatives, general practitioners and outcome after 60 days. *British Journal of Addiction*, **85**, 61–70.

Strang J (1990). Intermediate goals and the process of change. In *AIDS and Drug Misuse* (eds. J Strang and G Stimson). *The Challenge for Policy and Practice in the 1990s*. Routledge, London.

Strang J, Smith M and Spurrell S (1992). The community drug team. *British Journal of Addiction*, **87**, 5–14.

Strang J, Johns A and Caan W (1993). Cocaine in the UK – 1991. *British Journal of Psychiatry*, **162,** 1–13.

Strang J, Griffiths P, Abbey J and Gossop M (1994). Survey of use of injected benzodiazepines among drug users in Britain. *British Medical Journal*, **308**, 1082.

Swadi H (1988). Drug and substance use among 3,333 adolescents. *British Journal of Addiction*, **83**, 935–942.

Taylor C, Brown D, Duckitt A, Edwards G. Oppenheimer E and Sheehan M (1985). Patterns of outcome: drinking histories over ten years among a group of alcoholics. *British Journal of Addiction*, **80** 45–50.

Temple M T and Leino E V (1989). Long-term outcomes of drinking: a 20-year longitudinal study of men. *British Journal of Addiction*, **84**, 889–899.

Tober G (1991). Helping the pre-contemplator. In *Counselling Problem Drinkers* (eds. R Davidson, S Rollnick and I MacEwan). Routledge, London.

Tuchfield B S (1981). Spontaneous remission in alcoholics: empirical observations and theoretical implications. *Journal of Studies on Alcohol*, **42**, 626–641.

Vaillant G E (1973). A 20-year follow up of New York narcotic addicts. *Archives of General Psychiatry*, **39**, 127–141.

Vaillant G E (1983). *The Natural History of Alcoholism*. Harvard University Press, Cambridge, Mass.

Vaillant G E (1988). What can long-term follow-up teach us about relapse and prevention of relapse in addiction? *British Journal of Addiction*, **83**, 1147–1157.

Wagstaff A and Maynard A (1988). *Economic Aspects of the Illicit Drug Market and Drug Enforcement Policies in the United Kingdom*. Home Office Research Unit study, No. 95. HMSO, London.

Ward J, Darke S, Hall W and Mattick R (1992). Methadone maintenance and the human immunodeficiency virus: current issues in treatment and research. *British Journal of Addiction*, **87**, 447–453.

Wilkinson D A and LeBreton S (1986). Early indications of treatment outcome in multiple drug users. In *Treating Addictive Behaviors. Processes of Change* (eds. W R Miller and N Heather). Plenum, New York.

Winick C (1962). Maturing out of narcotic addiction. *Bulletin on Narcotics*, **14**, 1–7.

Woody G E, McLellan A T, Luborsky L and O'Brien C P (1987). Twelve-month follow-up of psychotherapy for opiate dependence. *American Journal of Psychiatry*, **144**, 590–596.

Zeitlin H and Swadi H (1991). Adolescence: the genesis of addiction. In *The International Handbook of Addiction Behaviour* (ed. I B Glass). Routledge, London.

11 Shifting into community focus: a pastoral perspective

M. R. Sutherland

Introduction

This volume contains widely differing perspectives on interprofessional cooperation in community mental health care. At the time of writing a significant shift in focus is moving mental health care away from its traditional base in hospital institutions towards the setting of the community. This chapter is organized against the background of this shift. I would contend that this is a shift which not only affects the nature and style of mental health care provision but will profoundly affect the dynamics influencing the interprofessional relationships between health care professionals.

My task in this chapter is to write about the pastoral contribution to the widening perspective of interprofessional cooperation in mental health. The focus is interprofessional working in the community and this introduces an immediate difficulty. The contribution pastoral care makes to interprofessional working in the community has been hampered by the exclusion of pastors and pastoral care from health care team settings. Generally speaking, there has been little cooperation between community-based pastors and mental health care teams in the community. Therefore, in this chapter I will focus on the contribution pastoral care has made to hospital-based interprofessional cooperation in mental health care, with particular reference to the way interprofessional dynamics are likely to change under the influence of the move from hospital to community focused care.

I employ the term 'mental health' to include the term psychiatry. This is not to confuse the two. While psychiatry may be the most dominant of the several disciplinary components of mental health care, it is essentially only one component and can be, and often is, viewed as separate. Behind any discussion of the pastoral contribution, it is necessary to bear in mind the still uneasy debate concerning the way psychiatry and other mental health care disciplines fit together.

Important, but hopefully complementary, distinctions continue to emerge within the debate about the pastoral contribution to mental health care. It is important to draw a distinction between the psychiatric chaplain as the mental health expert and the parochial pastor who, while not being a mental health expert, is often intimately concerned for, and involved with, persons with mental health issues. Some of these persons, though by no means all, will attract the attention of the community and hospital mental health services.

Before I turn to an exploration of the contribution which can be made by pastoral care to community mental health, some understanding of wider interprofessional dynamics is required. Existing interprofessional dynamics have been powerfully shaped by the institution of the hospital. Although the work of the hospital is distinct, its organization and social operation share characteristics which can be clearly associated with the structure of public institutions in our society. Institutions, by their nature and reason for existing, tend towards centralization and stratification of decision-making and task monitoring. This produces hierarchical and authoritarian relationships.

Institutional dynamics are complex examples of what happens to us when we encounter one another in collective or group experience (De Board 1978). Community dynamics, being no less complex, are in reality different. Therefore the setting in which the activity of care occurs imposes its own stamp upon the way interprofessional relationships are conducted.

Different schools of psychology and organizational theory offer alternative ways of understanding interprofessional dynamics (De Board 1978). The late James Mathers (1976) drew a simple analogy between the human body and human society. He describes how the human body's complex sensory neuron system coordinates motor neuron activity. This system collects, processes and communicates information via the central nervous system. In comparing biological and organizational communication systems, he noted that organizational life operates with a less developed and more primitive communication structure. Our social enterprises have developed a strong command structure designed for task performance. Nevertheless, highly complex tasks are accomplished through crude hierarchical and authoritarian command structures which exact a high toll in terms of psychological and emotional stress, pain and strain. Only in the face of a perceived threat to life does the biological communication system permit the body to risk levels of stress and exertion which could seriously damage it. It does this through marshalling an emergency communication (adrenalin) carried throughout the body. This adrenalin message overrides other kinds of stress and pain sensors. In our social organization intolerable (adrenalin) levels of stress are inflicted upon individuals as the cost paid for normal cooperative achievement. High levels of pain are tolerated in institutions because they have not yet evolved pain and stress sensors which operate independently of the command structure. Mathers (1976) notes that 'whenever power and information flow in the same channel, the information becomes distorted' (p. 10).

Enormous distortions occur within organizations which create levels of distress, which in turn result in the brutal way institutions deal with the people who inhabit them. This brutality is an everyday feature of institutional life and rather than serving the efficiency of task achievement, as is commonly believed, it diverts energy away from task performance toward attack and defensive activity. The diversion of energy in this way detracts from, and on occasion can bring to a halt, effective task performance. Usually this situation is masked from our attention through what Bion (1961) has termed basic assumption behaviour. In particular relation to health care activities, the work of Isabel Menzies-Lyth (1989) clearly demonstrates these processes in action.

Community mental health care inherits an interprofessional model based on the psychiatric hospital's institutional dynamic. My experience working in institutions is that conscious and unconscious layers of interprofessional rivalries lead to a taking up of professional roles in ways which either initiate or reinforce interprofessional conflicts. One of the significant aspects of my work as a psychiatric hospital chaplain has been in the area of consulting with interprofessional staff groups. Although an analysis of interprofessional dynamics within psychiatric institutions would take me well beyond the scope of the present chapter, this has been well documented elsewhere (Stanton and Schwarz 1954). It is sufficient for me to characterize the situation in my own hospital institution as one of interprofessional cohabitation rather than cooperation.

Interprofessional 'cooperation' is a term which we increasingly encounter. However, like collegiality (a term more familiar within church circles), the actual practice indicated is more difficult to specify. Interprofessional cooperation is often used by psychiatrists to mean the agreement or acquiescence of other professional groups within a medical model framework of treatment. I have heard nurses talk of cooperation in situations more appropriately described with reference to a lack of interference, or an attitude of indifference from other more powerful professions which avoids a situation of overt conflict. As a chaplain, I use the term to refer to the way professionals find it possible to take up their work-related roles within a shared operational and conceptual space. This is in recognition of both their separate links to the patient, and their links with one another through a sharing of the patient. The patient is not a divisible unit. The patient is an essential unity of differentiated needs which come to be reflected, and hopefully met, in the cooperative activity of the interprofessional team. The team can reflect this unity through its own sense of interconnectedness around the patient, or it can reflect an image of the patient distorted and fragmented along the lines of interprofessional demarcation.

Psychologically, the hope is for roles to be taken up in the service of the patient's mental health care needs rather than in defence against anxiety. I have mentioned that some of this anxiety is evoked through coming together for cooperative activity. These are the common anxieties of competition, rivalry and fear of difference. Anxiety in interprofessional working is also evoked by identification with patients and their experience of illness producing a spectre of dependency and the fear of being overwhelmed (Menzies-Lyth 1988). Cooperation aims at avoiding a situation in which the patient's needs are fragmented and parcelled out between competing professional activities. R D Laing (1967), identifying the mechanisms of depersonalization, reification, splitting, and denial, as characterizing psychiatric illness, noted that these mechanisms also come to characterize the attempts to treat illness. Lack of interprofessional cooperation leads to attempted therapeutic practices which tend in themselves to exhibit the symptoms with which they are attempting to deal.

The patient may instigate, exploit or collude with interprofessional and interpersonal rivalries. Main (1989) addresses the issues of rivalry arising within interprofessional situations and their relationship to issues of projection and identification between the care giver and the care receiver. Interprofessional conflicts also have deep roots in the experience of differentials in power between professions. Difference in function is represented by hierarchical status. Differentials in interprofessional power relate to the way society confers authority upon certain professional groups. Nowhere is this more clearly seen than in the degree to which society entrusts psychiatry with powers unprecedented outside the criminal justice system. In return for this authority, society requires a high degree of accountability from psychiatry for the policing of mental health safety. In the exercise of this responsibility psychiatry employs a medical model derived from the treatment of physical diseases. The problem, as I see it, is that this model continues to replicate the historical masculine/feminine relationship between male physicians and female nurses with all the attendant social constructions concerning the superiority of masculine modes of thought, organization and values. The historically and sociologically constituted relations between medicine and nursing remain appreciably unaltered by the fact that women are doctors and that, within nursing, men exercise considerable authority. Interprofessional working which fails to address the way interprofessional relationships replicate wider historical and social patterns of power inequality will be in danger of having its therapeutic aims diverted by conflict.

Current issues in interprofessional cooperation

Models of community-based mental health care are, for the most part, only recently being developed as a response to care in the community legislation. As this shift into community care gains momentum what will the model of interprofessional cooperation look like? Two crucial areas will require urgent exploration. The first concerns the nature and style of leadership within the community-based mental health care team. Is an institutionally derived style of medical leadership an appropriate model to translate into the community? The second area relates to the relationship between preexisting community-based primary care agencies and new community mental health care structures. Within the scope of this chapter I do not attempt to address the first of these areas. However, the second area directly raises issues likely to be of more direct concern when considering the contribution made by a pastoral component to interprofessional cooperation in community mental health care.

After seven years' experience in parish ministry I moved from the community into the institutional setting of psychiatric hospital chaplaincy. This could be seen as a move in the opposite direction to the current shift away from hospital-based care. My experience has nevertheless highlighted for me some of the differences between the dynamics of care in the two different settings. Hospital chaplaincy provides a location from which to comment on the pastor's role and the contribution made by pastoral care to the wider interdisciplinary context of existing mental health care provision. I am not advocating hospital chaplaincy as a model for community pastoral care, but it does provide a particular flavour of the issues raised by the inclusion of a pastoral and spiritual contribution within cooperative interprofessional working in community mental health care.

The shift towards community-based care

The shift from the hospital to the community is a complex matter. What is involved is little short of a revolution in conceptions concerning the way care is to be delivered. Something of this revolution can already be seen in the changing relationship between providers and recipients of care, as patient groups politicize into user movements. This shift signifies a different power relationship between people with mental health problems and the mental health services. In my own hospital this is an area in which there is already an extensive degree of pastoral care involvement.

The chaplaincy has facilitated the meeting of a patient group for many years. This group, under the title of 'Faith and Doubt', has met once a week to discuss and argue the widest range of issues and experiences occasioned by the experience of mental health problems. After 15 years the group's weekly meetings are currently in abeyance, and it is unclear to me whether this is a temporary state or a more permanent one. The group's life has ebbed and flowed considerably over the years. However, what had been clear to me for some time is that this traditional hospital-based group was no longer meeting the same needs it once did. In the past, it may have been appropriate for a largely in-patient group to meet in this format. Such a group arose from within the strictly limited circumstances of a hospital setting in which the chaplaincy provided one of the few locations for the expression of dissent. By contrast, the present situation reflects an increasingly politicized group of mental health service users who now have access to their own local user forums and other community advocacy agencies.

It is my view that change between care-taker and user reflects the way in which more egalitarian community dynamics are already successfully challenging the institutional models of care. This makes inevitable the need for a recognition of a similar process of revolutionary change occurring within the arena of interprofessional cooperation, although in such an arena revolutionary change may be slower to take effect.

Institutional projections upon community-based professionals

The hospital represents a power base for the medical and nursing professions. Hospitals are places for medical speciality and expertise. This reflects the tendency in the West for excellence to be institutionally rather than community focused. The most powerful professions are those who have built strong institutional power bases: lawyers, doctors and to a lesser extent nurses and university teachers.

Compared with hospital-based medical specialists, GPs are seen as less skilled and less competent. Within medicine, as in many other branches of learning and skilled endeavour, a hierarchy exists between those based within the institutional centres of excellence and those members of the profession who choose to be community-based generalists.

Perhaps this model originally began in the church with its prestigious monasteries and humble community-based parishes. The prestige of the monasteries in some cases was passed on to the university and the cathedral. But in most cases the monastery legacy faded away, unable to adapt to social and political change, leaving behind the less powerful, yet more adaptable, parish structure. Is there a lesson for other institutions to learn here?

Nursing resembles medicine in reproducing a split between institutional and community-based groups. It is interesting to note the fate of community psychiatric nurses (CPNs) within the organization of community sector teams. In my own hospital these teams have been disbanded. Although there was a need to rework CPNs into new integrated nursing teams, the impression is easily formed that in the eyes of hospital-based professionals the CPN ethos, developed and successfully employed for use in community settings, was perceived as time costly, excessively therapeutic as opposed to managerial, and too highly graded, i.e. expensive.

Against which criteria are these judgments made? Such judgments do not reflect the values of the community into which the CPNs ventured. The CPNs experienced the frustrations and pains of their clients without the protection of the hospital clinic. Exercising one's professional skill in the squalor and poverty of an inner city bedsit can be a frightening and humbling experience which can make one feel extremely vulnerable. Foskett (1994) writes movingly of his experience of working with this group of professional nurses. He seems to suggest that it was their success in adapting their working models to the values of their clients which singled them out for the fearful projections of an elitist, institutionally-based psychiatry, frightened to get its hands dirty: 'They have forsaken the wisdom of hospital medicine. Is it expedient that they die? They certainly wonder what has become of them.' There is a sense that existing community-based psychiatric nursing, regarded as a costly experiment, has now been brought back into line.

The anxiety communicated to me as a chaplain surrounding the role of CPNs reminds me of the colonial anxiety concerning those who lived away from the centres of colonial life. They were said to have 'gone native'. Behind this expression lies the fear about 'difference' and the maintenance of rigid and artificial distinctions between people. Up country, the distinction between colonial masters and colonized was more difficult to maintain because it seemed to make much less sense.

Something similar seems to operate in the shift from hospitals to community care. Professions or groups within professions who are community-based are tainted by being seen to be closer to lay ways of thinking than professional colleagues who remain within the protected and artificial environment of the hospital. Community care engenders more intimate, less formal relationships between care giver and care receiver. For some professions this will be easier to manage than for others. The questions raised earlier about the nature of leadership in interprofessional teams and the relationship between the new secondary sector and primary care agencies will form an important focus for understanding evolving dynamics and ensuing interprofessional conflicts. Foskett writes of the CPNs that 'They have made friends with the sick and the general practitioners, the minor officials of the priestly caste.' The minor official of the priestly caste can be interpreted as both a reference to lowly GPs and the parochial clergy. Both share the odium of a perceived lowliness which, I believe, is largely the consequence of their community work setting.

The *'parson'* is an old English word literally meaning the 'person'. The parson remains the only professional intimately associated with the community in which they work. The increasing 'professionalization' of the 19th century which distanced the professions from their community positions left the clergy behind. Consequently, along with those other groups of the sick, women and, more recently, the unemployed, the clergy bear the taint attached to all groups left at home after the men have gone away to work.

The pastor and formal mental health care

In the early years of this century Richard Cabot, professor of medicine at Harvard, followed his pioneering development of medical social work with *A Plea for a Clinical Year in the Course of Theological Study*. When published in 1925, this treatise laid the foundations for clinical pastoral education (Hall 1992).

Anton Boisen, known as the 'father of clinical pastoral theology' (Eastman 1951), further developed this educational method within the specific context of the psychiatric hospital. Strongly influenced by William James and Sigmund Freud, Boisen (1930) developed a method of theological enquiry for pastors working with persons suffering from mental illness, which he called the study of 'living human documents'. In Britain, the inclusion of hospital chaplaincy within the over-arching vision of the National Health Service brought the clergy into formal relationship with health care. Chaplains once more became part of hospital establishments, many of which were originally the creation of religious houses dedicated to the church's ministry to the sick. However, the chaplain's association with the church, a community-based institution, has always carried a serious disadvantage for them in negotiation with other health care professions.

Depending on one's perspective, the position of the chaplain within the mental health care team is both unique and also anomalous. No matter how involved a chaplain may be with a particular patient or group of patients, among all the other professionals who make up the health care team he or she is alone in not being responsible for any aspect of the patient's treatment. The chaplain is concerned with the overall well-being of the patient as a human being. The 'living human document' is one in which the spirit, mind and body cannot be treated separately. They form an essential unity of personhood and can only be understood together, within as much of the patient's emotional and social history as can be discovered.

Soon after my appointment as a hospital chaplain I encountered a particular consultant who always insisted that his patients had the right not to see the chaplain. This was not an opinion as much as a policy statement. I was ready to receive this as an expression of psychiatric hostility. However, I came to see that the psychiatrist's attitude was a recognition of the value of having a professional who had no power to force himself upon the patient. This enabled my position to be highlighted in a way which communicated to the patient that I was someone who could be approached and related to in quite a different way.

The confidentiality still attaching to communications with the clergy and my distance from the enforcement of treatment decisions opened up the possibility for a more informal and flexible relationship between myself and the patient. While I had a responsibility not to interfere with the treatment, I could afford to be less defensive in the face of patient complaints and distress resulting from elements within the treatment itself.

This consultant genuinely wanted his patients to have a friend at court. By insisting that the chaplain participate in team decisions concerning the patient only with the permission of the patient, he was making it clear that the power to involve me somehow rested with the patient.

This example can be balanced by others in which the attitude among health care professionals towards my involvement has been one of uncertainty and insecurity. This will often reflect a situation in which all interprofessional relationships are tainted with suspicion, in attempting to divide the patient up into autonomous areas for the exercise of professional expertise. The area allowed to me will be the patient's spirituality, narrowly confined so as to prevent me from connecting spirituality with psychological, emotional and social aspects of the patient's experience. Confidentiality is a central issue in these instances. Confidentiality is often misused by health care professionals to exclude chaplains and pastors. However, the anxiety is not that we cannot be trusted but that we are likely to enjoy particular confidences which patients deliberately keep from their doctors and nurses.

This raises the important question: does the chaplain, and even more so the parish pastor, come within the boundary of the team's shared confidentiality or not? I have often been left with the feeling that other team members do not know if I can be trusted. To an extent I understand this anxiety; it is based on the recognition that there is a difference between us. If the patients control their access to me, might they also control me? In any conflict between the team and the patient it is not a foregone conclusion whose side I would be on. This was often presented as staff uncertainty about confiding in me which I felt masked their envy concerning the way patients communicate very private matters to the chaplain. While this often will be quite appropriate, such communications can also be a secret attack upon the health care team. In the above example, the consultant and his team displayed an implicit trust in my knowing the difference between communications from patients which specifically related to their relationship with me and those which may have had another purpose. These are often prefaced by, 'You won't tell this to anyone else will you?'

The chaplain is under a strict duty not to withhold information which could relate to the treatment of the patient. How is this duty to be reconciled with the ancient obligation of confidentiality invoked by the patient? In the reported instance above, I endeavoured to offer the patient opportunities to disclose significant treatment-related information directly to the team while preserving their capacity to trust me. The boundary of confidentiality surrounds all those whose professional duty involves working with the patient and that includes the pastoral worker. However, the channel of communication is not necessarily as direct between the pastor and the team as between other team members. My role is to help the patient have the confidence to communicate directly with those who carry responsibility for knowing.

Pastoral professionalism

The chaplain/pastor occupies a position on a demarcation line between the professionals concerned with the patient's treatment and rehabilitation from illness and the person of the patient, his or her relatives and friends.

I recently questioned a number of chaplains about their attitudes to patients and there was a considerable variation in their response. One group clearly saw themselves as trained mental health professionals. These were the chaplains who either possessed a health care background prior to becoming chaplains or who had acquired additional expertise in the form of psychologically-based understanding and training in order to equip themselves better in their role as chaplains. Others were very adamant that while they considered themselves professionally skilled people, this was as pastors and not as health care professionals. This group understood their role in patient care to centre on the emotional and spiritual support given in the course of remaining present alongside the patient undergoing treatment.

All the chaplains saw themselves as offering an advocacy role on behalf of the patient. The function and content of their advocacy varied, with some taking on a mild form of personal advocacy emphasizing the humanity and spiritual integrity of the patient. For others, advocacy involved emphasizing the patient as a complex psychosocial being in protest against what they felt to be the reductionist medical view held by many psychiatrists. For a smaller group of chaplains, advocacy meant political advocacy, involving taking the patient's side in the unequal power relationship between patient and professionals. Those who held a more politicized view of advocacy maintained strong community orientations.

Two aspects emerge from this cross-section of chaplain opinion. The first, concerns the distinction I have made between institutional and community dynamics. It is possible to break down the responses as representing two different groups within chaplaincy. The first group were full-time hospital chaplains whose work was completely bounded by the institution. Sharing the coinage of health care professionalism was important to them. The second group were mainly part-time chaplains whose work was split between hospital and the community. In comparison to the full-time chaplains, the part-time chaplains considered it a hindrance to know too much about psychiatry or psychology.

The second aspect to emerge concerns the likelihood that the chaplain will hold a view of experience which is in many ways closer to the one held by the patient and his or her relatives and friends. This is even more likely to be so for pastors whose contact with the person with mental health difficulties arises out of the context of their life in the community, or at the very least, life beyond the consulting-room door. Whatever the personal view of his or her own work a particular chaplain holds, not 'treating' the patient sharply distinguishes the pastoral relationship with the patient from that of the medical, nursing and therapeutic members of the mental health care team. Even where the chaplain is knowledgeable about psychiatry and engages with the process of diagnosis and treatment, it remains essential to repeat that he or she does not 'treat' the patient, neither is he or she understood to be responsible for any aspect of carrying out the treatment.

A theology of mental health leading to collaboration

The pastoral presence reminds other mental health professionals of the uneasy and sometimes disturbing and mysterious connections between the symptoms of psychosis and spirituality.

Boisen (1926) pointed out that two-thirds of the cases which came to the attention of psychiatrists did not have a discernible cause despite a growing reliance upon physogenic explanations. He also noted that in the majority of cases a religious element existed. From this he drew support for his contention that psychosis and religious experience shared a number of common characteristics.

The traditional Christian approach to questions of psychotic experience has tended to view it as evidence for profound spiritual and emotional conflict. St Paul spoke of the war between his desires and his intentions bringing about a state of intense conflict. For Paul, the Gospel, which literally translated means the good news, provided him with a context within which to make sense of his conflict, as well as offering him a way of creatively living with conflict. This has been equally true for many of the writers and exponents of Christian living throughout the centuries, especially those whose example has been taken as a source of encouragement to others.

From our narrow 20th century perspective, prominent religious figures from the past appear to have gone in and out of periods of experience containing powerful psychotic elements. These periods of 'madness' functioned to enable a reorganization of the spiritual, psychological and emotional life to take place and, as such, constituted a transition from one phase of living to another. Boisen himself experienced bouts of mental illness requiring hospitalization and it is clear that behind much of his writing lies an immediate familiarity with the psychotic levels of mental functioning. For the clinician, this may seem a scandalous admission. However, the unique perspective which the Christian tradition offers modern mental health disciplines is one in which the psychotic levels of mental functioning are seen as a counterpart to rational functioning. There is no rubicon line between them. Instead, rational and psychotic mental functioning lie in relationship to one another which makes an up-and-down or in-and-out movement between them possible. Reed (1978) following psychoanalytic thinking about the relationship between psychotic and rational levels of mental functioning, recognized a free movement from one to the other and back again as being a prerequisite for all successful mental functioning at both the level of the individual and the collective. His studies in this area formed the basis of his book, *The Dynamics of Religion* (1978), in which he coined the term 'oscillation' to describe this process. An example of this oscillation process occurs both collectively as well as individually. For the Christian, worship is a dynamic process in which collective identifications which belong to psychotic levels are contained within, and used to refresh, the continued capacity for rational reflection. Boisen (1926) describes the same process in the life of an individual as follows:

It would follow, then, that functional mental disorders and religious conversion experience may have a relationship which is at once very close and very far apart. They may each be solutions to a common situation, a conflict within the personality. But one is a happy solution and the other an unhappy solution or else no solution at all, but a condition of unstable equilibrium with the issue still in the balance ... mental disorders concern the religious worker quite as much as they do the medical worker, and religious experiences are quite likely to have pathological elements.

(Asquith 1992, p. 20)

For Boisen, the function of the religious worker was to liaise with other mental health professionals in an early assessment of the character of the disturbance leading to an identification of the function of the psychotic phenomenon in the overall pattern of a personality's development. He criticized the church for neglecting the development of its natural expertise in this area. More significantly, he criticized the church's lack of interest in the mentally disturbed:

We have therefore this truly remarkable situation – a Church which has always been interested in the care of the sick, confining her efforts to types of cases in which religion has least concern and least to contribute [physical illness] while in those types in which it is impossible to tell where the domain of the medical workers leave off and that of the religious worker begins, there the Church is doing nothing.   (Asquith, p. 21)

Psychiatry and mental health, unlike general medicine, is where the spiritual specialist has a real contribution to make.

Keenly aware of the resistance he provoked in both religion and psychiatry, Boisen suggested that the religious worker offered three elements to the interprofessional work of mental health care:

- The religious worker is concerned for the ultimate realities of life which when addressed bring great comfort to the sufferers from mental health problems.
- The activity of prayer is a proper engagement with the re-education of an individual's attitude in living.
- The religious worker represents a social community able to magnify greatly his or her activities and provide for the sufferer a social context for acceptance and rehabilitation.

The philosopher and theologian Tillich (1952) wrote about the distinction between existential anxiety and pathological anxiety. The first was the concern of the pastor, the second the psychiatrist. Pathological anxiety, by which I take him to be referring to mental illness, resulted from an incomplete or unsuccessful attempt to face the terror of the anxiety of simple existence. In Tillich's (1952) terms these were people who did not have the 'courage to be'. Fear of death caused a striving towards security and a use of those aspects of civilization which served to provide safety against the attacks of fate and death. However, no complete security is possible and time and again 'we are called to surrender some or even all security for the sake of full self-affirmation' (p. 78).

The church plays an important role in the attempt to reduce the threat of death as much as possible. In cases of existential anxiety, the church, through its beliefs, rituals and communal solidarity, is able to provide a means for effectively containing anxiety and reducing it to a level which can be tolerated (Reed 1978). This opens up the possibility for sublimation, a device which Freud identified as the necessary basis for social achievement and cultural advance.

By comparison Tillich (1952) described pathological anxiety about fate and death as that which 'impels towards a security of the prison'. Once entered the person is held captive within the prison of increasing self-limitation. This limitation is not based on reality, for the psychotic 'fears what is not to be feared and feels safe what is not safe' (p. 79). Images are produced (fantasies and phobias) which have no basis in reality. Misplaced fear is a consequence of the pathological form of the anxiety of fate and death.

Tillich (1952) considers the relationship between the pastor and the doctor. Medicine cannot heal disease without a doctrine of humanity. It must cooperate with those professions whose central object is humanity, i.e. those whose task it is to help people achieve their potential as human beings. The product of such a cooperation is nothing less than an empowering of distressed human beings towards the pursuit of their essential self-affirmation. This is what Tillich means by the phrase 'courage to be'. In its pathological form anxiety is the subject of psychiatry. In its existential form it is the subject of pastoral and spiritual care. Between the two is an area of considerable overlap. Tillich suggests that 'neither the medical nor the priestly function is bound to its vocational representatives'. Out of a true cooperation different disciplines overlap in their capacities for response. This is not to confuse their distinctiveness, nor to lead one to try to replace the other. Instead, cooperation leads us to realize that the nature of the human being does not easily give rise to clear severable areas for autonomous professional operation.

Contribution of the pastor in interprofessional mental health care

The pastor lives and works among the people he or she serves. Compared with the highly developed specialisms which hospital care promotes, the pastor's way of working can be seen as amateur and unfocused. Yet this is the most valuable element the pastor provides to any interprofessional setting. He or she already knows the community into which the health care professionals are only now beginning to venture. The unit of the church he or she heads is already in place and, likely as not, has been dealing with a wide variety of mental health problems. The pastor will know of many people with a variety of mental health problems who are unknown to the mental health services. Of those known to mental health professionals, a proportion will identify with a religious congregation or community.

A recent survey (Hambridge 1990) quotes a number of interesting statistics. There are, according to this survey, some 49 500 Christian churches with 39 300 pastors. There are 1300 general adult psychiatrists each responsible for 43 000 persons of whom 5300 will be regular church attenders.

Psychiatrists each year see around 1 per cent of the general population of whom 50 will be regular church attenders. Pastors on average minister to 176 persons of whom 22 will have a significant psychiatric syndrome. Hambridge concludes:

> there may be considerable overlap between the population served by the religious and psychiatric communities ... and that an awareness of each other's existence and philosophies is important in providing maximum care to those individuals presenting with psychiatric disorders. Therefore it would seem important for ministers of religion and psychiatrists to have some awareness of each other's philosophical understanding of life and how each approaches the problems of everyday living.

While not being an expert in mental health the pastor knows about the ordinary lives and social contexts of persons whom the health care professional has only had the opportunity to know in the rather limited context of the clinic or ward. In addition the pastor stands within a tradition which has ordinary common sense insights into the wider context and experiences which health care professionals come to see only within an area bounded by the borders of their clinical gaze. It would be a mistake if community mental health care teams did not relate to local pastors in the same way as they relate to local GPs. Together the GP and the pastor form the bedrock of good mental health promotion and containment at the primary care level.

As chaplains to a hospital which is in the process of developing community mental health care models, my colleagues and I have been keen to establish relationships between the new community mental health care sectors and the local church and faith communities within their areas. Establishing communication and working relationships between local pastors and mental health care workers is not always an easy matter. Mutual suspicion needs to be quietly chipped away. Past attitudes and experiences have made for a high degree of mistrust especially among pastors, many of whom have felt disregarded when persons who look to them for major support have come into contact with statutory services.

The 1993 Second Biennial Conference in Religion and Psychiatry, hosted jointly by the Maudsley Hospital Chaplaincy and the Institute of Psychiatry, debated the relative weight given to different areas of a patient's life in psychiatric history-taking. The willingness of psychiatrists to take a detailed sexual history from the patient but not even consider taking a religious history was questioned. It was felt that many patients have unremarkable sexual histories, while often having quite significant historical associations with religious groups.

Strategy for early pastoral involvement in community sectorization

I want briefly to recount my involvement and that of my colleagues with the setting up of four community mental health care sectors. The first step in setting up links was to inform the health care sectors of the presence and whereabouts of local church and faith communities. The sector teams were then in a position to invite local pastors and other religious leaders to meetings held with primary care agencies. Chaplains were instrumental in encouraging the pastors to attend. As a result, quiet confidence in one another has been built up between local pastoral workers and the health care teams. It has now become possible for health care workers and religious group representatives to negotiate a range of matters face to face.

The shift to community care has brought about a revaluing of the roles of the two least clinically-orientated members of the hospital-based mental health care team. The role of the chaplain as pastor and mental health care specialist is one of liaison and information giver. In this capacity, after the initial process of establishing links and building up mutual confidence, one of my colleagues has continued to facilitate a liaison group where representatives of local church and faith communities regularly meet with members of the mental health care team.

Links which in the first instance were established by the chaplains between the two groups are now carried on via the occupational therapist member of the health care team. The interests of occupational therapy and pastoral care are often very similar. Both concern themselves with life skills and tend to focus on the mental health service user's capacity for effective living at a practical everyday level. At this practical level the church is able to offer buildings, space and an extended network of community relationships. These are resources which occupational therapists are considerably skilled in drawing upon as a basis for their extended activities.

A number of churches who can count trained counsellors and psychotherapists among their members or pastors have begun to form small befriending and counselling training groups to better equip people interested in supporting mental health service users. The capacity and resources of such groups vary from the ability to run a drop-in centre on one afternoon a week to offering professionally-based counselling aimed at providing long-term support and containment for persons with mental health difficulties. Talking therapies, long regarded as ineffective and cost inefficient within the institutional care setting, are versatile and very cost effective in community settings when compared with institutional alternatives. Research is needed to document what many in the community already feel to be true, that it is possible to contain chronic mental health problems through regular and sustained counselling contact.

As a chaplaincy department we are attempting to respond to this area of neglect. We are in the process of creating a fellowship in Mental Health and Community Care. This post will be filled by a practical theologian. The fellow will spend half of his or her time in psychiatric chaplaincy and half in conducting research into more effective models of pastoral care as a real contribution to community and mental health care. I have recently written in more detail concerning the role of the pastor as counsellor. I provide a theoretical and case discussion of how a psychodynamic psychological working framework is able to provide a disciplined space within which traditional theological, spiritual and pastoral understandings can be used in meeting the containment needs of persons with manic depressive conditions (Sutherland 1995).

Into the future

Today our major social institutions are in trouble. In education, social work, local government as well as in health care, rapid change and restructuring prevent us from seeing whether this is simply a reorganizing period in a prolonged phase of social and economic decline or a turning-point laying new foundations for future development. As a social institution the church has been in decline for much of the present century. Serious study of the demise in the church's wider political and social influence reveals something rather surprising. Amid sustained decline in its power and influence as an institution, the church has rediscovered its roots in small local communities existing within a highly pluralist context.

What really lies behind current governmental strategy towards community-based mental health care is hard to fathom. While mental health care workers increasingly recognize in community care a superior care philosophy, other interpretations of government strategy abound. Not least among these is the fear of an attack upon the kind of professionalism which is centred around a strong institutional dynamic. What is clear is that the shift away from institutionally-based responsibility will change the dynamic of interprofessional working. As the large psychiatric institutions decline, community psychiatry will take on many of the characteristics hitherto despised in GPs, CPNs and the clergy.

As governmental responsibility for health and welfare declines, a shifting of some of the burden towards the private sector can already be detected. The church and other religious organizations re-emerge as a focus for the expressions of local community concern and practical help. The legacy of a national church in England, Wales and Scotland means that no area of the country falls outside the responsibility of a local pastor who exists to serve the needs of all the people within the extent of a locality. In the complex and pluralistic environments of the inner city, these parochial communities are often the only place where a sense of belonging together extends beyond the narrower confines of single interest groups. These small church and religious communities form a nationwide, coordinated network of local communities with good community-orientated material and human resources. They represent a rich tradition of community experience. If tapped appropriately, they offer a well-tempered wisdom and experience concerning the nature of community care and support. The ability of community mental health care professionals to perceive this as a resource will depend upon their capacity for a genuine community-orientated evolution in the area of interprofessional attitudes and working.

Interprofessional cooperation in community mental health capable of including and using the pastoral care element offered by local pastors will require a capacity in both pastors and mental health professionals to face the anxiety aroused by a sense of competition. Psychiatry and mental health is an arena within which religious and medical workers have more in common than either are prepared to recognize (Boisen 1926). In between health care and pastoral workers, mental health chaplains on the one hand, and mental health workers who understand the importance of religious beliefs on the other, provide that which Tillich (1952) recognized as an area in which both groups overlap in their capacities for response.

Hambridge (1990), commenting on the relationship between psychiatrists and pastors, comments that:

> Both philosophies tend to agree that human existence is frequently coloured by unhelpful and puzzling experiences such as fear, anger, depression, and guilt as well as abnormal mental phenomena such as hallucinations and delusions. Where the two philosophies differ so markedly is on their perception of the causation of these abnormal experiences, and, based on the causation, effective ways to try and help overcome them.

I have suggested that the shift from institutional to community care must involve a change in the dynamics between care givers and care receivers. From this it is not unreasonable to assume a similar change in the way care givers relate towards one another. The engine for this change is the dynamic of the community setting itself. In the area of professionalism, community is tainted with negative images in comparison with institutionally-based models of expertise. It is therefore, all the more important to consider the positive side to community dynamics. Egalitarian dynamics more characteristic of community settings replace hierarchical patterns of structuring interprofessional relationships.

When consultation replaces an authoritarian line of command, from one perspective this can seem very fuzzy. Yet, the advantage for interprofessional relationships is that consultation more accurately reflects the process of negotiation employed by psychologically healthy individuals. Such individuals seek to reconcile the conflicting psychological and social demands, that is demands which originate within the psyche as well as those between the psyche and external reality, through negotiation rather than authoritarian command. Laing (1967) has already been cited concerning the danger which may arise when health care systems designed to combat pathological patterns in the individual unconsciously recreate the very dynamics as an inherent aspect of the treatment. The lack of a capacity in individuals for negotiation in the face of a number of different, conflicting and competing psychological or social demands will not be served by a similar inability between the interprofessional components within the health care team.

The pastor brings to the mental health team some of the strengths of the community work setting. Added to this, the pastor represents a rich humanitarian tradition of mental health understanding and experience. Between this tradition, and the mental health disciplines, especially the psychiatric pole of mental health care, there remains considerable difference. It is to be hoped that the strengthening of community-based mental health care structures will, along with the adoption of a more egalitarian cooperative model of care and professional working, prove the setting for a less defensive recognition that in difference and diversity lies richness.

References

Asquith G H Jr (1992). *Vision of a Little Known Country: A Boisen Reader*. Journal of Pastoral Care Publications, Dectur, Ga.

Bion W R (1961). *Experiences in Groups and other Papers*. Tavistock Publications, London.

Boisen A (1923). Experience and mental disorder. In *Vision of a Little Known Country: A Boisen Reader* (ed. G H Asquith 1992). Journal of Pastoral Care Publications, Dectur, Ga.

Boisen A (1926). The challenge to our seminaries. In *Vision of a Little Known Country: A Boisen Reader* (ed. G H Asquith 1992). Journal of Pastoral Care Publications, Dectur, Ga.

Boisen A (1930). Theological education via the clinic. In *Vision of a Little Known Country: A Boisen Reader* (ed. G H Asquith 1992). Journal of Pastoral Care Publications, Dectur, Ga.

Eastman F (1951). Father of the clinical pastoral movement. In *Vision of a Little Known Country: A Boisen Reader* (ed. G H Asquith 1993). Journal of Pastoral Care Publications, Dectur, Ga.

De Board R. (1978). *The Psychoanalysis of Organisations.* Tavistock Publications, London.

Foskett J (1994). Seeing is believing. *Journal of Pastoral Care*, **48**(4), 363–369.

Hall C (1992). *Head and Heart: The Story of the Clinical Pastoral Education Movement*. Journal of Pastoral Care Publications, Dectur, Ga.

Hambridge D (1990). *Survey in Cross-Training in Psychiatry and Religious Belief.* Christian Psychiatric Counselling, Ashtree House, The Moors, Bramton Borth, Lincoln LN4 1JE.

Laing R D (1967). *The Politics of Experience*. Pantheon Books, New York.

Main T (1989). *The Ailment and other Psychoanalytic Essays* (ed. J Johns). Free Association Books, London.

Mather J (1976). *A Brain of Brains*. Reprinted in *Contact*, The Interdisciplinary Journal of Pastoral Studies, 1988, **3**, 9–14.

Menzies-Lyth I (1970). The functioning of social systems as a defense against anxiety. In *Containing Anxiety in Institutions*, Vol. 1. Free Association Books, London.

Menzies-Lyth I (1989). A personal view of groups. In *The Dynamics of the Social*. Free Association Books, London.

Reed B (1978). *The Dynamics of Religion*. DLT, London.

Stanton A and Schwartz M (1954). *The Mental Hospital.* Tavistock Publications, London.

Sutherland M (in press). Mental illness or life crisis: a Christian pastoral counselling contribution. In *Psychiatry and Religion* (ed. D Bhugra). Routledge, London.

Tillich P (1952). *The Courage To Be*, 12th edn 1980, Chapter 3. Fount Paperbacks, Collins, Glasgow.

12 Interventions with families: dealing with psychosis

E. Kuipers

Introduction

As care in the community is implemented as government policy, and as hospital beds close, family care is becoming even more essential for people with psychosis. There are advantages and disadvantages in this. First, there is now clear evidence that for schizophrenia and manic depression the quality of the home environment has a significant effect on promoting recovery (Kavanagh 1992; Kuipers 1992). Second, the evidence on social networks shows that those with long-term mental health problems have severely reduced networks (Creswell *et al.* 1992). This can make family contacts even more crucial. Third, families are a potential resource (Kuipers and Bebbington 1985). Family contact is important for most people. Whereas professional staff move on and are not always available, family contact is likely to be lifelong. Moreover, families potentially provide 'normal' rather than institutional care. However there are also disadvantages. Families can feel exploited, unsupported, and may feel that care for the client is at a cost to themselves (Lefley 1987). The families' own social networks can become reduced as well as the patients' (Anderson *et al.* 1984). Issues such as the stigma of mental illness and the difficulty of discussing any problems can exacerbate their isolation (Kuipers *et al.* 1989). Thus it is necessary to balance the demands and costs of the caring role (Noh and Turner 1987) with its undoubted possible benefits for clients in terms of support, company and social recovery.

While there are no definite figures, estimates of the number of relatives involved in the care of adults with schizophrenia show that families remain essential to this care. Up to 60 per cent of first admissions (MacMillan *et al.* 1986) and 50 per cent if subsequent admissions are included (Gibbons *et al.* 1984), return to live with relatives. In the long-term group, between 40 and 50 per cent live with, or are in high contact with, a relative, or have other patients in their network who take on the caring role (Creer *et al.* 1982).

In schizophrenia, carers can be parents, spouses or, occasionally, siblings or children. While most carers who are parents are mothers, in the other categories there will be a substantial number of male carers. In depression, carers are more likely to be spouses and will again be of either sex (Fadden *et al.* 1987*a*).

If patients do not live with families and are not homeless, they are likely to live in hostels, or alone. Some hostels act as 'families' and staff in them can share similar attitudes to relatives (Ball *et al.* 1992; Moore *et al.* 1992). Thus the majority of those with psychosis are likely to be in contact with carers.

Burden

The burden of care can be defined in various ways. Platt (1985) says it is 'the presence of problems, difficulties or adverse events which affect the life (lives) of the psychiatric patients' significant others' (e.g. members of the household and/or family) (p. 385). More simply it can be stated as 'the effect of the patient upon the family' (Goldberg and Huxley 1980, p. 127).

Since Hoenig and Hamilton (1966), researchers have tended to distinguish between 'objective burden' – the potentially verifiable disruptions such as loss of income and isolation – and 'subjective burden' – the personal feelings or distress that relatives attribute to the caring role. More recently there have also been attempts to distinguish between an event and its perceived cause; what has been called patient relatedness (e.g. Platt *et al.* 1983).

Burden in relatives of those with schizophrenia and depression has been assessed since the 1950s (e.g. Yarrow *et al.* 1955) and has been reviewed recently (e.g. Fadden *et al.*, 1987*b*; MacCarthy 1988; Kuipers 1992, 1994). Studies vary as to which criteria they use but there is considerable agreement that families are extensively burdened by the demanding and often unsupported role of caring for psychosis, both objectively and in terms of the emotional impact of these disorders. The degree of burden may be severe and can affect the carers' own well-being, particularly as caring is likely to last for a lifetime (Lefley 1987; Stevens 1972) without respite (MacCarthy *et al.* 1989).

Specific burdens

It is now well documented that the caring role in psychosis is likely to affect most aspects of family functioning.

Effect on social and leisure activities

Carers are likely to face restrictions in their social activities (e.g. Mandelbrote and Folkard 1961*a* and *b*; Wing *et al.* 1964; Waters and Northover 1965), have reduced social networks of their own (Anderson *et al.* 1984), and may remain isolated in their own homes with few other social contacts (MacCarthy 1988). The stigma of mental illness in the family is still widespread and may contribute to their social isolation (Kuipers *et al.* 1989).

Financial and employment difficulties

These are emphasized in a number of studies (e.g. Hoenig and Hamilton

1966, 1969; Stevens 1972). Because schizophrenia typically occurs in early adulthood and is likely to affect long-term earning and employment capacity, higher levels of burden occur if the patients had been earning (e.g. if carers are spouses) than in families where earning capacity and commitment were not yet established (e.g. parental carers). The loss of *potential* earnings is easy to underestimate, but at the very least is likely to lead to a more impoverished lifestyle than otherwise.

Burdensome symptoms

Behaviour problems in patients are major correlates of burden (Lefley 1987). The two areas that cause most difficulties are socially disruptive behaviour and negative symptoms such as social withdrawal (e.g. Creer and Wing 1974; Gibbons *et al.* 1984; MacCarthy *et al.* 1989). In depression the most burdensome symptoms are sleeplessness, followed by misery, worry and the inactivity of patients (Fadden *et al.* 1987*a*).

Emotional impact of care on families

A wide range of emotional responses can be expected from relatives in the caring role. This has been most extensively assessed by the measure of expressed emotion (EE) (Leff and Vaughn 1985). Relatives make various attributions about patients in an attempt to deal with day-to-day issues (Brewin *et al.* 1991). The most common of these is to decide an individual is being difficult and blame them for their behaviour. An alternative is to feel extremely worried and upset and attempt to alleviate this by treating the patient as a child again. The latter two attitudes, while entirely understandable, are encapsulated by ratings of criticism and over-emotional involvement. The latter, either singly or together have been found to be reliable predictors of outcome in schizophrenia, and patients returning to live with high EE families are found to have a poorer outcome in the next nine months (Kavanagh 1992). In depression, criticism, rather than over-involvement, has tended to be the main predictor of poorer outcome (Hooley *et al.* 1986), at even lower levels than that found in schizophrenia.

Surprisingly, the relationship between burden and EE in relatives has not been examined in any detail. However, preliminary studies confirm that high levels of burden and EE co-exist (Jackson *et al.* 1990; Smith and Birchwood 1992; Scazufca and Kuipers 1995).

Other feelings include anger, grief, guilt and rejection. The grief has been likened to a bereavement process in the length of time it can take to accept the patient as they are now (Lefley 1987; Kuipers *et al.* 1989). Things may not become easier over time, as objective hardships may increase (e.g. Lefley 1987). So also can resignation, which is associated with less objective stress, but may be detrimental to patient functioning (MacCarthy *et al.* 1989).

The psychological impact of caring has only recently been assessed for relatives. When standard measures such as the general health questionnaire (GHQ) (Goldberg and Hillier 1979) or the present state examination (PSE) (Wing *et al.* 1974) are used there is a consistent finding that around one-third of relatives are likely to have raised levels of anxiety or depression connected to the caring role (Creer *et al.* 1982; Fadden *et al.* 1987a; MacCarthy *et al.* 1989).

Unmet needs

The only study to look specifically at how services cater for families' needs was by MacCarthy *et al.* (1989). She found unmet needs in three areas: the provision of information and advice, emotional support and respite care. Practical needs, e.g. for housing or help with benefits, were more often met. Relatives were confirmed as having a demanding role, finding it difficult to articulate what help they wanted and being unlikely to complain.

Intervention

Therapists proposing to intervene with family members have to be well aware of the burden of care that families are coping with. This starting-point is essential in terms of offering services because any offer of help which tries to deny or minimize burden is likely to be rejected. Interventions, particularly those in people's homes, have to be credible and acceptable. It is obvious that no intervention is possible if a family rejects help because therapists are insensitive to these issues.

The partnership model

There is now an extensive literature on successful family intervention, which includes social and pharmacological treatments. This focuses on families coping with schizophrenia. While a similar model could potentially be used for depression, such treatment is still being evaluated. However the work published so far emphasizes the need for professionals, carers and clients to work together to maximize the likelihood of a good outcome (Leff *et al.* 1982, 1985, 1989, 1990; Falloon *et al.* 1982, 1985; Hogarty *et al.* 1986, 1987; Tarrier *et al.* 1988, 1989). The intervention studies evaluated have used the measure of EE, which by definition stresses the importance of family attitudes on the course of recovery in schizophrenia (reviewed by Kuipers and Bebbington 1988, 1990; Lam 1991). All the research groups have now published manuals which specify the techniques used (Falloon 1985; Anderson *et al.* 1986; Kuipers *et al.* 1992; Barrowclough and Tarrier 1992). Family sessions of at least a year are usually recommended.

A collaborative stance allows professionals to take carers' viewpoints seriously and to act preventatively rather than only in a crisis. Some recent work shows that carers and patients themselves are well able to assess early signs of relapse, and this information can be used with clinicians to prevent more serious symptoms from developing (Birchwood *et al.* 1989). It is likely that integrating this work with specific family interventions is another way of improving outcome.

Overall, the outcome for these studies has reduced relapse rates to around 10 per cent in the first nine months, compared with around 50 per cent in the control groups. Studies which have measured broader outcomes have also found improvements in social performance in clients (Doane *et al.* 1985;

Hogarty *et al.* 1986) and in the subjective burden of carers (Falloon and Pederson 1985). In follow-ups, relapse has tended to be delayed, though not prevented, and improvements in outcome in the intervention groups are still detectable at two years. This is in contrast to three other published studies where outcome did not differ significantly from that of control groups (Kottgen *et al.* 1984; McCreadie *et al.* 1991; Vaughn *et al.* 1992). It is not entirely clear what this might have been due to, although in the latter two studies a lack of specific staff training may have been contributory. It is likely that successful family interventions do need particular staff skills and the quality of family sessions may well need to be monitored in the future. Work in this area is already under way (Lam *et al.* 1993).

Essential features of successful interventions

From the published literature, successful interventions with families are characterized by broadly similar input which seems to be essential. These include:

- a positive attitude – from therapist towards carers and clients, rather than blaming families for problems
- education – offering information in various formats, as a precondition for later therapeutic input
- problem solving – a focus on current problems in the family and on improving communication skills in order to begin to solve them
- emotional processing – sometimes called cognitive behavioural strategies, or dealing with stress (Barrowclough and Tarrier 1992), or is referred to as part of problem solving (Falloon 1985), but some aspects of the upset, distress and burden carried by families is usually tackled
- medication – all studies help patients to remain on optimum medication levels while receiving social treatments.

The interventions that our research group have developed are discussed in our manual (Kuipers *et al.* 1992). In this we discuss practical issues and then more emotional ones, although often these issues are intertwined and cannot be so neatly separated. No more than an outline of the interventions suggested can be summarized here.

Engaging families

One of the key aspects of work with families is how necessary it is to spend time at the beginning ensuring the family accepts the need for help. However skilled an intervention, unless a family is willing to take it up it cannot be effective. Many families have a history of what they perceive as unhelpful or inadequate professional help in the past and may have very low expectations of things being different this time. Other families are unwilling to risk the uncertainty of new help, in case things become worse. Seeing families initially at a crisis point, such as admission to hospital, can be a useful starting-point, as things have obviously not been going well. Families at this stage may be more willing to begin to discuss coping and prevention than at a time when things are 'as normal'. Potential therapists have to be flexible and persistent. Early refusal, or difficulties keeping to an initial appointment, can often be coped with by continuing to offer alternatives. It is certainly not helpful to be rigid about the timing or place of an early meeting with relatives. We have found that pleasant but persistent offers of help at this stage, are more likely to lead to long-term engagement in later intervention.

Education

One of the most useful ways to engage a family is to offer education, and most studies have endorsed this. Education by itself does not impart much information or lead to long-term behaviour change (Tarrier *et al*. 1988; Smith and Birchwood 1987) but does help families feel more optimistic about the future (Berkowitz *et al*. 1984) and helps relatives' feelings of mastery and self-esteem (Lam 1991). Offering information also has high face validity and overtly satisfies relatives' consumer demands. The way in which information is provided seems less important. Various studies have offered workshops (Hogarty *et al*. 1986), relative groups (Smith and Birchwood 1987) or individual home visits (Leff *et al*. 1982, 1989). A number of leaflets are now available to back up spoken information (e.g. from the National Schizophrenia Fellowship). The crucial part of an information session appears to be when some sort of active learning takes place, i.e. when relatives ask questions and receive specific information as a result. Education needs to be given flexibly and not according to some rigid format. This allows disagreements to be aired and dealt with. For instance, clients and families may not accept the diagnosis but may well accept there is a problem, and will be encouraged to know that they are not alone in having to deal with it. The use of clients as the 'expert' in these situations is worth fostering. It can be suggested that relatives ask clients to describe some of their psychotic experiences and clients can then tell relatives how they might help.

Relatives' groups are also very useful in encouraging carers to discuss common themes, ask each other questions and exchange information, so that feelings of isolation and fear of the unknown can diminish (Kuipers *et al*. 1989; Kuipers and Westall 1992; Kuipers *et al*. 1992).

Specific interventions

These will differ depending on the type of family, the range of members (e.g. spouses or a parental family, one, two or three generations), the stage of the illness (first onset, or many years afterwards) and the diagnosis. However, there are some overall strategies that will need to be used. Even families who have lived with problems for many years may not have begun to sort out the problems and resemble a new onset family in terms of having unsuccessful coping skills and unrealistic expectations of progress.

Communication skills

The first task in any family meeting is to help participants to improve their communication skills. This may in fact take many sessions and have to be reiterated. Family members may have to practise listening to each other, not interrupting, and talking directly to each other, not about each other. This helps to defuse negative statements in itself, and encourages everyone's participation in a session. For example, 'He is very difficult', has to be rephrased and is usually toned down if said directly to the person: for example, 'You are difficult at home sometimes'.

In some families, communication patterns may be disrupted or dysfunctional. Talking to each other may always lead to an argument and so may be avoided. Therapists may have to make and enforce 'ground rules', such as turn taking and listening, and be prepared to intervene to prevent arguments or negative comments. Having a co-therapist in the session can be particularly useful, as they are an ally and can help model constructive dialogue.

Problem solving

One of the key vehicles of behaviour change in these interventions, and one that each research group has stressed, is some sort of family consensus followed by action taken around a particular task, normally called problem solving. Family members are encouraged to take turns in offering a list of current problems. These are then prioritized by the family and some specific alternative solutions are arrived at. Proposed solutions are then negotiated, agreed to and hopefully practised as homework before the next session. This emphasis on the 'here and now', allows families to feel that current problems are being dealt with and encourages engagement and participation. It is also the case that however menial or prosaic the problem decided upon, the very fact that it has not been resolved so far points out other problems of family functioning which can be dealt with in due course. The fact that clients are (for example) not allowed on a bus, to buy the shopping, to be left alone, are not trusted to spend money sensibly or take medication, can then begin to be dealt with. This allows more constructive approaches to be practised and helps family members begin to experience success and then optimism, rather than failure and resignation.

Emotional issues

Living with psychotic disorders can give rise to a wide variety of emotional responses, ranging from grief, guilt, anger, rejection, hopelessness, resignation, to unrealistic denial that there are any problems. In manic depression, the family may find their emotions 'see sawing' as the client switches from high to low mood. Clients will experience similar feelings, including despair and loss of confidence after many years of illness. The stress and burden of care and the resultant guilt that both clients and carers feel may also need to be tackled. Therapists need to know how to deal with these if intervention is to progress. While problem solving may be part of this process, in some families the feelings are so intense or long lasting that emotional issues have to be dealt with before any other work can be done.

Therapists can start the process off by normalizing even extreme emotional upset. Virtually all families will feel some aspects from the possible emotional range; it would be surprising if they did not, given the difficulties that many have to cope with. Finding out from therapists that such reactions are commonplace rather than unusual can be very reassuring and allay fears such as 'I started to feel I was the one who should be in hospital'. Relatives' groups and other opportunities for carers to talk to each other can also help this, as it becomes obvious that such feelings are universal. A relatives' group can also provide a vivid demonstration of the fact that it is possible to cope with and survive some of carers' worst fears.

A strategy that we have found useful for emotional issues is called positive reframing. This is where the meaning underlying even hurtful or extreme emotional statements is made clear by the therapists. Thus even comments such as 'I wish he was dead' or 'I can't stand living with you' can be reframed to demonstrate that it is only because the person cares at all that such extreme sentiments are uttered. Often the way that illness has disabled or changed an individual is the cause of the feeling, and this too can be discussed; i.e. 'I wish he was dead' might mean that it is unbearably upsetting to watch a loved one suffer or behave differently, and probably reflects the unspoken grief over the loss the illness may have caused, for both client and relative. In most family sessions, the fact that relatives and clients are trying to sort out the problems can be drawn upon, plus the fact that family members would not be attending if they were totally indifferent.

This is not to deny that in some family situations it may be impossible for care to continue. In some settings (particularly with a spouse) it may be true that a partner does want to leave and to reject the caring role. If these factors are prominent then even they can be reframed as a clear indication of strong feelings. An attempt can then be made, perhaps in the session, perhaps separately, to discuss how the caring role might be modified or, if necessary, how alternative care might be offered.

From the research on EE it is obvious that criticism and over-involvement are particularly likely to have to be dealt with in family settings. With critical relatives, negative emotions are usually due to anger, frustration, and (typically) a misunderstanding of negative symptoms. Education and continuing discussion, particularly of the causes of negative symptoms can alleviate these feelings. Carers can then begin to restructure their expectations and to notice progress even if it is slow. A clearer attribution of causes and reframing of the time scale for change, will be likely to reduce many critical aspects of relationships.

Over-involvement is a more complex set of emotional responses; often surrounding guilt and unresolved grief. Parents are the most likely to exhibit it in an attempt to care for the patient, and offer help with perceived disabilities. Over-involvement can be seen as a protective parental response similar to that made when the client was a child and needed high levels of care. While this is a helpful reaction to acute illness, in the long term it locks a client into the 'sick' role, removes adult responsibilities and roles, and can impede social recovery. At its most damaging it can place a client in a permanently childlike role. If the carer is also unable to set limits on unacceptable behaviour, this can at times lead to overtly demanding or even violent behaviour on the client's part. At other times it may just mean that a client is shielded from normal adult decisions and roles. This is not only unrealistic for the client, preventing the normal practice of these roles, but also places unrealistic burdens on a carer.

A useful strategy with an over-involved carer is for therapists to examine 'the worst outcome'. What would happen, for example, if the client was left alone for half an hour? Sometimes the worst outcome has actually happened and this is why the carer is so worried; but even then, the likelihood of it being repeated may be small, and safeguards might be possible. Often, how-ever, the fear is not well founded and carers are worried about 'what if?' Some testing out of this, in a very careful and graded way as part of task setting and in consultation with the client, may not only begin to help a client take responsibility and become more independent, but may also demonstrate that the 'catastrophe' is not inevitable.

Therapists may also give relatives 'permission' to take some time off from the caring role, and take up old friends and interests. This can allow a client to function in a more adult way. Again, practising these ideas and finding out that both carer and client may feel or manage better as a result is the most effective way of beginning to help family functioning to change.

Implications for services

As well as the above interventions, typically offered by staff in the commu-nity, there are other family needs which must be considered if the burden of care is to be lightened.

Continuity of care

Hopefully the new emphasis on care in the community and a designated key worker at discharge will make continuity of care more likely. However one of the more frustrating aspects of offering care to a psychotic member of the family, is having to deal with new and different staff, to negotiate with dif-ferent agencies and receive a consistent approach. Typically a family will be involved with the GP, a mental health multidisciplinary team, possibly a CPN. In some instances, for example if children are involved, or a client has been 'sectioned', social services will be called in. For other families the housing department, or a 'resettlement team' may be asked for advice. There may also be contacts with police, probation officers, legal services and the courts. As care is likely to continue for many years and through most of the stages of the life cycle, these aspects need to be considered carefully when inter-ventions are offered, and at the very least the involvement of other agen-cies needs to be checked, and coordinated. In future a care manager from one agency should take a lead role and liaise and coordinate with others as necessary.

Respite

One of the needs of families that was least likely to be offered for long-term mental health clients was respite care (MacCarthy *et al.* 1989). Now that the need has been identified there is some awareness from services that it is a legitimate requirement for families who take on the caring role. However, provision is often dependent on local and charitable initiatives. As hospital beds become a scarcer resource, emphasis is now being put on 'respite houses' in the community. These services will have to be developed more routinely if they are to offer effective, planned help to families.

A range of structured activities easily and locally available, such as day care, sheltered workshops and drop-in centres, also provide some 'respite' for relatives, both in terms of hours out of the house, and opening up other roles apart from that of 'patient' to help social recovery to progress.

Relatives themselves may need help to take time off from caring, to take up other interests and to increase their social networks. This can both alleviate the isolation and burden of the caring role, provide other contacts for support and give some perspective on difficulties.

In some cases, carers and relatives will not be able to live together, however much respite is provided. In these situations it is much better as part of a family intervention for staff to help negotiate reasonable alternatives such as supported accommodation for a client rather than insist on a deteriorating relationship continuing. If alternatives are faced and discussed before problems become intractable, independence can be fostered and carers' worries about the future may be alleviated. However, for many families caring for a long-term client, facing this before you need to is very difficult.

Involvement with clinical decision-making

When asked, families often request that clinical teams involve them in at least some of their decision-making. As part of a partnership approach this should follow naturally, but many clinical teams still practise keeping considerable distance between 'professionals' and 'carers'. While teams do not always like to acknowledge the collaboration that long-term care requires between staff, carers and clients, it is essential that it is offered so that families feel supported and valued and not exploited.

A collaborative style between staff, carers and client implies more openness and equal respect given to 'consumer' views rather than just to staff opinion. This is part of the new legislation, and the patients' charter, which advocate access to patients' notes, and canvassing client and carers' views. Including clients and carers routinely in team meetings, reviews and discharge planning is to be encouraged and is quite possible. This not only helps a team to make more realistic decisions but because of better participation means that these decisions are more likely to be carried out. Offering meetings with relatives can be mutually beneficial (Mullen *et al.* 1992) and many of the voluntary associations organize this routinely (Kuipers and Westall 1992).

Summary

The burden of the caring role in psychosis is considerable, and is likely to affect most aspects of family functioning. Furthermore care is likely to continue over many years. In order to support those families who wish to offer the caring role, despite its costs to themselves, practitioners must be sensitive to families' needs and be prepared to offer interventions that attempt to meet them. This has become even more essential as relatives are once more in the front line of care in the community.

Families can be offered effective help that not only improves the outcome for clients but can reduce the burden and improve the family's quality of life. This is likely to maximize the potential for social recovery that exists in family settings. Successful social interventions include education, problem solving, and emotional support. Other services that need to be offered are continuity of care, respite care and involvement of carers and clients in multidisciplinary team decision-making. None of these elements are difficult to provide, and overall they are extremely cost effective in reducing admissions to hospital and limiting the number of damaging crises. Offering families as a whole an integrated service, rather than only considering clients' needs, is going to be increasingly required if community care is to be a reality.

References

Anderson C M, Hogarty G, Bayer T et al. (1984). EE and social networks in parents of schizophrenic patients. *British Journal of Psychiatry*, **144**, 247–255.

Anderson C M, Reiss D J and Hogarty G E (1986). *Schizophrenia in the Family: A Practical Guide to Psycho-education and Management*. Guilford Press, New York.

Ball R A, Moore E and Kuipers E (1992). EE in community care facilities: a comparison of patient outcome in a 9 month follow-up of two residential hostels. *Social Psychiatry and Psychiatric Epidemiology*, **27**, 35–39.

Barrowclough C and Tarrier N (1992). *Families of Schizophrenia Patients: Cognitive Behavioural Intervention*. Chapman and Hall, London.

Berkowitz R, Eberlein Fries R, Kuipers E and Leff J (1984). Educating relatives about schizophrenia. *Schizophrenia Bulletin*, **10**, 418–429.

Birchwood M, Smith J, MacMillan F et al. (1989). Predicting relapse in schizophrenia: the development and implementation of an early signs monitoring system using patients and families as observers, a preliminary investigation. *Psychological Medicine*, **19**, 649–656

Brewin C R, MacCarthy B, Duda R and Vaughn C E (1991). Attribution and Expressed Emotion in the relatives of patients with schizophrenia. *Journal of Abnormal Psychology*, **100**, 546–554.

Creer C and Wing J K (1974). *Schizophrenia at Home*. National Schizophrenia Fellowship, Surbiton.

Creer C, Sturt E and Wykes T (1982). The role of relatives. Long term community care, experiences in a London Borough (ed. J K Wing). *Psychological Medicine Monograph* (Suppl 2), pp. 29–39.

Cozzolino L J, Goldstein M J, Nuechterlein K S et al. (1988). The impact of education on relatives varying in levels of EE. *Schizophrenia Bulletin*, **14**, 675–686.

Cresswell C M, Kuipers E and Power M (1992). Social networks and support in long-term psychiatric patients. *Psychological Medicine*, **22**, 1019–1026.

Doane J A, Falloon I R H, Goldstein M J and Mintz J (1985). Parental affective style and the treatment of schizophrenia: Predicting course of illness and social functioning. *Archives of General Psychiatry*, **42**, 34–42.

Fadden G B, Kuipers E and Bebbington P E (1987a). Caring and its burdens: a study of the relatives of depressed patients. *British Journal of Psychiatry*, **151**, 660–667.

Fadden G B, Bebbington P E and Kuipers E (1987). The burden of care: the impact of functional psychiatric illness on the patient's family. *British Journal of Psychiatry*, **150**, 285–292.

Falloon I R H (1985). *Family Management of Schizophrenia*. Johns Hopkins Press, University Press, Baltimore.

Falloon I R H and Pederson J (1985). Family management in the prevention of morbidity of schizophrenia. Adjustment of the family unit. *British Journal of Psychiatry*, **147**, 156–163.

Falloon I R H, Boyd J L, McGill C W, Razani J, Moss, H B and Gildersman, A M

(1982). Family management in the prevention of exacerbations of schizophrenia. A controlled study. *New England Journal of Medicine*, **306**, 1437–1440.

Falloon I R H, Boyd J L, McGill C W, Williamson M, Razani J, Moss H B, Gilderman A M and Simpson G M (1985). Family management in the prevention of morbidity of schizophrenia. Clinical outcome of a two-year longitudinal study. *Archives of General Psychiatry*, **42**, 887–896.

Gibbons J S, Horn S H, Powell J M *et al.* (1984). Schizophrenic patients and their families. A survey in a psychiatric service based on a district general hospital. *British Journal of Psychiatry*, **144**, 70–77.

Goldberg D P and Hillier V G (1979). A scaled version of the GHQ. *Psychological Medicine*, **9**, 139–146.

Goldberg D and Huxley P (1980). *Mental Illness in the Community*. Tavistock, London.

Hoenig J and Hamilton M W (1966). The schizophrenic patient in the community and his effect on the household. *International Journal of Social Psychiatry*, **12**, 165–176.

Hoenig J and Hamilton M W (1969). *The Desegregation of the Mentally Ill*. Routledge and Kegan Paul, London.

Hoffman H and Hubschmid T (1989). The social dependence of the long-term patient: a study in social psychiatric ambulatory care. *Psychiatrie Paxis*, **16**, 1–7.

Hogarty G E, Anderson C M, Reiss D J, Kornblith S J, Greenwald P, Javna C D and Madonia M J (1986). Family psycho-education, social skills training and maintenance chemotherapy in the aftercare treatment of schizophrenia. I. One year effects of a controlled study on relapse and Expressed Emotion. *Archives of General Psychiatry*, **43**, 633–642.

Hogarty G E, Anderson C and Reiss D J (1987). Family psycho-education, social skills training, and medication in schizophrenia: the long and the short of it. *Psychopharmacology Bulletin*, **23**, 12–23.

Hooley J M, Orley J and Teasdale J (1986). Levels of EE and relapse in depressed patients. *British Journal of Psychiatry*, **148**, 642–647.

Jackson H T, Smith N and McGorry P (1990). Relationship between EE and family burden in psychotic disorders: an exploratory study. *Acta Psychiatrica Scandinavica*, **82**, 243–249.

Kavanagh D J (1992). Recent developments in Expressed Emotion and schizophrenia. *British Journal of Psychiatry*, **160**, 601–620.

Kottgen C, Sonnichsen I, Mollenhauer K and Jurth R (1984). Group therapy with the families of schizophrenic patients: result of the Hamburg Camberwell Family Interview Study III. *International Journal of Family Psychiatry*, **5**, 84–94.

Kuipers E (1992). Expressed Emotion in Europe. *British Journal of Clinical Psychology*, **31**, 429–443.

Kuipers E (1994). The measurement of expressed emotion: its influence on research and clinical practice. *International Review of Psychiatry*, **6**, 187–199.

Kuipers E and Bebbington P (1985). Relatives as a resource in the management of functional illness. *British Journal of Psychiatry*, **147**, 465–470.

Kuipers E and Bebbington P (1988). Expressed emotion research in schizophrenia: theoretical and clinical implications. *Psychological Medicine*, **18**, 893–909.

Kuipers E and Bebbington P (1990). *Working in Partnership: Clinicians and Carers in the Management of Long-standing Mental Illness*. Heinemann Press, Oxford.

Kuipers E and Westall J (1992). The role of facilitated relative groups and voluntary self-help groups. In *Principles of Social Psychiatry* (ed. D Bhugra and J Leff). Blackwell, London.

Kuipers E, MacCarthy B, Hurry J, *et al.* (1989). Counselling the relatives of the long-term adult mentally ill: (ii) a low cost supportive model. *British Journal of Psychiatry*, **154**, 775–782.

Kuipers E, Leff J and Lam D (1992). *Family Work for Schizophrenia: A Practical*

Guide. Gaskell, London.

Lam D H (1991). Psychosocial family intervention in schizophrenia: a review of empirical studies. *Psychological Medicine*, **21**, 423–441.

Lam D, Kuipers E and Leff J (1993). Family work with patients with schizophrenia. *Journal of Advanced Nursing*, **18**, 233–237.

Leff J and Vaughn C (1985). *Expressed Emotion in Families*. Guilford Press, London.

Leff J, Kuipers E, Berkowitz R *et al.* (1982). A controlled trial of social intervention in the families of schizophrenic patients. *British Journal of Psychiatry*, **141**, 121–134.

Leff J, Kuipers E, Berkowitz R *et al.* (1985). A controlled trial of social intervention in the families of schizophrenic patients. Two year follow up. *British Journal of Psychiatry*, **146**, 594–600.

Leff J, Berkowitz R, Shavit N *et al.* (1989). A trial of family therapy versus a relatives' group for schizophrenics. *British Journal of Psychiatry*, **154**, 58–66.

Leff, J, Berkowitz R, Shavit N, Strachan A, Glass I and Vaughn C (1990). A trial of family therapy versus a relatives' group for schizophrenia: a two year follow-up. *British Journal of Psychiatry*, **157**, 571–577.

Lefley, H P (1987) Ageing parents as care givers of mentally ill adult children: an emerging social problem. *Hospital and Community Psychiatry*, **38**, 1063–1070.

MacCarthy B (1988). The role of relatives. In *Community Care in Practice* (eds. A Lavender and F Holloway). John Wiley, Chichester.

MacCarthy B, Lesage A, Brewin C R *et al.* (1989). Needs for care among the relatives of long-term users of day-care. *Psychological Medicine,* **19**, 725–736.

McCreadie R G, Phillips K, Harvey J A, Waldron G, Stewart M and Baird D (1991). The Nithsdale Schizophrenia Surveys VIII. Do relatives want family intervention and does it help? *British Journal of Psychiatry*, **158**, 110–113.

McMillan J F, Gold A, Crow T J *et al.* (1986). The Northwick Park Study of first episodes of schizophrenia: IV. Expressed emotion and relapse. *British Journal of Psychiatry*, **148**, 133–143.

Mandelbrote B M and Folkard S (1961*a*). Some problems and needs of schizophrenics in relation to a developing psychiatric community service. *Comprehensive Psychiatry*, **2**, 317–328.

Mandelbrote B M and Folkard S (1961*b*). Some factors related to outcome and social adjustment in schizophrenia. *Acta Psychiatrica Scandinavica*, **37**, 223–235.

Moore E, Ball R A and Kuipers E (1992). Expressed emotion in staff working with the long-term adult mentally ill. *British Journal of Psychiatry*, **161**, 802–808.

Mullen R, Bebbington P and Kuipers E (1992). A workshop for relatives of people with chronic mental illness. *Psychiatric Bulletin*, **16**, 206–207.

Noh S and Turner R J (1987). Living with psychiatric patients: implications for the mental health of family members. *Social Science and Medicine*, **25**, 263–272.

Platt S (1985). Measuring the burden of psychiatric illness in the family: an evaluation of some rating scales. *Psychological Medicine,* **125**, 383–393.

Platt S, Weyman A and Hirsch S (1983). *Social Behaviour Assessment Schedule* (SBA), 3rd edn. NFER, Nelson, Windsor, Berks.

Scazufca M and Kuipers E (1995). Expressed Emotion, Burden of Care and Coping Styles in Adults Suffering from Schizophrenia. Paper presented at the conference of the World Psychiatric Association, New York.

Smith J and Birchwood M J (1987). Specific and non specific effects of educational intervention with families living with a schizophrenic relative. *British Journal of Psychiatry*, **150**, 645–652.

Smith J, Birchwood M, Cochrane R and George S (1992). The needs of high and low expressed emotion families: a normative approach. *Social Psychiatry and Psychiatric Epidemiology*, **28**, 11–16.

Stevens B (1972). Dependence of schizophrenic patients on elderly relatives. *Psychological Medicine*, **2**, 17–32.

Tarrier N, Barrowclough C, Vaughn C, Bamrah J S, Porceddu K, Watts S and Freeman

H (1988). The community management of schizophrenia: a controlled trial of a behavioural intervention with families to reduce relapse. *British Journal of Psychiatry*, **153**, 532–542.

Tarrier N, Barrowclough C, Vaughn C, Bamrah J S, Porceddu K, Watts S and Freeman H (1989). Community management of schizophrenia in a two year follow-up of a behavioural intervention with families. *British Journal of Psychiatry*, **154**, 625–628.

Vaughan K, Doyle M, McConathy N, Blaszcynski A, Fox A and Tarrier N (1992). The relationship between relatives' EE and schizophrenic relapse: an Australian replication. *Social Psychiatry and Psychiatric Epidemiology*, **27**, 10–15.

Waters M A and Northover J (1965). Rehabilitated long-stay schizophrenics in the community. *British Journal of Psychiatry*, **111**, 258–267.

Wing J K, Monck E, Brown G W et al. (1964). Morbidity in the community of schizophrenic patients discharged from London mental hospitals in 1959. *British Journal of Psychiatry*, **110**, 10–21.

Wing J K, Cooper J E and Sartorius N (1974). *Measurement and Classification of Psychiatric Symptoms*. Cambridge University Press, Cambridge.

Yarrow M, Schwartz C G, Murphy H S et al. (1955). The psychological meaning of mental illness in the family. *Journal of Social Issues*, **11**, 12–24.

13 Liaison psychiatry and primary health care settings

G. Strathdee and K. Sutherby

Introduction

This chapter reviews the interface between primary and secondary care. First, the range of the psychiatric morbidity encountered in primary care is described and the historical patterns of liaison between primary and secondary services reviewed. Second, the impact of community care on the role of general practice is delineated. The third section sets out the models of liaison and attachment of a variety of mental health workers to primary care settings. The fourth section delineates the range of needs of individuals with mental health disorders and reviews the research evidence of where and how these can best be met in the interface of primary and secondary care. Finally, issues which are likely to be of concern and influence for the future will be discussed.

The extent and nature of mental health disorders in primary care

With few exceptions Great Britain leads the world in the strength of its primary health care teams. Ninety-eight per cent of the British population is registered with a GP, and of these, 60 per cent will consult at least once a year. The average GP has 2010 patients on their personal list and over the course of any two-year period can expect to see 90 per cent of their entire registered population (Sharp and Morell 1989). On an average working day 750 000 people visit their GP nationally. Between one-fifth and one-quarter of all consultations in the average GP's daily surgeries are undertaken by individuals who have a mental health problem either as the sole, or a major component of their problems (Shepherd *et al.* 1966). In the average consultation time of six minutes, just under a half of these problems are recognized by the doctors (Goldberg and Bridges 1988). While the majority of mental health disorders fall within the less severe or 'neurotic' areas (Table 13.1), one-tenth have a chronic disorder defined as continually present for one year or requiring prophylactic treatment (Strathdee and Sutherby 1993). Primary care has always dealt with the bulk of mental health morbidity within its own team. Only one in 20 people are referred on for specialist care. General practice consultations are in a ratio of 10:1 for psychiatric out-patient attendances and 100:1 for psychiatric admissions (Sharp and Morrell 1989).

Table 13.1 Mental health morbidity in primary care

Diagnosis	Rates per 1000 population per year	Number of patients in an average practice of 2010 per year
Schizophrenia	2.0	4–5
Affective psychosis	3.0	6–7
Organic dementia	2.2	5–6
Depression	28.0	65
Anxiety and other neuroses	35.7	80–85
Situational disturbances/ other diagnoses	26.7	60–65
Drug/alcohol disorder	2.7	6–7
Personality disorder	1.1	2–3

Historical patterns of liaison

Until the past two decades the main form of liaison between secondary and primary care took place surrounding the few patients who were either referred for a consultant opinion in a domiciliary visit or those referred to psychiatric out-patient clinics in large mental health institutions or local district general hospitals (Sutherby *et al.* 1992). In the original terms and specifications of the NHS, domiciliary visits by consultants to patients' homes were to take place in the company of general practitioners for the assessment of those individuals whose physical or mental health condition made it impossible for them to attend for hospital care (NHS Act 1948). However, in recent years joint visits between consultants and GPs have become increasingly rare and opportunities for liaison have been lost.

The factors influencing referral of patients are idiosyncratic and have no systematic relationship to need (Coulter and Bradlow 1993). Three factors are thought to influence the referral decision (Goldberg and Huxley 1980). These are the nature of the patient, the attitude and training of the GP and the nature of the service. Referral practices among general practitioners vary enormously with larger numbers in urban areas, among older doctors and practices with attached mental health professionals. Patients are more likely to be referred for specialist care if they are male, if they are young, if referral is requested by them or their relative, if they have not responded to GP treatment, or if they are suicidal or presenting behavioural difficulties in the community. Even for those patients who get referred to hospital out-patient clinics, satisfaction with the service is not universal. Patients' and referrers' criticisms include long waiting lists, delay in communications and disappointment with treatment strategies.

Even written forms of liaison have not been universally successful. Communication difficulties have been one of the major areas of discord between GPs and hospital-based doctors (Williams and Wallace 1974; Strathdee 1990; Pullen and Yellowlees 1985). Disagreements centre around the frequency of communication, especially for individuals with longer-term disorders (Myers *et al.* 1993), speed of receipt of assessment letter after an out-patient referral, content and format of information contained in letters and lack of clarity about the relative roles and responsibilities of hospital and GP staff.

Relationship between psychiatric services and primary care

In recent years both psychiatry and general practice have undergone more structural change than any other specialties (Strathdee 1994). Much of their growth and development has been in parallel. The status of both has improved relative to the rest of medicine, they have developed the concept of working in teams more than other specialties and both have a strong community orientation. The role which primary care plays in providing care for those with mental health difficulties is influenced by the nature of the general practice and the type and organization of the local mental health teams. For example, larger practices, especially those based in larger and purpose-built health centres, are more likely to be in less deprived social areas and attract attached specialists. At least one of a larger pool of partners is also likely to have undertaken post-graduate training in psychiatry. The orientation of the local mental health services in working with primary care is also important. In some areas, the model is one of integration where work is always undertaken through and with the primary workers, supervision and direction being provided. In other areas the model is of collaboration where, at one extreme, secondary care staff are based in, for example, a community mental health centre and work in parallel with local GPs. Specialists in other districts act as the first-contact workers dealing directly with the families in the community but liaising and communicating with primary care.

Effect of community care on primary care

In psychiatry the move towards deinstitutionalization and community care has placed an increased burden on GPs and the primary care team (see Table 13.2) (Thornicroft and Bebbington 1989; Strathdee 1992). As hospital beds have decreased, the numbers of resettled patients on GPs' lists have increased. This occurs particularly where the practice is near a large hospital which is being closed, where the GP has undertaken a post-graduate training in psychiatry, or if there is an attached psychiatrist visiting the practice on a regular basis (Kendrick 1992).

Without the provision of suitable crisis or respite facilities in the community, or of established care management teams undertaking home-based treatments as an alternative to hospital care, GPs are increasingly providing more care and support for those with acute disorders.

Table 13.2 The effect of community care on general practice

Community care practice	Effect on primary care
Closure of large psychiatric institutions	• More patients with long-term disorders on GPs' lists
More sheltered houses/group homes in the community	• GP roles and responsibilities increased in provision of physical, mental and continuing care to residents • GP role in providing care and support to housing workers increased
Fewer available acute hospital beds	• More patients treated at home, therefore requiring GP enhanced skills in the assessment and management of acute disorders • Need for GPs to work with carers and families
Less access to respite facilities	• GPs engaged in increased support of families/carers • Need for GPs to be involved in service planning and development of alternative respite in the community
Short length of stay in acute wards	More acute illness treated at home: • GPs need to use increased psychotropic medication • GPs need to train in acute psychiatric care in the community • Increased need for GPs to liaise with care management and assertive outreach teams doing home-based treatment
First point of contact with the severely ill	• GP engaged in crisis intervention • GP increased use of the Mental Health Act
Patients with more severe disorders and 'challenging behaviours' in the community	• GPs need to work with secondary care to develop case registers and assertive outreach mechanisms
Decrease in specialist responsibility	• Clear role of GP in providing physical care to patient • GP's need to get involved in care programme approach

Role of the primary care team

As the point of first contact for most British patients, the GP is in a prime position to undertake *detection and assessment of mental health disorders*. Just under half the individuals with severe and continuing mental health disorders fall out of contact with the mental health services and only their GP provides *continuing care* (Pantellis *et al*. 1988; Lee and Murray 1988). As Johnson and Thornicroft (1992) found, the vast majority of mental health services provide only emergency care within routine working hours. Casualty departments and consultant domiciliary visits are the unsatisfactory alternatives in the vast majority of districts. The primary care team thus provides *first contact crisis care*, even for individuals in contact with specialist services. The GP, by virtue of his/her continuing role and knowledge of families and individuals, is well placed to *practise prevention and health education*. Individuals often present their psychological distress with physical symptoms. The GP's skills are needed to meet the *physical health care* needs associated with the increased physical morbidity of the severely mentally ill. With the increasing pressure to ensure that services are prioritized to meet the needs of the most severely ill, the role of the GP as *gate-keeper* can ensure that specialist services are targeted appropriately.

Mental health professional liaison

In the development of community mental health services in recent years, rational planning based on needs has not been a major feature. In many areas, services have arisen piecemeal, with members of secondary care teams developing individual attachments to primary care practices in an idiosyncratic and autonomous, rather than needs-led way.

Attached professionals in primary care

The numbers of mental health professionals working in primary care have increased across all the disciplines from the mid-1970s to the following levels (Thomas and Corney 1992; Strathdee and Williams 1984; Gilchrist *et al*. 1978):

- In 1985 there were 3000 CPNs in the UK projected to increase to 4500 in 1990 and 7500 by 1995.
- By 1982 between 1 in 3 and 1 in 5 psychiatrists were working in a primary care setting.
- Between 1977 and 1986 the proportion of clinical psychologists working with GPs rose from 14 per cent to 27 per cent.
- In 1978, 60 per cent of social workers were working in primary care although the numbers have since declined with the cutbacks in local authorities in the 1980s.

There has been a tendency for some practices to have many links while others have few, raising questions about the efficiency and equity of these schemes. Thus, of individual practices in 1991:

- 48 per cent had a link with a CPN
- 21 per cent had a link with a social worker
- 17 per cent had a link with a counsellor
- 15 per cent had a link with a clinical psychologist
- 16 per cent had a link with a psychiatrist.

Psychiatrists working in primary care

First reports of members of secondary care teams developing closer liaison with the primary care sector came from the psychiatric literature. In 1966 Alexis Brook, a psychotherapist, first reported undertaking a clinic in a GP surgery (Brook 1967). Throughout the 1970s the numbers grew, until by 1984 19 per cent of all consultant general adult psychiatrists in England and Wales (Strathdee and Williams 1984) and half the Scottish psychiatrists (Pullen and Yellowlees 1988) worked in this way. The impetus for such clinics came from grass-roots psychiatrists dissatisfied with the lack of coordination of care exemplified in the hospital out-patient setting, accompanied by the determination to establish and expand community services and to improve liaison and communication between primary and secondary care (Strathdee 1988).

The clinics are conducted in a variety of formats (Strathdee and Williams 1984; Mitchell 1985). General practitioners have expressed a preference for the 'consultation' style wherein the psychiatrist and referrer jointly make an assessment, and the primary care professional undertakes the treatment with supervision. In the 'shifted out-patient model' the specialist sees the patients from the immediate catchment area in the local surgery rather than at the often distant psychiatric hospital. This enables them to provide crisis intervention and carry out assessment and short-term treatment. In longer standing arrangements the liaison attachment model evolves with an integrated approach between the specialist and primary care teams in the management of patients. This model is regarded as being cost effective in that the psychiatrists can contribute to the care of more patients by providing advice on patients not seen, treating others through supervision and enhancing the skills of the primary care team (Creed and Marks 1989; Darling and Tyrer 1990).

An early criticism of the clinics was that specialists in the primary care setting would inevitably, as with the American community mental health centres, drift towards seeing the 'walking well'. However, a number of authors have demonstrated that the proportion of patients with serious and long-term mental illness seen is at least equal to that encountered in hospital out-patient clinics. In fact there is evidence to suggest that the clinics provide for the previously unmet needs of chronic patients reluctant to attend hospital follow-up clinics, especially women, those with paranoid illnesses, those with schizophrenia (Tyrer 1984; Browning *et al.* 1987; Brown *et al.* 1988; Strathdee *et al.* 1990) and the homeless (Joseph *et al.* 1990).

Referral practices among Scottish GPs are different. Low and Pullen (1988) in a Scottish case-register study, found that when a range of services is available GPs tend to refer along a spectrum of severity. Psychotic patients were preferentially referred for emergency care in the form of domiciliary consultation. This finding has been replicated in England where approximately one-third of referrals to domiciliary visits and crisis intervention services are for the treatment of the seriously ill with psychotic illnesses (Boardman 1987; Sutherby *et al.* 1992). In contrast to England, the Scottish group found that only the neurotic end of the spectrum were referred to psychiatrists working in the primary care setting.

Psychologist liaison to primary care

Clinical psychologists working in primary care are significantly more likely than CPNs or practice counsellors to be referred patients with the following disorders, which are usually treated with behaviour therapy: psychosexual problems, eating disorders, phobias and obsessive compulsive disorders (Robson *et al.* 1984; Earll and Kincey 1982; Deys *et al.* 1989). Patients report a high degree of satisfaction with behavioural treatment, and, as happens with other professionals involved in counselling, the result is decreased drug prescribing. One study indicated that 28 per cent of the psychologists' salaries could be found from drug savings alone. Where psychologists have used their specialist training in cognitive therapy to treat depression, studies have found a significantly greater improvement compared to GP treatment alone, but no difference three months after completion of treatment (Teasdale *et al.* 1984). It has been advocated that the most important roles for clinical psychologists are to provide education and consultative liaison for the GP and consultation for self-help or other voluntary sector organizations.

Community psychiatric nurse attachments

The attachment of community psychiatric nurses to particular general practices has followed two general models. In those services where the nurses are hospital based and work as members of the secondary care team, 80 per cent of their referrals are from psychiatrists and are of individuals with severe and continuing mental health disorders. In the second model, that of the nurses, although employed by secondary care services being attached to particular general practices, the referral pattern shifts with 80 per cent of their referrals coming directly from GPs. The latter model is characterized by large caseloads, composed of patients with neurotic and adjustment disorders with large numbers of patients receiving care from the CPN as the sole involved discipline. Although the caseloads of both the hospital-based and primary-care-based CPNs remain similar in terms of the numbers of individuals with schizophrenia in the latter, the mean time in contact with psychotic patients is a third of the time spent with non-psychotic patients and almost entirely limited to the administration of injections (Cumberledge Report 1986; Wooff *et al.* 1989).

Research evidence indicates that CPNs trained in psychosocial interventions with the families of individuals with schizophrenia produce significantly greater improvements in negative symptoms, social adjustment and family satisfaction compared with controls. CPN (Brooker *et al.* 1992) treatment of neurotic patients produces similar results in terms of symptoms, social adjustment and family burden as that of psychiatric out-patient clinics. Nurse behaviour therapists, with their focused training, have better post-treatment outcome than treatment given by GPs (Paykel *et al.* 1982; Marks *et al.* 1985).

Counsellors working in primary care

In a study in 1992, Sibbald and her colleagues identified that 1 in 20 practices in England and Wales consider themselves to have a counsellor working on site (British Association of Counselling 1990; Sibbald *et al.* 1993;

Irving 1993). In 1992, half of the employed counsellors had specialist training in counselling, but one-fifth of the employing GPs were unaware of the qualification of the counsellors in their practices. Counsellors have referred to them a wide variety of problems ranging from family and relationship difficulties to drug and alcohol abuse and psychiatric illness. The introduction of counsellors into primary care has been demonstrated to reduce psychotropic drug prescribing, GP consultation rates and referrals to psychiatrists, as well as providing patient and GP satisfaction. There are, however, increasing concerns expressed by counsellors themselves (Irving 1993) that their role in primary care is not clearly defined. Many counsellors work without supervision or pay for supervision themselves. Many counsellors are also interested in working more closely with secondary care mental health teams in order to obtain peer support and ongoing training.

Social workers in primary care

Two models of primary care liaison have been described. The medical social work model is implemented when the social worker uses the practice premises as a base. This results in greater collaboration and coordination, and more appropriate referrals, although social workers report that they suffer from professional isolation and inadequate clerical backup. The more common social services model occurs when the social worker visits the practice to collect referrals or discuss patients, and passes these referrals on to colleagues. In this model the opportunities for mutual education and trust are reduced, feedback can be delayed and case discussions are infrequent (Corney 1984, 1985).

Social workers in primary care can provide practical help such as arranging day nursery placements, accommodation and benefit claims, as well as counselling. Studies have shown that practical help, as well as emotional support, is beneficial and studies of clients' views support this finding. General practitioners tend to regard social workers as solely involved with practical tasks, whereas with liaison, the skills of mental health social workers can be used appropriately as more patients with mixed psychological and social problems are referred. Women with acute or chronic depression and relationship difficulties show long-term benefits from social worker intervention. Mental health social workers are more likely than CPNs to examine patients' relationships, to undertake some service or task and offer support, reassurance or guidance (Wooff *et al.* 1988; Scott and Freeman 1992).

Models of primary-care-orientated community mental health services

As indicated above, in the organization of community mental health care, the central issue is the extent to which the community mental health services can integrate with primary care teams or work as collaborative parallel services. A number of integrated models have been described.

Model 1   The relocation of out-patient clinics

This relocation from hospital to community sites is the most minimal form of liaison between secondary and primary care as described above.

Model 2   The hive model

This model, in which the primary care liaison clinics form an important component, is described by Tyrer (1985). He proposes that comprehensive care can only be achieved by a system which integrates community psychiatry with the hospital base which should be sited within reach of all parts of the catchment area. Closely coordinated sub-units of care such as day hospitals, community clinics, or mental health centres should be located in the areas with the greatest psychiatric morbidity. Links can then be made with all the actual and potential psychiatric services, including the primary care teams in the locality. In Nottingham, where the 'hive' model has been developed, Tyrer found that with GP clinics incorporated into the sub-unit structure, there was a 20 per cent fall in admissions to hospital. He perceived additional benefits to be the earlier detection of psychiatric illness and a greater ability to prevent relapse in those patients who traditionally are poor attenders at hospital clinics, such as the young and those who feel stigmatized by the process.

Model 3   The Falloon model

This model was developed in a rural area where every practice has an attached nurse who undertakes an assessment within 24 hours of referral and has access to the skills of a multidisciplinary team if necessary. An important aspect is that the team worked using problem-solving techniques with families (Falloon *et al.* 1990).

Model 4   The Hansen model

This model in Scandinavia involves an even greater degree of integration with primary care, including not only primary health care but also social and other agencies. The community mental health team, based in a large primary care health centre, is regarded as an integral part of the primary care tier and refers to the hospital services as a secondary level. Hansen (1987) developed his model after finding primary care dissatisfaction with a hospital-based system of care. The main reasons included too little contact with mental health professionals for consultation on difficult cases, too few possibilities for direct referral to specialist services and too few patients discharged back to primary care after discharge from in-patient status.

Referrals from both community and hospital agencies were accepted only if a primary care agency assumed responsibility for the future continuity of care. Both day and night emergencies were dealt with by the primary care teams who had rapid access to the psychiatric services if they felt this to be necessary. Referrals for admission were always undertaken by the primary care coordinator even when the judgment that it was necessary had come from the psychiatric team. The three main aims formulated for the service were that it should replace admissions with consultation and treatment within primary care, provide access to consultation for all primary care workers and agencies regardless of profession and execute ambulatory treatment without the patient being disconnected from the primary care provider. An 18 per cent reduction in admissions was achieved over a two-year period.

Hansen, commenting on the experiment, considered that the role of primary care must be a core concern in any attempt to shift the emphasis of psychiatric treatment from an institution to the community.

Model 5   The Nunhead sector model

This model (Strathdee *et al.* 1993) has been developed in a sector with 45 000 population in the Nunhead area of south London. The sector mental health services are developed with an emphasis on integration with primary care. Current initiatives have included:

- joint case registers of the long-term mentally ill in the practices
- development of good practice protocols for the treatment of common mental health conditions
- out-patient clinics relocated to GP surgeries
- joint audit of care using the good practice protocols
- specific liaison nurses attached to practices
- proposals to develop locality commissioning service models along mental health sector boundaries.

In summary, models which integrate primary and secondary care have been demonstrated to have the following benefits:

- reduction of hospital admissions and length of stay
- earlier detection of psychiatric illness
- a greater ability to promote relapse prevention
- provision of care for those who are poor attenders at hospital clinics
- increased patient and carer satisfaction.

The needs of individuals with mental health disorders

In this section we examine how a more systematic approach to the development of liaison services might come from adopting a needs-led approach. Two major dichotomies are involved in the delivery of mental health services in primary care today. First is the matter of equity of access to both quality and quantity of specialist services. The majority of practices which have attached professionals are the larger, better resourced ones which can offer accommodation to specialist teams. The patients of smaller single-handed or small group practices are at a disadvantage in that their teams are smaller, and their premises are inadequate to house additional workers. In addition, they are often based in areas with the highest levels of deprivation and, therefore, likely psychiatric morbidity. Their patients therefore have less access to specialist care.

The second dichotomy is the difference in priority given to individuals with different mental health disorders. In theory, secondary care services give the long-term mentally ill priority, while hard-pressed general practice more often wants immediate help for individuals with short-term difficulties. In many ways this dilemma seems unnecessary. Table 13.3 identifies the range of needs of those with both severe and 'minor' disorders and demonstrates that the *needs differ in degree rather than in the total range.*

Table 13.3 The range of needs of individuals with mental health disorders

Needs	The long-term mentally ill	Common primary care disorders
Case identification and case register recall	+++	+
Crisis intervention (including for suicide and parasuicide)	+++	++
Medication	+++	+
Respite and crisis community beds	+++	+
Family education and support	+++	++
Marital/sexual counselling	+	+++
Behavioural/cognitive therapies	+	+++
Supportive counselling	++	+++
Case management and assertive outreach	+++	+
Physical care	+++	++
Social skills and stress management	+++	+++
Day care	+++	+
Welfare benefits advice	++	++
Housing	++	++
Assessment	+	+
Support group/self-help group	++	+++
Information and education about illness and services	+++	+++

Research into practice

This table of needs and a review of models of good practices from the literature suggest future directions for liaison in the interface of primary and secondary care. This section examines the research evidence for the form of liaison which will produce an optimal interaction, and explores possible models.

Users' views of primary care services

In addition to professional views about the shape of provision, the political strength of the service user or consumer has gained increasing respect and authority. A major study of the views of 516 users of mental health services nationally (Pilgrim and Rogers 1993*a*) found that the profile of primary care services was high on the agenda. Their key findings were that users regard GPs as the most important gate-keepers to health and social services. In contrast to expressed views about secondary services, the majority found GPs helpful and to have a positive attitude, being regarded as 'pathologizing' behaviour less than psychiatrists. The accessibility, flexibility and lack of stigma of primary care services were seen to contrast favourably with those of secondary care. GPs were seen to offer continuity of care in contrast to rotating hospital doctors. Dissatisfaction with GPs centres on their use of drugs at the expense of referral for counselling or other specialist help. Lack of information on problem definition and treatment also formed a cause for concern. The problem of GPs perceiving individuals as 'mental' cases and therefore treating their physical illnesses less seriously was highlighted

(Rogers 1993). Users of mental health services in a crisis are highly critical of the unsuitable environment and attitudes, experience, and management offered by casualty staff. They value rapid response in crisis situations and ask for continuity of care by known and experienced health workers. Increasingly they seek alternative facilities to in-patient hospital admission such as crisis houses in the community, crisis flats and user-run sanctuaries.

General practices: equity of access and referral practices of GPs

General practitioners are, in general, enthusiastic about community mental health teams and having access to them (Ingham *et al.* 1972; Brown and Tower 1990). However, two models would appear to be necessary depending on the sort of general practice that exists.

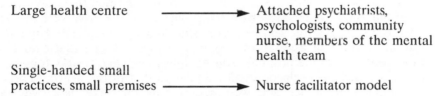

Large health centre ⟶ Attached psychiatrists, psychologists, community nurse, members of the mental health team

Single-handed small practices, small premises ⟶ Nurse facilitator model

In the text above we have alluded to the difficulties of providing equity of access for patients coming from small, poorly resourced practices compared with those in a large well-rounded group practice or health centre. In the latter, the sessional attachment, either of individual members of the community teams or of the community team as a whole is feasible. For the former, the model must be one of provision of a nurse facilitator (Sutherby *et al.* 1994). In a recent survey of over 1000 individuals involved in the care of people with mental health difficulties in the area of Southwark, many general practitioners and psychiatrists argued that, for this sort of practice, it was important to provide facilitators whose role could be the setting up of resource directories of all services in the area and negotiating sessional inputs for patients of small practices. These staff could possibly be based at a local community mental health centre.

Agreeing priorities in the liaison

It is important that primary and secondary care services and the various disciplines work together to prioritize the most vulnerable individuals with severe disorders. This makes planning sense for a number of reasons. First, this group tends to be 'needy, rather than noisy' and it is important that practitioners advocate their needs. Second, unless the needs of this group are prioritized and met, with the provision of care plans including care management and assertive outreach, they will continue to be heavy users of inappropriate services. For example, they are over-represented in police stations, courts, and prisons; they are frequent consulters of their GPs; have a high level of physical morbidity and use the most expensive mental health resource – hospital beds. There is clear evidence that once these patients have adequate care, their use of hospital beds decreases significantly, allowing a redeployment of staff and other resources to the community. The priorities have to be agreed as it is clear that no one discipline can effect change single-handed.

The skills and expertise of the multidisciplinary team including nurses, occupational therapists, social workers, psychologists and psychiatrists are necessary (Marks *et al*. 1988).

Service and primary care liaison for the long-term mentally ill

Research clearly indicates that this group falls away from contact with the specialist services. Murray Parkes *et al*. (1962), following up a cohort of schizophrenic patients discharged from London mental hospitals, found that almost three-quarters had seen their GP in the year after discharge with more than half consulting over five times. Just less than 60 per cent of the sample had attended hospital out-patient clinics in the same time and, of these, over half had been seen less than five times. Similarly, Pantellis *et al*. (1988) in the South Camden Schizophrenia Study identified that only three-fifths of the known individuals with schizophrenia in the area were in contact with the psychiatric services. Lee and Murray (1988), studying the long-term outcome of a group of depressed patients, found that over half had lost contact with the hospital services. Johnstone *et al*. (1984), following a cohort of discharged schizophrenics similar to that of the Murray Parkes group, found that 24 per cent were seeing only their GP in a five-year follow-up period.

It is therefore crucial that secondary and primary services join together in an agreed service plan and timetable to improve the quality of care for the long-term mentally ill. General practice is no stranger to the management of chronic disorders. It has been demonstrated that in primary care settings the quality of care of individuals with continuing disorders such as diabetes and asthma is significantly improved by a six-part strategy. For the severely mentally ill, this could involve (Strathdee and Kendrick 1994):

- Stage 1 – establish a practice case register of the severe long-term mentally ill (SLTMI)
- Stage 2 – work with social services to arrange for comprehensive holistic needs assessments
- Stage 3 – develop agreed, feasible good practice guidelines in consultation, review and care planning with local mental health services
- Stage 4 – develop and participate in specific training programmes
- Stage 5 – define clearly agreed roles and responsibilities for primary and specialist services
- Stage 6 – develop a practice policy as the basis of joint audit and evaluation.

The development of registers of vulnerable individuals can form a practical focused first step to the development of good liaison between primary and secondary care services. Such initiatives are facilitated by practices having computerized age/sex registers with repeat prescribing lists and by local mental health services having care programme approach registers. Without registers of the most vulnerable individuals, GPs are at risk of being unaware of the needs or existence of this client group until they present in crisis. The care programme approach policy (Kingdon 1994) requires that vulnerable individuals are known through a register which prevents them being neglected by services. Having identified such individuals, the joint development of practice policies in optimal care offers a useful strategy for the organization of practices to maximize care of this client group. From secondary care the growing development of care management and assertive outreach teams is a welcome initiative. Home-based community care by experienced community teams has been demonstrated to be as effective as hospital care in both the management of acute episodes and rehabilitation services for this group of people (Hoult *et al.* 1983; Stein and Test 1980; Dean and Gadd 1989, 1990).

Communication and discharge practices

As has been indicated above, the patterns of communication between GPs and mental health services are unsatisfactory to both parties and rarely meet minimum standards. Clear guidance on the optimal form and content of communications emerges from studies (Williams and Wallace 1974; Pullen and Yellowlees 1985). Psychiatrists want specific items of information in referral letters. These include: background family and social history, details of presenting problems, details of interventions tried and effects noted, the reason for referral, the service the GP expects the psychiatrist to offer and their own view of their continuing or transferred responsibilities.

General practice

GPs expect specific items of information in letters back from a mental health assessment. These include: a clear management plan, indication of suicide risk, what the patient has been told about their condition, the prognosis and likely continuing disabilities and influence on the patient's lifestyle, the role the GP and primary care team is expected to play in the management plan and the role to be played by the specialist staff, and an indication of prescribing roles and responsibilities. In the management of patients with continuing disorders, GPs want: six-monthly management plans, indications of treatment time scales, effects, possible side effects, outcomes, defined roles and responsibilities of primary and specialist teams. Clearly, local differences exist in different areas and such 'want lists' should form the basis of negotiation and contracting.

Education and information

In a study of 154 GPs in Camberwell, Strathdee (1990) found that information and education were considered important in ensuring effective liaison by general practitioners. Specific requests included: a directory of all local services and resources for their practices with details of services/interventions offered, criteria for referral, details of time and scope of treatments, expected outcomes and difficulties of therapies, named contact and telephone number in each department to discuss appropriateness of referral, and rapid communication about appointments and assessments. Users are also increasingly asking for additional information about their condition, treatment models and the range of services available to them (Pilgrim and Rogers 1993*b*).

Physical care

Liaison is particularly important in terms of defining clear roles and responsibility in relation to individuals who have physical health care needs. Physical morbidity often co-exists with psychiatric morbidity. Forty-five per cent of individuals with long-term mental health disorders have physical morbidity with standard mortality rates significantly higher than the general population (Brugha *et al.* 1989; Mortensen and Juel 1993). Such disorders most commonly affect the cardiovascular and respiratory systems but also include obesity and anaemia secondary to undernourishment. Often patients, particularly those who have difficulty in forming trusting relationships or who experience articulation problems, may be helped in their consultations by the presence or support of a key worker or care manager.

Family and carer education and support

The GP is often the point of main contact for the families of individuals, whether it is a patient presenting in crisis, or individuals with continuing mental health disorders. In some areas, it is clear that where GPs work well with families and the secondary care services, the liaison can have an advantageous effect for patients. The most apposite work for family intervention has come from Falloon (Falloon *et al.* 1984; Falloon 1989) who has developed an effective, family-based treatment package for schizophrenia. The patient-orientated management combines optimal neuroleptic drug therapy, rehabilitation, counselling, problem-solving psychotherapy, crisis intervention, and practical assistance with problems such as finances and housing. This approach seeks to enhance the stress reducing capacity of the individual and family through improved understanding of the illness, and training in behavioural methods of problem-solving. Falloon *et al.* (1990) advocate the application of this approach to the primary care setting with referrals processed initially by community psychiatric nurses based in general practices.

Responsibility for community homes and hostels

With the decrease in psychiatric beds in hospital settings many residents are placed in sheltered accommodation in the community. Horder (1991) studied the establishment of three hostels and group home facilities for patients discharged from Friern hospital. Her aim was to establish the burden of extra responsibility placed on the local GPs and to ascertain the nature of the medical care needed. She found that the residents had a relatively high sickness rate and had higher rates of consultation than the population at large (an average of 7–8 per year, compared with the population norms of 4). Despite this, the unanimous opinion of the GPs involved was that the work had not been unduly arduous or difficult, and that off-duty work was minimal. Three-quarters of the doctors had no regrets about taking on the patients and several were spontaneous in commenting on its interest and value. She concluded that the amount of work devolved to GPs in community facilities depends on such factors as age and health of residents, staffing levels, training, experience and morale in the homes, the standard of local community services and the involvement and interest of the GPs and psychiatrists.

Crisis services

Surveys of Camberwell GPs (Strathdee 1990) and national replications have found that GPs value: rapid response on a 24-hour, seven-day-a-week basis by crisis intervention outreach teams, assessment by experienced staff, outreach assessment and treatment of suicidal and parasuicidal patients, and easily accessible approved social worker services. Nationally the majority of crisis intervention services are provided only on a nine-to-five basis by experienced mental health staff. Out of hours, casualty departments are the commonest form of service (Johnson and Thornicroft 1992). There is, therefore, a clear discrepancy between what GPs and patients think is effective crisis care and that currently provided by secondary care services around the country. Other elements of shared care are important in further developing the liaison, for example, the development of crisis cards and contracts as a possible liaison initiative which improves joint working by helping individuals prevent crises or identify their own individualized optimal response to crisis.

Even when the patients are in contact with the secondary care services, the GP is often the point of first contact in crisis. In his follow-up study of schizophrenics in the community Murray Parkes concluded that 'while the hospitals and out-patient clinics were responsible for initiating most of the treatment required for maintaining the patients' health, it was the general practitioners who played the major role in dealing with the crises and relapses that occurred in over half the cases'. Eighty per cent of Kendrick's GPs (Kendrick 1992) asserted that often patients with long-term mental health problems only came to their attention when a crisis arose. In keeping with the thrust of primary care to move to health promotion and health gain, rather than reactive treatment, for their more stable population general practitioners are well placed to practise prevention as they can use their frequent contacts with patients to recognize changes in behaviour or consultation habits (Widmer and Cadoret 1979). Over time they can play a key role in working with patients, carers and relatives in establishing premorbid patterns of relapse and enabling timely, tested and individually appropriate levels of medication to be instituted (Birchwood *et al.* 1989). GPs have themselves identified a need for training in the implementation of the Mental Health Act (Phelan *et al.* 1993) and clarification of their role in relation to social workers.

Suicide prevention in primary care

Liaison in training between primary and secondary care teams has a major role to play in working to achieve the *Health of the Nation* (Department of Health 1993) suicide targets. Sixty per cent of individuals who kill themselves will have visited their GP in the month before the act. However, this is not the case for individuals below the age of 35 and it may be that there is a growing number of individuals who do not find it appropriate to discuss emotional or psychological problems with a doctor. An alternative explanation is the greater degree of impulsiveness in these suicide attempts (Vassilas and Morgan 1993). In every sector of 50 000: 6–12 people kill themselves annually, of whom 3–5 will be known to the psychiatric services, and 8–10 will be known to GPs.

GPs may not recognize when patients suffer from depression and are at risk of suicide, and often do not ask patients about suicide plans or previous suicide attempts. Patients are at particular risk of suicide during the first month after discharge and when they discharge themselves against medical advice. The GP has a crucial role in monitoring the patient and providing continuity of care (Vassilas and Morgan 1993).

The attitudes of professionals and relatives have been shown to have a significant influence on patterns of repeated self-harming behaviour in vulnerable individuals (Pierce 1986; Patel 1975). GPs often feel anxious about the management of suicidal patients, as they believe they lack the skills to deal with them. Specific training in suicide prevention for GPs has been shown to be effective (Rutz *et al.* 1992) and should consist of:

* basic facts about suicide and risk factors
* clear guidelines for assessment of suicide risk
* defined role of staff in recognizing and treating suicide risk
* practical guidelines for the management of patients
* specific safeguards for the community management of individuals at risk.

Fund-holding and mental health services

The general practice fund-holding scheme was introduced as part of the organizational reforms of the NHS in 1991. This scheme offered general practitioners control over their budgets to cover prescriptions, allowed them to negotiate for specialist out-patient consultations and elective surgical procedures for their patients. The fund-holding scheme was thought to be a key strategy in forcing secondary care to take the needs of primary care more seriously in their strategic planning and service delivery. Concern has been expressed by many that the reforms would lead to a two-tier service in which the advantages gained by fund-holders for their patients would be achieved at the expense of patients in other practices (Coulter and Bradlow 1993). To date, the implications would appear to be as follows: referral patterns among fund-holding GPs remain as idiosyncratic and unrelated to need as those by non-fund-holders and differ little from the pre-fund-holding implementation. General practitioners are thought in fund-holding to have negotiated for quality measures to be included in the contracts of patients by out-patient clinic staff. These relate particularly to the availability of patients' notes in out-patient clinics, respect shown to general practitioners in telephone communications by hospital doctors, the availability and supply of medicines after discharge, the clarity of patient management plans for general practitioners, the earlier arrival of discharge notification, the seniority of hospital doctors seeing new out-patients and the avoidance of unnecessary duplication investigations (Bowling *et al.*).

Summary of the way forward for liaison between primary and secondary care

We have outlined above many areas which particularly focus on the practical interface between primary and secondary care for the future. It is hoped that many of these areas, including the realms of communication patterns, patterns of service delivery and mutual teaching and training, will form the basis of discussions between local primary care and community mental health teams. If effective liaison is to be established, we would suggest that there needs to be a two-tiered approach with purchasers becoming more sophisticated in the nature and quality of services, which they require providers to deliver. Providers need to take ownership of developing good practice protocols, jointly agreed guidelines, and the development of high-quality and cost effective services.

References

Balestrieri M, Williams P and Wilkinson G (1988). Specialist mental health treatment in general practice, a meta-analysis. *Psychological Medicine*, **18**, 711–717.

Birchwood M, Smith J, Macmillan F *et al.* (1989). Predicting relapse in schizophrenia: the development and implementation of an early signs monitoring system using patients and families as observers, a preliminary investigation. *Psychological Medicine*, **18**, 649–656.

Boardman J (1987). *The Mental Health Advice Centre in Lewisham. Service Usage Trends from 1978–1984*. Research Report No. 3. The National Unit for Psychiatric Research and Development, Lewisham.

British Association of Counselling (1990). *Guidelines for the Employment of Counsellors*. Information sheet 9. British Association of Counselling, Rugby.

Brook A (1967). An experiment in GP/psychiatrist co-operation. *Journal of the Royal College of General Practitioners*, **13**, 127–131.

Brooker C, Tarrier N, Barrowclough B and Goldberg D (1992). Skills for CPNs working with the seriously mentally ill: report of a pilot trial of psycho-social intervention. In *Community Psychiatric Nursing: a Research Perspective* Vol. 11 (eds. C Brooker and E White). Chapman and Hall, London.

Brown L and Tower J (1990). Psychiatrists in primary care: would general practitioners welcome them? *Journal of the Royal College of General Practitioners*, **40**, 369–371.

Brown R, Strathdee G, Christie-Brown J and Robinson P (1988). A comparison of referrals to primary care and hospital outpatient clinics. *British Journal of Psychiatry*, **153**, 168–173.

Browning S M, Ford M F, Goddard C A and Brown A C (1987). A psychiatric clinic in general practice; a description and comparison with an outpatient clinic. *Bulletin of the Royal College of Psychiatry*, **11** (4), 114–117.

Brugha T S, Wing J K and Smith B L (1989). Physical ill-health of the long-term mentally ill in the community. Is there an unmet need? *British Journal of Psychiatry*, **155**, 777–782.

Corney R (1984). The effectiveness of attached social workers in the management of depressed female patients in general practice. *Psychological Medicine*, **14** (monograph suppl. 6), 47.

Corney R H (1985). Social work in general practice. *Journal of the Royal College of General Practitioners*, **35**, 291–292.

Coulter A and Bradlow J (1993). Effect of NHS reforms on general practitioners' referral patterns. *British Medical Journal*, **306**, 433–437.

Creed F and Marks B (1989). Liaison psychiatry in general practice: a comparison of the liaison-attachment scheme and the shifted outpatient clinic models. *Journal of the Royal College of General Practitioners*, **39**, 514–517.

Cumberledge Report (1986). *Neighbourhood Nursing – a Focus for Care*. Report of the Community Nursing Review, HMSO, London.

Darling C and Tyrer P (1990). Brief encounters in general practice: liaison in general practice psychiatry clinics. *Psychiatric Bulletin*, **14**, 592–594.

Dean C and Gadd E M (1989). An inner city home treatment service for acute psychiatric patients. *Psychiatric Bulletin*, **13**, 667–669.

Dean C and Gadd E M (1990). Home treatment for acute psychiatric illness. *British Medical Journal*, **301**, 1021–1023.

Department of Health (1993). *The Health of the Nation*. HMSO, London.

Deys C, Dowling E and Golding V (1989). Clinical psychology: a consultative approach in general practice. *Journal of the Royal College of General Practitioners* **39**, 342–344.

Earll L and Kincey J (1982). Clinical psychology in general practice. *Journal of the Royal College of General Practitioners*, **32**, 32–37.

Falloon I R H (1989). Behavioural approaches in schizophrenia. In *Scientific Approaches on Epidemiological and Social Psychiatry. Essays in Honour of Michael Shepherd* (eds. P Williams, G Wilkinson and K Rawnsley). Routledge, London.

Falloon I, Boyd J L and McGill C W (1984). *Family Care of Schizophrenia*. Guilford Press, New York, pp. 355–375.

Falloon I R H, Shanahan W, Laporta M and Krekorian H A R (1990). Integrated family, general practice and mental health care in the management of schizophrenia. *Journal of the Royal Society of Medicine*, **83**, 225–228.

Gilchrist I C, Gough J B, Horsfall-Turner Y R *et al.* (1978). Social work in general practice. *Journal of the Royal College of General Practitioner*, **28**, 675–686.

Goldberg D and Bridges K (1988). Somatic presentation of psychiatric illness in primary care settings. *Journal of Psychosomatic Research*, **32**, 137–144.

Goldberg D P and Huxley P (1980). *Mental Illness in the Community. The Pathway to Psychiatric Care*. Tavistock Publications, London.

Hansen V (1987). Psychiatric service within primary care. Mode of organisation and influence on admission rates to a mental hospital. *Acta Psychiatrica Scandinavica*, **76**, 121–128.

Horder J (1991). Care for patients discharged from psychiatric hospital. *British Journal of General Practice*, **4**, 399–400.

Hoult J, Reynolds I, Charbonneau-Powis M, Weekes P and Briggs J (1983). Psychiatric hospital versus community treatment: the result of a randomised trial. *Australian and New Zealand Journal of Psychiatry*, **17**, 160–167.

Ingham J, Rawnley K and Hughes D (1972). Psychiatric disorder and its declaration in contrasting areas of South Wales. *Psychological Medicine*, **2**, 281–292.

Irving J (1993). Practical and training issues. In *Counselling in General Practice* (eds. R Corney and R Jenkins). Routledge, London.

Johnson S and Thornicroft G (1992). *A Survey of Mental Health Emergency Services in England and Wales*. Unpublished research report, Institute of Psychiatry, London.

Johnson S and Thornicroft G (1993). The sectorisation of psychiatric services in England and Wales. *Social Psychiatry and Psychiatric Epidemiology*, **28**, 45–47.

Johnstone E C, Owens D G C, Gold A *et al.* (1984). Schizophrenic patients discharged from hospital – a follow-up study. *British Journal of Psychiatry*, **145**, 586–590.

Joseph P, Bridgewater J A, Ramsden S S and El Kabir DJ (1990). A psychiatric clinic for the single homeless in a primary care setting in inner London. *Psychiatric Bulletin*, **14**, 270–271.

Kaeser A C and Cooper B (1971). The psychiatric out-patient, the general practitioner and the out-patient clinic; an operation study: a review. *Psychological Medicine*, **1**, 312–271.

Kendrick T (1992). The shift to community health care: the impact on general practitioners. In *The Primary Care of Schizophrenia* (eds. R Jenkins, V Field and R Young). HMSO, London.

Kingdon D (1994). Care programme approach. Recent government policy and legislation. *Psychiatric Bulletin*, **18**(2).

Lee A S and Murray R M (1988). The long-term outcome of Maudsley depressives. *British Journal of Psychiatry*, **153**, 741–751.

Low C B and Pullen I (1988). Psychiatric clinics in different settings: a case register study. *British Journal of Psychiatry*, **153**, 243–245.

Marks I (1985). Controlled trial of psychiatric nurse therapists in primary care. *British Medical Journal*, **240**, 1181–1184.

Marks I, Connolly J and Muijen M (1988). The Maudsley Daily Living Programme. *Bulletin of the Royal College of Psychiatrists*, **12**, 22–24.

Mitchell A R K (1985). Psychiatrists in primary health care settings. *British Journal of Psychiatry*, **147**, 371–379.

Mortensen P B and Juel K (1993). Mortality and causes of death in first admitted schizophrenic patients. *British Journal of Psychiatry*, **163**, 183–189.

Murray Parkes C, Brown G W, and Monck E M (1962). The general practitioner and the schizophrenic patient. *British Medical Journal*, **1**, 972–976.

Myers S N, Nazareth I D and King M B (1993). Care of schizophrenia in general practice: 4. Psychiatric, social and service utilization profiles. (In preparation).

Pantellis C, Taylor J and Campbell P (1988). The South Camden schizophrenia survey. *Bulletin of the Royal College of Psychiatrists*, **12**, 98–101.

Patel A (1975). Attitudes towards self poisoning. *British Medical Journal*, **2**, 426–430.

Paykel E S, Mangen S P, Griffiths J H and Burns T P (1982). Community psychiatric nursing for neurotic patients: a controlled trial. *British Journal of Psychiatry* **140**, 573–581.

Phelan M, Strathdee G and Holden A (1993). *A General Practitioner's Guide to the Mental Health Act*. The Maudsley Practical Handbook Series No. 1. Boots Pharmaceuticals in Association with PRiSM, London.

Pierce D (1986). Deliberate self-harm: how do patients view their treatment? *British Journal of Psychiatry*, **149**, 624–626.

Pilgrim D and Rogers A (1993a). *A Sociology of Mental Health and Illness*. Open University Press, London.

Pilgrim D and Rogers A (1993b). Mental health service users' views of medical practitioners. *Journal of Interprofessional Care*, **7**(2), 167–176.

Pullen I M and Yellowlees A (1985). Is communication improving between general practitioners and psychiatrists? *British Medical Journal*, **153**, 663–666.

Robson M H, France R and Bland M (1984). Clinical psychologists in primary care: controlled clinical and economic evaluation. *British Medical Journal*, **288**, 1805–1808.

Rogers S (1993). *Primary Care and Mental Health. 'On tap: Not on top'. Consulting Mental Health Service Users about Primary Care Services in South-East London (Lewisham)*. London School of Economics and Political Sciences, London (unpubl. thesis).

Rutz W, Von Knorring L and Walinder J (1992). Long term effects of an educational programme for general practitioners, given by the Swedish Committee for the Prevention and Treatment of Depression. *Acta Psychiatrica Scandinavica*, **85**, 83–88.

Scott A I F and Freeman C P L (1992). Edinburgh primary care depression study: treatment outcome, patient satisfaction and cost after 16 weeks. *British Medical Journal*, **304**, 883–887.

Sharp D and Morrell D (1989). The psychiatry of general practice. In *Scientific Approaches on Epidemiological and Social Psychiatry. Essays in Honour of Michael Shepherd* (eds. P Williams, G Wilkinson and K Rawnsley). Routledge, London.

Shepherd M, Cooper B, Brown A and Kalton G (1966). *Psychiatric Illness in General Practice.* Oxford University Press, Oxford.

Sibbald B, Addington Hall J, Brenneman D and Freeling P (1993). Counsellors in English and Welsh general practices: their nature and distribution. *British Medical Journal,* **306**, 29–33.

Stein L I and Test M A (1980). Alternative to mental hospital treatment. I: Conceptual model, treatment program, and clinical evaluation. *Archives of General Psychiatry,* **37**, 392–397.

Strathdee G (1988). Psychiatrists in primary care: the general practitioner viewpoint. *Family Practice,* **5**(2), 111–115.

Strathdee G (1990). The delivery of psychiatric care. *Journal of the Royal Society of Medicine,* **83**, 222–225.

Strathdee G (1992). The interface between psychiatry and primary care in the management of schizophrenic patients in the community. In *The Primary Care of Schizophrenia* (eds. R Jenkins, V Field and R Young). HMSO, London.

Strathdee G (1994). Mental health services and primary care. In *Psychiatry in General* (eds. G Pereira, A Wright, G Wilkinson and I Pullen). Gaskell, London.

Strathdee G and Sutherby K (1993). *Literature Review for the Development of a Primary Care Strategy for Mental Health.* (Unpubl. report.)

Strathdee G and Thornicroft G (1994). Community psychiatry and service evaluation. In *The Essentials of Psychiatry* (eds. R Murray, P Hill and P McGuffin). Oxford University Press, Oxford.

Strathdee G and Williams P (1984). A survey of psychiatrists in primary care: the silent growth of a new service. *Journal of the Royal College of General Practitioners,* **11**, 615–618.

Strathdee G, King M B, Araya R *et al.* (1990). A standardised assessment of patients referred to primary care and hospital psychiatric clinics. *Psychological Medicine,* **20**, 219–224.

Strathdee G, Perry M and Wood H (1993). Pencis, Making Community Care a User-Centered Service: Openmind, **67**, 16–17.

Sutherby K, Srinath S and Strathdee G (1992). The domiciliary consultation service: outdated anachronism or essential part of community psychiatric outreach? *Health Trends,* **24**(3), 103–105.

Teasdale J, Fennell M J V, Hibbert GA *et al.* (1984). Cognitive therapy for major depressive disorder in primary care. *British Journal of Psychiatry,* **144**, 400–406.

Thomas R V R and Corney R H (1992). A survey of links between mental health professionals and general practice in six district health authorities. *British Journal of General Practitioners,* **42**, 358–361.

Thornicroft G and Bebbington P (1989). Deinstitutionalisation: from hospital closure to service development. *British Journal of Psychiatry,* **155**, 739–753.

Tyrer P (1985). The 'hive' system: a model for the psychiatric service. *British Journal of Psychiatry,* **146**, 571–575.

Tyrer P, Sievewright N and Wollerton S (1984). General practice psychiatric clinics: impact on psychiatric services. *British Journal of Psychiatry,* **145**, 15–19.

Vassilas C A and Morgan H G (1993). General practitioners' contacts with victims of suicide. *British Medical Journal,* **307**, 300–301.

Widmer R B and Cadoret R J (1979). Depression in family practice: changes in pattern of family visits and complaints during subsequent developing depressions. *Journal of Family Practice,* **9**, 1017–1021.

Williams P and Wallace B (1974). General practitioners and psychiatrists – do they communicate? *British Medical Journal,* **1**, 505–507.

Wing J K. (ed.) (1989). *Health Services Planning and Research: Contributions from Case Registers.* Gaskell, London.

Wooff K, Goldberg D P and Fryers T (1988). The practice of community psychiatric nursing and mental health social work in Salford. Some implications for community care. *British Journal of Psychiatry*, **152**, 783–792.

Wooff K, Rose S and Street J (1989). Community psychiatric nursing services in Salford, Southampton and Worcester. In *Health Services Planning and Research: contributions from case registers* (ed. J K Wing). Gaskell, London.

14 Long-term medication and the responsibilities of the team

M. Peet

Introduction

In recent decades, there have been significant advances in the psychological and social management of people with mental disorder. Nevertheless, drug treatment remains an essential component of treatment for many patients. If drug treatment is to be used, then this should be done with the highest possible level of knowledge and skill in order to maximize benefits and minimize adverse effects. Drug treatment is not a matter for the psychiatrist alone, and other team members have an essential part to play. In this chapter, the proper use of long-term medication will be outlined, and the role of multidisciplinary team members in relation to long-term medication will be discussed.

Antipsychotic medication

Antipsychotic drugs are also commonly known as neuroleptics or major tranquillizers. The primary use of antipsychotic drugs is to treat symptoms of psychosis, that is delusions, hallucinations and related phenomena. Antipsychotic drugs are important in the short-term treatment of psychotic conditions such as schizophrenia, mania and delusional depression. The only well-established indication for long-term antipsychotic medication is schizophrenia.

Types of drug

The available standard drugs such as haloperidol and chlorpromazine have differing chemical structures but all have similar efficacy. Side effects vary somewhat between drugs, and this may form the basis for choosing one antipsychotic drug over another. For example, haloperidol has more neurological side effects but less cardiovascular side effects than chlorpromazine.

For long-term treatment, depot preparations are often used. These are oily esters of the drugs which are given by deep intramuscular injection. The drug is slowly released from the injection site over a period of one to four weeks.

It is often said that the use of depot neuroleptic medication aids compliance with treatment. Against this, controlled trials comparing depot with oral medication have shown no difference in efficacy (Rifkin *et al.* 1977; Schooler *et al.* 1980). However, compliance is always better in research studies than in real life, and experience does suggest a higher relapse rate in people taking oral antipsychotic medication than in those on depot medication (Johnson 1990). A drawback of using depot antipsychotic drugs to improve compliance is that responsibility for medication is taken away from the patient and the treatment can become coersive. This can be damaging to the therapeutic relationship. Also, dosage adjustments take longer with depot than with oral medication.

Efficacy

Davis (1975) reviewed 24 placebo controlled clinical trials of antipsychotic drug maintenance therapy in schizophrenia and found an average relapse rate of 65 per cent when no medication was used, compared with 30 per cent when antipsychotic drugs were given. However, this gives too positive a picture of the benefits of antipsychotic medication, because some studies were only a few months in duration. Most schizophrenic patients will relapse even whilst taking medication, if they are followed up for long enough. A study which followed first episode patients with schizophrenia for up to two years from hospital discharge showed relapse rates of 46 per cent with drug treatment, relative to 62 per cent with placebo treatment (Crow *et al.* 1986). Antipsychotic drugs are in no sense curative. A further disadvantage of antipsychotic drugs is that they are not effective against chronic negative symptoms such as emotional blunting and loss of spontaneity and motivation. Indeed, high doses of neuroleptics produce side effects which mimic negative schizophrenic symptoms (Van Putten *et al.* 1990; Lader 1993). It is these negative symptoms which are responsible for much of the social morbidity of chronic schizophrenia. Some of the newer antipsychotic drugs such as risperidone are claimed to be more effective against negative symptoms, but available clinical data give little support to this claim (Drug and Therapeutics Bulletin 1993*b*). An exception is clozapine, which does appear to improve negative symptoms (Kane *et al.* 1988).

For patients who remain symptomatic despite long-term antipsychotic medication, a number of alternative drug treatments are available. The addition of lithium or carbamazepine may be helpful if there is prominent mood disturbance or aggression associated with the schizophrenia (Christisen *et al.* 1991). A notable recent introduction is the novel antipsychotic drug clozapine which is effective in treating 30 to 60 per cent of patients who have failed to respond to conventional antipsychotic drugs (Kane *et al.* 1988). When effective, clozapine is continued as a long-term treatment. The main drawback of clozapine is blood toxicity with a 1 to 2 per cent incidence of agranulocytosis. This causes susceptibility to infections so that a sore throat or other infection in a patient on clozapine should be taken seriously. At present, clozapinetreatment can be initiated only in hospital by a psychiatrist, with frequent blood testing to measure the white cell count.

Dosage and duration of treatment

There is increasing emphasis on the need to minimize exposure to antipsychotic drugs, particularly in view of the long-term side effects which are discussed later. For some antipsychotic drugs there is evidence of a 'therapeutic window'. This is a dose range providing maximal efficacy, with doses higher or lower than the window being less effective. An analysis of all studies of long-term treatment with fluphenazine decanoate suggested a therapeutic window of between 10 and 30 mg fortnightly (Baldessarini *et al.* 1988). The same authors reviewed 33 studies of high-dose long-term antipsychotic treatment and concluded that it was unusual to obtain significant additional benefit from megadose treatment but that the risk of neurological side effects was substantially increased.

The Royal College of Psychiatrists (1993) has published a consensus statement on the use of high-dose antipsychotic medication. They define high dose as exceeding the upper limit recommended in the British National Formulary. Such high dosages are not uncommon in British psychiatric practice. Included in the guidelines is the need to discuss high-dose treatment with the multidisciplinary team; to obtain valid consent for high-dose treatment; and to reduce the dose back to normal levels after a three-month period if there has been no improvement. All too often, patients are left on high-dose antipsychotic medication for long periods of time, even when lack of efficacy is demonstrable by continuing symptoms.

Because of the concern about high-dosage treatment, a number of very low-dosage strategies have been investigated. These have recently been reviewed (Schooler 1993). The two main strategies are continuous very low-dose depot medication (for example 5 mg every two weeks of fluphenazine decanoate), or 'targeted' neuroleptic medication which is given only when there are early warning signs of a relapse. Overall, the results of this work show that very low-dose and targeted neuroleptic treatment are less effective in preventing relapse than standard treatment, particularly during the second year of follow-up. However, patients on minimal neuroleptic treatment have fewer side effects. The balance between risk of relapse and severity of side effects is something which needs to be discussed with individual patients. It is possible that very low-dose neuroleptic treatment would be adequate if it was combined with effective psychosocial treatment, and research on this topic is currently in progress (Schooler 1993).

The studies of low-dose medication all included patients already stabilized on moderate doses, who have had their medication reduced at random. So far, there have been no adequately controlled trials of dosage reduction in people taking high dosages, although anecdotal evidence suggests that reduction from high to moderate dosage can be clinically beneficial (Cohen *et al.* 1989).

There is a problem as to when, if ever, antipsychotic medication can be safely discontinued. In some patients, careful review shows that they were started on long-term medication for inadequate reasons, possibly when primarily suffering from a mood disorder rather than schizophrenia. In such cases, long-term antipsychotic drugs can and should be gradually withdrawn. If the diagnosis of schizophrenia is sustained, then evidence from drug withdrawal studies suggests that only 20 per cent of patients will remain free of relapse even if they have been mentally stable for up to four years (Johnson *et al.* 1983). Drug withdrawal should be attempted only if every other factor, such as family and social environment, is optimal, and then only after discussion with the patient and family about the high risk of relapse. Withdrawal should be gradual over several months and closely monitored for signs of early relapse (Drug and Therapeutics Bulletin 1987). Even if complete withdrawal is not possible, at least a lower dosage can usually be attained. However, early success should not give rise to complacency. The peak time for relapse after discontinuing depot antipsychotic drugs is about five months.

Long-term side effects

The commonest long-term side effects of antipsychotic drugs are neurological, the so-called extrapyramidal side effects or EPS. The three commonest EPS are parkinsonism, akathisia and tardive dyskinesia (Bristow and Hirsch 1993). A recent Scottish survey of neuroleptic-treated schizophrenic patients found parkinsonism in 27 per cent, akathisia in 18 per cent, tardive dyskinesia in 29 per cent, and only 44 per cent of patients with no movement disorder (McCreadie *et al.* 1992).

Parkinsonism is characterized by muscle stiffness, tremor, shuffling walk and lack of facial movement. Many patients are prescribed long-term anticholinergic medication such as procyclidine or orphenadrine, to control parkinsonian symptoms but these extra drugs are often unnecessary (Double *et al.* 1993), especially when the dosage of antipsychotic medication is minimized.

Akathisia is a sensation of motor restlessness, particularly in the legs, which causes patients to fidget, walk around and march in one place. It is more common with higher dosages. A potential error is to confuse akathisia with agitation and to respond by increasing the dose of antipsychotic drug, when the appropriate response would be to reduce medication. Akathisia is a distressing experience which can lead to anxiety and depression, and non-compliance with medication (Van Putten 1974).

Tardive dyskinesia is probably the most serious long-term side effect of antipsychotic drugs, because in some patients it is irreversible even after antipsychotic medication is stopped. The main feature consists of abnormal movements of the mouth and tongue, including smacking and pouting movements of the lips and writhing of the tongue which may protude from the mouth. The hands and other parts of the body can also be affected. It has a prevalence of 15–20 per cent in patients on long-term antipsychotic drugs (Casey 1991) and is particularly prevalent in the elderly. It can follow a fluctuating course, so that the symptoms can appear and disappear even when antipsychotic medication is continued. Paradoxically, increasing the dose of antipsychotic medication can temporarily suppress tardive dyskinesia, whereas the movements may emerge for the first time only when dosage is reduced. Many patients with tardive dyskinesia do not realize that they suffer from the condition. Clearly any patient on long-term antipsychotic drugs should be warned about and monitored for tardive dyskinesia, but practice in this respect is very variable.

Psychosocial treatments and antipsychotic medication

The outcome of schizophrenia is markedly affected by social environment, and social environment has a substantial impact on the effectiveness of antipsychotic drugs. For example, high levels of expressed emotion (EE), with such features as excessive criticism, hostility and emotional over-involvement amongst family members, is associated with a high relapse rate in schizophrenia. Leff and Vaughn (1981) showed that, over a two-year period, patients treated with antipsychotic drugs had a 43 per cent relapse rate if they lived in high EE homes, but there were no relapses for those who lived in low EE homes. For those on no drugs, relapse rates were 50 per cent in low EE homes and 71 per cent in high EE homes. Thus, it appears that a high EE environment can largely negate the benefit of long-term antipsychotic medication.

There have been many studies on the interaction between drug treatment and various psychosocial interventions, including educational programmes about illness and treatment, exploration of potential stressors, and social skills training. Falloon and Brooker (1992) have reviewed ten controlled studies with adequate research design and follow-up for at least one year. The overall results are shown in Table 14.1. It is clear that social skills training and family- (or carer)-based management can substantially enhance the efficacy of antipsychotic medication. It should be noted that psychosocial treatment appears to be effective only against a background of effective antipsychotic drug treatment.

Lam (1991) reviewed studies of psychosocial family interventions in schizophrenia, and found that there were several common components of the various packages reported. These components are: a positive approach and genuine working relationship; avoiding the attribution of blame to family members; providing a structured, stable and dependable care package which in some cases included out of hours contact points; a focus on 'here and now' relationships and coping strategies; a focus on the family unit with respect for interpersonal boundaries; education about the nature and symptoms of schizophrenia; a behavioural approach; and improving communication between family members. One of the most standardized family approaches is that described by Falloon *et al.* (1984) which emphasizes a focus on family problem solving, structured education of the entire family unit about schizophrenia and its management, and home-based sessions. In a trial comparing this family treatment with a patient-orientated approach of similar

Table 14.1 The additive effects of drugs and psychosocial treatment in schizophrenia, percentage of patients relapsing at one and two years. Combined results of nine controlled studies (figures taken from Falloon and Brooker 1992).

	One year	Two years
Drugs and support	50%	64%
Drugs and social skills training	30%	37%
Drugs and family approaches	15%	37%

intensity, it was found that family treatment led to fewer exacerbations of schizophrenia, reduced symptomatology, and fewer hospital admissions over a two-year follow-up period (Falloon *et al*. 1985).

The most comprehensive study of social skills training in the after-care of schizophrenic patients is that of Hogarty *et al*. (1986, 1991). They studied patients living in high EE households and compared the effects of family treatment, social skills training and no psychosocial intervention. All patients were medicated. Over the first year, both family treatment and social skills training reduced relapse rate by half and the two approaches had an additive benefit. Benefits were maintained for most of the two-year treatment period, though patients given social skills training started to relapse at the end of the second year of follow-up. The effects of psychosocial interventions on social adjustment were minimal in this group of patients. Overall, it appears that long-term psychosocial input is necessary, and even then relapse may be delayed rather than prevented.

Several intervention strategies include education about medication. Simply giving information about current medication using a written factsheet is not an effective educational strategy. A behaviourally orientated programme for teaching medication management skills has been developed by Eckman *et al*. (1990). This programme not only gives information about medication and an understanding of its effects, but also gives the skills necessary to evaluate response to medication and side effects, the action to be taken when side effects occur, and how to negotiate medication issues with health care providers. Techniques include the use of video, role play, homework assignments and real-life exercises. The programme can be applied by a variety of mental health professionals including psychiatrists, psychologists, social workers, nurses and occupational therapists. A controlled trial of the programme has demonstrated its lasting effectiveness in improving knowledge and skills relating to medication (Eckman *et al*. 1992).

Lithium

Lithium salts, usually taken as lithium carbonate, have had several different uses in medicine over the centuries. Natural spring waters containing lithium were reputedly used by the ancient Greeks as a treatment of 'ill humour' and 'excitement'. The current use of lithium in psychiatric disorders has recently been reviewed by Peet and Pratt (1993). Lithium is effective in the short-term treatment of mania, and in combination with antidepressant drugs for treatment-resistant depression. However, the main use of lithium is in the long-term treatment of manic depressive disorder and recurrent depression.

Effectiveness of long-term lithium treatment

Recurrent mood disorder, whether bipolar (manic depressive) or unipolar (recurrent depression), tends to recur with increasing frequency over the years. Lithium is the treatment of choice for prevention of mood swings in manic depressive patients. Efficacy has been confirmed in many double blind trials (e.g. Coppen *et al*. 1971; Prien *et al*. 1973, 1984). However, the effect is not complete. The response rate to lithium is approximately 65 per cent. Of the patients who do respond, only some 20 per cent will have complete remission with no further episodes of mood disorder. The remainder will show reductions in severity and frequency of mood swings ranging from good to negligible (Prien and Gelenberg 1989). Episodes of depression or mania occurring during long-term lithium treatment can be treated with antidepressant or antipsychotic drugs added to the lithium as appropriate. For patients who fail to respond to lithium, particularly those with rapid cycling manic depressive disorder (greater than four episodes per year), carbamazepine may be effective, although the evidence supporting this is less secure than that for lithium (Prien and Gelenberg 1989). There is no good evidence that long-term antipsychotic medication is of benefit to patients with manic depressive disorder.

In the past there has been disagreement as to the effectiveness of lithium for preventing recurrent episodes of depression in the absence of manic episodes. However, the accumulated evidence now shows clearly that lithium is at least as effective as long-term antidepressant treatment in preventing relapses of recurrent depression (Souza and Goodwin 1991). In practice, the choice of whether to use lithium or an antidepressant for long-term preventative treatment depends upon the tolerability of the drug for individual patients. In most cases an antidepressant is easier to use because there is no need to monitor blood levels. Often, whichever antidepressant has been beneficial to treat the acute episode of depression is then continued for long-term preventative treatment (see section on antidepressants).

Practical management of lithium treatment

Practical aspects of patient selection and initial stabilization on lithium treatment have been reviewed by Peet and Pratt (1993). For patients established on long-term lithium treatment, regular monitoring is necessary. The blood level of lithium should be maintained at 0.5–0.8 mmol l⁻¹ in a blood sample taken 12 hours after the last dose. At one time, higher blood levels of 0.7–1.2 mmol l⁻¹ were recommended, but lower levels are just as effective for most patients (Coppen *et al.* 1983; Hullin 1980). Lower levels also give less risk of side effects and toxicity. Nevertheless, some individuals may require higher levels for optimum efficacy.

When therapeutic serum levels of lithium are established, these usually remain constant over time if the dosage is unaltered, except for the gradual reduction in dosage which may be necessary due to decreasing kidney function as patients become elderly. In physically healthy, well-informed and motivated patients who are aware of the signs of lithium toxicity, regular monitoring will contribute little to the safety of their treatment. However, regular contact with the prescriber is important and lithium estimations every four to six months will reinforce compliance and give both the patient and the prescriber confidence that lithium concentrations are stable (Schou 1988*b*). More frequent monitoring will be necessary under circumstances which can predispose to lithium toxicity, which are described later.

Lithium can cause reduced thyroid function, so that blood tests for thyroid hormones on an annual basis can be helpful in detecting early hypothyroidism (Myers and West 1987). Other routine tests during lithium treatment are unnecessary unless the patient has some known complicating physical disorder such as kidney or heart disease.

Lithium side effects and toxicity

Minor side effects such as tremor and loose stools tend to be seen more at the start of treatment and decrease with prolonged treatment (Vestergaard *et al.* 1988). Long-term side effects include weight gain and increased production of urine with resulting thirst. These effects are worse at higher dosages. Previous concern that lithium treatment might lead to kidney failure is not supported by careful review of the available evidence (Schou 1988*a*). Hypothyroidism is an uncommon complication of long-term lithium treatment which is reversible by stopping the lithium treatment or by adding a small dose of thyroxin.

By far the most important complication of lithium treatment is acute intoxication which occurs when the blood level rises too high. It is essential that both specialist and primary care team members, as well as the patients themselves, should be well aware of the circumstances which predispose to lithium toxicity, and the symptoms which occur with impending toxicity. Elevation of serum lithium concentrations giving rise to intoxication occurs because some factor affecting either lithium ingestion or excretion has changed (Schou 1989). Some cases are a result of intentional overdose, others because of patients taking extra lithium in the mistaken belief that this would be helpful to them. Circumstances which predispose to lithium intoxication include feverish illness, low salt diet, diarrhoea and vomiting, sudden slimming diets, and coadministration of certain drugs including diuretics and nonsteroidal-anti inflammatory drugs such as ibuprofen which can be bought over the counter in many countries including Britain. Symptoms of impending lithium intoxication include vomiting and diarrhoea, coarse tremor, sleepiness, poor concentration, slurred speech and unsteady walking. With more fully developed lithium intoxication, clouding of consciousness occurs, leading to coma with increased muscle tone and twitching, and fits (Thomsen and Schou 1975). Death or permanent brain damage can result.

To put the risks of lithium therapy into context, it is important to note that there is a high death rate, primarily from suicide, associated with recurrent mood disorder. It has been shown in two studies that the high death rate associated with recurrent mood disorder is reduced down to, or even below, that of the general population when effective long-term lithium treatment is used (Coppen *et al.* 1991; Muller-Oerlinghausen *et al.* 1991).

Mood disorder clinics

Specialist lithium clinics were started in the 1960s and have been established in increasing numbers. Some clinics are aimed primarily at optimizing lithium treatment, whereas others are mood disorder clinics which offer a broader spectrum of treatment (Fieve and Peselow 1987). The more developed clinics use specific monitoring systems with rating scales for mood disorder and side effects. Arrangements are made for monitoring lithium concentrations and other biochemical variables in a systematic fashion so that valuable information does not get lost or delayed. The clinic, with regular staff skilled in the management of affective disorder, provides a contact point for patients and relatives who may be worried about early signs of relapse or lithium intoxication. Well-run clinics have an established contact and follow-up system for any patient who may default from an appointment. The lithium clinic is also a good focus for support groups and self-help groups (Rook 1987), as well as facilitating patient education about their treatment.

Studies have shown that patients attending a lithium clinic are monitored more regularly and are less likely to experience undue elevation of serum lithium concentration than are patients treated with lithium by their family doctors (Kehoe and Mander 1992; Masterton et al. 1988).

Psychosocial approaches

All patients with manic depressive disorder will require supportive counselling as individuals. The disorder has severe consequences in all areas of psychosocial functioning including family and marital relationships and employment prospects. Group support for both sufferers and their relatives can be offered in the mood disorder clinic or other settings. However, there is no good evidence that psychosocial approaches will alter the course of manic depressive illness.

Educating lithium-treated patients about their medication brings significant benefits in both compliance and safety of lithium treatment. A simple educational programme, including a videotape and a written handout, has been shown to produce substantial and sustained improvement in patient knowledge about their lithium treatment as well as a more favourable patient attitude towards lithium and improved compliance with treatment (Peet and Harvey 1991; Harvey and Peet 1991). Of particular interest is the finding in this study that there was a substantial improvement of awareness concerning the hazards of lithium treatment including ways of avoiding lithium toxicity and recognizing early symptoms of toxicity when they occur. Knowledge of lithium treatment was also tested in three groups of mental health professionals. It was found that social workers had a very poor knowledge base which was similar to that of the patients before they had been educated. After the patients had been educated, their level of knowledge rose to a level similar to that of community psychiatric nurses. Doctors training in psychiatry had consistently higher levels of knowledge than the other mental health professionals. It appears that non-medical multidisciplinary team members may themselves require further training on medication issues before they can adequately educate the patients.

Antidepressants

Antidepressant drugs are an effective treatment for the symptoms of various mental disorders: not only depression, but conditions as diverse as anxiety, obsessive-compulsive neurosis and eating disorders. However, the most common use of long-term antidepressant treatment is for chronic or recurrent depression.

When using antidepressant drugs to treat an episode of depression, the two commonest errors in practice are inadequate dosage and inadequate duration of treatment. When treating a single episode of depression, antidepressant medication should be continued for up to six months (Paykel and Priest 1992). This reduces the relapse rate from 50 per cent down to 20 per cent. If only a single episode of depression is being treated, the antidepressant medication can be discontinued at the end of this six-month period. However, many patients experience either chronic symptoms or recurrent episodes of depression. Long-term preventative (prophylactic) treatment should be considered for any patient who has had two or more severe episodes of major depression within a five-year period (WHO 1989). Both antidepressants and lithium are effective for long-term prophylaxis, though antidepressants are commonly preferred because of their relative ease of administration.

Efficacy of long-term antidepressants

Most of the research evidence relating to the efficacy of prophylactic antidepressant medication comes from studies of the tricyclic antidepressants and the newer selective serotonin reuptake inhibitor (SSRI) drugs (Montgomery and Montgomery 1992). The most investigated drug has been the tricyclic antidepressant imipramine. A recent study of the efficacy of imipramine in long-term prophylactic treatment is that of Frank *et al.* (1990). Over a three-year period, recurrence of depression occurred in 22 per cent of patients treated with imipramine relative to 78 per cent of patients treated with placebo. Those patients who completed three years of drug treatment were then re-randomized to receive either continued imipramine or placebo for a further two years. This demonstrated continuing efficacy in preventing recurrence of depression, for the full five-year treatment period (Kupfer *et al.* 1992).

There is increasing evidence that the new SSRI drugs are effective in the prophylaxis of recurrent depression. Thus, fluoxetine reduced the relapse rate from 57 per cent on placebo treatment down to 26 per cent in a one-year study (Montgomery *et al.* 1988).

Although the long-term efficacy of antidepressants has been clearly demonstrated in a research setting, naturalistic studies in 'real-life' situations have shown that depression managed by conventional medical treatment has a rather poor long-term outcome. Brugha *et al.* (1992) showed that over a four-month period, patients who were prescribed antidepressant medication did not improve to a greater degree than those who were not given drugs. Follow-up studies of patients treated in a medical setting for depression have demonstrated a very poor long-term outcome (Kiloh *et al.* 1988). It is likely that many real-life failures of medication are caused by either inadequate prescribing (too low a dose, too short a duration) or by poor patient compliance with medication. Again in real-life situations, there is evidence that the risk of serious consequences of depression such as suicide is much less in patients treated adequately with antidepressants than in those given inadequate or no antidepressant treatment (Peet 1992).

Side effects with long-term antidepressants

The side effects of the tricyclic antidepressants are well known. They include 'anticholinergic' effects such as dry mouth and blurred vision, cardiovascular side effects such as impaired electrical conduction in the heart and lowered blood pressure, and nervous system effects including tremor, sedation and subtle impairment of memory. Other side effects such as impaired liver function and blood abnormalities are much less common (Rouillon *et al.* 1992). Usually, side effects are most troublesome at the start of treatment but are reduced in severity with longer-term treatment. However, side effects can become chronic, particularly when higher dosages are used. Persistent dry mouth is associated with the development of dental cavities and other disorders of the mouth and gums (Pollack and Rosenbaum 1987). These effects are worsened by the carbohydrate craving caused by tricyclic antidepressants which also leads to weight gain (Paykel *et al.* 1973). Continuing sedation and subtle memory impairment can potentially interfere with concomitant psychological treatment.

The side effect profile of the SSRI drugs is quite different. These drugs are not sedative and have no demonstrable adverse effect on information processing, so they may be preferable for combination with psychological treatment. The main side effects of these drugs are gastrointestinal, particularly nausea which can occur in up to a quarter of the patients treated with these drugs but which usually settles with long-term treatment.

Antidepressants are not addictive like benzodiazepines, but sudden withdrawal of high-dose tricyclic antidepressant treatment can cause withdrawal symptoms lasting several days in up to 20 per cent of patients. These symptoms include nausea, diarrhoea, flu-like symptoms, anxiety and sleep disturbances (Rouillon *et al.* 1992). Tricyclic antidepressants should therefore be discontinued gradually. Withdrawal symptoms do not appear to be a problem with the SSRI drugs. There is some evidence that true addiction can occur with monoamine oxidase inhibitors such as phenelzine.

Psychological treatment for recurrent depression

The two main psychological treatments which have been investigated for long-term effectiveness are cognitive therapy and interpersonal therapy (Frank *et al.* 1992). Antidepressants are only effective whilst patients are taking them. The hope has been that psychological treatment might have benefits which extend beyond the phase of active treatment.

In short-term treatment, cognitive therapy appears to be as effective as antidepressant drug treatment for mild to moderate states of depression, but more severe or psychotic depressive states respond better to medication (Elkin *et al.* 1989). Though some studies have shown an additive effect between cognitive therapy and antidepressant drugs, other well-designed studies have shown no advantage of combined treatment over either treatment individually (Hollon *et al.* 1992).

Long-term studies of cognitive therapy have been of two types. First, there are long-term naturalistic studies of outcome of patients who have been given short-term cognitive therapy during an acute episode of depression. Other studies have included longer-term continuation of cognitive therapy or at least booster sessions during the follow-up period. Overall, naturalistic studies show that treatment with cognitive therapy reduces relapse rate by around half during follow-up for two years after treatment, relative to patients who were treated with drugs for their acute episode of depression

(Evans *et al.* 1992). This is similar to the level of gain achieved by long-term antidepressant medication. Booster sessions (Blackburn *et al.* 1986) and long-term cognitive therapy (Thase *et al.* 1991) also appear to be associated with a low relapse rate. Despite methodological criticisms of some studies (Frank *et al.* 1992), it does appear that cognitive therapy provides longer-term coping strategies which can reduce the risk of depressive relapse. How intensive or long term the cognitive therapy needs to be is as yet unanswered.

Treatment with interpersonal psychotherapy during an episode of depression has not been shown to lead to long-term advantages in symptom reduction when compared with medication, though this form of psychotherapy may have long-term benefits on social adjustment (Frank *et al.* 1992). Long-term treatment with monthly sessions of interpersonal psychotherapy is substantially less effective than long-term drug treatment in reducing recurrences; psychotherapy appears to delay rather than prevent recurrence of depression (Frank *et al.* 1990).

In summary, it appears that cognitive therapy may have lasting benefits in preventing recurrence of depression, but there is no good evidence for the long-term effectiveness of other forms of psychotherapy.

Drugs for anxiety and insomnia

The drugs which have been most widely used to treat anxiety are the benzodiazepines such as diazepam (Valium) and lorazepam (Ativan). Some benzodiazepines are marketed for daytime anxiety, and others (such as temazepam) for night sedation. There is no difference in pharmacology between benzodiazepines used as anxiolytics or night time hypnotics. The difference is merely one of dosage: low-dose benzodiazepines relieve anxiety and high doses induce sleep. There are differences in duration of action between benzodiazepines. Thus, nitrazepam and diazepam are long-acting whereas temazepam and lorazepam are short-acting.

Problem of benzodiazepine dependence

It is ironic that benzodiazepines were originally introduced into clinical practice in the 1960s as the non-addictive alternative to barbiturates. Benzodiazepines increased in popularity during the 1970s, and there was a widely held expert opinion that abuse of benzodiazepines was not a significant problem, despite growing evidence to the contrary (Peet and Moonie 1977). More definitive research studies (Petursson and Lader 1981; Tyrer *et al.* 1981) and the advent of litigation (Ashton 1987) have substantially increased awareness of benzodiazepine addiction.

There are several reasons for this delay in recognizing benzodiazepine dependence. First, and contrary to popular belief, most people taking long-term benzodiazepines do not become dependent on them (Tyrer 1990). Second, anxiety is a long-term problem and stopping medication can often be associated with a recurrence of the patient's own symptoms. Third, milder withdrawal symptoms such as anxiety and insomnia can be indistinguishable from symptoms of a true anxiety state. Emergence of such symptoms readily leads to repeated re-prescription of the drug.

A true withdrawal syndrome includes symptoms which are not those of an underlying anxiety state, which peak after drug withdrawal and then. gradually attenuate. Double blind trials in which patients have been withdrawn from benzodiazepines on to placebo treatment have demonstrated that the acute withdrawal syndrome typically lasts for about a month (Petursson and Lader 1981). There are, however, reports of withdrawal symptoms apparently lasting for much longer periods of time (Ashton 1984).

Severe withdrawal symptoms which are rare during benzodiazepine withdrawal but which are never seen in simple anxiety include epileptic seizures, delirium and hallucinations. Other symptoms, more common with benzodiazepine withdrawal but less likely to be associated with simple anxiety, include perceptual changes such as itching and other sensations in the skin, feeling of things moving (including the floor, chair or bed), and abnormalities of taste and smell. Other common withdrawal symptoms are similar to those widely found in anxiety states, and include anxiety, tension, tremor and insomnia. A rating scale is available for recording and quantifying benzodiazepine withdrawal symptoms (Tyrer *et al.* 1990).

In the management of patients on long-term benzodiazepine treatment, simple measures should be tried first. A useful booklet has been produced by the Mental Health Foundation (Russell and Lader 1993). Up to 40 per cent of patients will stop or at least halve their intake of tranquillizers if this step is simply suggested to them. For more dependent patients, management will generally involve several members of the multidisciplinary team (Editorial, *Lancet* 1987). The elements of treating benzodiazepine dependence are shown in Table 14.2. The first stage is a full explanation of the problem. Many patients are now motivated to discontinue their medication by media coverage or by friends and family. The rate of dosage reduction depends on the duration of treatment, current dosage and a judgment of the probable severity of dependence. Sudden discontinuation is more likely to result in severe and potentially dangerous withdrawal symptoms such as fits. For people who have been on long-term medication, slow reduction over a period of months is generally necessary. Patients on short-acting benzodiazepines, particularly lorazepam, may have difficulty with dosage reduction and may experience withdrawal symptoms between doses. It can therefore be helpful to change them on to a long acting benzodiazepine such as diazepam which gives a smoother withdrawal. All patients require supportive counselling during the withdrawal period. Many patients have long-stand-

Table 14.2   Elements of the management of benzodiazepine dependence

1 Explanation and motivation
2 Gradual dosage reduction
3 Change from short- to long-acting drug
4 Supportive counselling
5 Self-help books and tapes
6 Psychological treatments for ongoing anxiety
7 Benzodiazepine withdrawal group
8 Medication (propranolol, antidepressant)

ing problems with anxiety quite apart from any withdrawal symptoms, and psychological treatments for anxiety are helpful in such cases. Such treatment is commonly included in the programmes offered by benzodiazepine withdrawal groups which have the added advantage of offering peer group support. Some individuals benefit greatly from self-help books (Tyrer 1986) and organizations such as TRANX (Tranquillizer Recovery And New eXistence). Additional or alternative medication should only be offered as a last resort. However, there is evidence that treatment with the beta receptor blocking drug propranolol can reduce the severity of benzodiazepine withdrawal symptoms (Tyrer *et al.* 1981) and some patients become sufficiently depressed to warrant the use of antidepressant medication during the withdrawal period. Low-dose neuroleptic drugs, and the new anti-anxiety drug buspirone, are not effective in the treatment of benzodiazepine withdrawal and should not be used for this purpose.

Because of the problem of benzodiazepine dependence, these drugs are now indicated only for the short-term relief (two to four weeks only) of anxiety that is severe, disabling or subjecting the individual to distress. In general, new prescriptions of benzodiazepine should be avoided.

There remains the thorny problem of patients who are either unmotivated or unable to discontinue their benzodiazepines. In such patients, it may be justified to continue with the benzodiazepine in the lowest attainable dose whilst carefully recording the fact that this was not the preferred option.

Alternative drug treatments for anxiety

There is good evidence that antidepressant drugs are effective in the treatment of anxiety. Three studies have compared a tricyclic antidepressant, a benzodiazepine and a placebo in the treatment of neurotic patients with predominant anxiety (Khan *et al.* 1986; Johnstone *et al.* 1980; Tyrer *et al.* 1988). Overall, the tricyclic antidepressants were more effective than the benzodiazepines, and the benefit of the benzodiazepine treatment was short lasting. These studies were of four to eight weeks duration. Long-term efficacy has been demonstrated for imipramine in the treatment of panic disorder (Schweizer *et al.* 1993). Antidepressants appear to be effective for the various subtypes of anxiety including generalized anxiety disorder (Rickels *et al.* 1993). A number of non-tricyclic antidepressants including trazodone (Rickels *et al.* 1993) and fluvoxamine (Black *et al.* 1993) also appear to be effective anti-anxiety agents.

Beta-receptor blocking drugs, particularly propranolol, are effective in the short-term treatment of anxiety (Peet 1988) but long-term efficacy has not been established. Buspirone is a new non-benzodiazepine anti-anxiety drug which at present is recommended only for short-term use.

Psychological treatment for anxiety

Psychological treatments for anxiety can broadly be categorized as counselling, cognitive therapy and behavioural therapy (Drug and Therapeutics Bulletin 1993*a*). Elements of all these approaches are included in various types of 'anxiety management training'. Much of the research has been short term and uncontrolled, but a number of long-term follow-up studies are available.

Catalan *et al.* (1984) investigated the short- and long-term benefits of counselling for patients seen by their general practitioners with minor emotional disorders who would normally have been prescribed a benzodiazepine. They used brief counselling which included explanation of the nature of symptoms, exploration of underlying personal or other problems and ways of dealing with them, and reasons why drugs were not being prescribed. Patients were randomly allocated to either counselling or to routine treatment which included medication. Outcome at one month and follow-up at seven months showed that counselling was as effective as drug treatment, and that the group given no initial drug treatment did not make increased demands on the doctor's time.

The long-term benefits of anxiety management have also been investigated (Butler *et al.* 1987). Patients with generalized anxiety of duration six months to two years were randomly allocated to anxiety management or to a no-treatment waiting list. Anxiety management in this case was a self-help programme giving information about the nature and manifestations of anxiety, and how to deal with anticipatory anxiety, avoidance and loss of self-confidence. A tape-recorded relaxation procedure was also provided, and all patients were encouraged to reduce their consumption of anxiolytic drugs. This led to highly significant improvement which was maintained over a six-month follow-up period.

There is evidence from several studies that behavioural treatment for agoraphobia/panic leads to sustained improvement over follow-up periods of four to eight years. In contrast, relapse is frequent when long-term drug treatment is discontinued (Marks and O'Sullivan 1988). A recent study compared the benzodiazepine alprazolam with exposure therapy alone, and in combination, in the treatment of panic disorder with agoraphobia (Marks *et al.* 1993). Eight weeks of treatment was followed by eight weeks of drug tapering and a six-month follow-up. Measures of panic improved on all treatments, including those given placebo only. On non-panic measures, exposure treatment had doubled the effect of the benzodiazepine, and during the six-month follow-up period the improvement with benzodiazepine treatment was lost whereas the improvement after exposure treatment was maintained.

Cognitive therapy has also been used to treat anxiety, particularly panic disorder. Cognitive therapy is effective in the short-term treatment of mild to moderate panic disorder and there is preliminary evidence of sustained long-term improvement, though definitive studies of long-term outcome after cognitive therapy have not yet been carried out (Black *et al.* 1993).

Treatment of persistent insomnia

Most benzodiazepine hypnotic drugs lose their efficacy within weeks of treatment; dependence and withdrawal symptoms occur as with other benzodiazepines. These drugs are therefore unsuitable for long-term treatment of chronic insomnia. Several non-pharmacologic treatments for insomnia are available (Bootzin and Perlis 1992). These include simple advice relating to daily activities which affect sleep, such as avoiding daytime naps and excessive use of caffeine and alcohol, and having a comfortable bed. 'Stimulus control instructions' are also used. These are primarily aimed at establishing the bed and bedroom as cues for sleep and reducing their association with activities that might interfere with sleep. For example, patients are told to lie down to sleep only when feeling sleepy, and not to use bed for reading, watching television or eating. Sex is the only permitted activity in bed apart from sleep. Various other techniques include relaxation training, meditation and cognitive therapy. In a controlled trial comparing behavioural treatment with the benzodiazepine triazolam in persistent insomnia, it was found that the effect of triazolam wore off over a one-month follow-up period but the benefits of behavioural treatment persisted (McClusky *et al.* 1991). Behavioural treatment is therefore a clearly preferred option for chronic insomnia. One of the newer hypnotic drugs, zopiclone, is not a benzodiazepine but does act on the benzodiazepine receptor and withdrawal effects have been reported. Nevertheless, both benzodiazepines and zopiclone may be useful drugs for very short-term use at times of stress-induced insomnia.

Drugs for epilepsy

There are two sets of circumstances in which mental health workers might become involved with patients on long term anticonvulsant medication. First, patients may suffer from psychiatric disturbances in association with epilepsy. Such psychiatric problems can be the result of the epileptic process itself, secondary to the psychosocial consequences of epilepsy, or caused by long-term anticonvulsant drug therapy. Second, long-term anticonvulsant medication is increasingly used for the treatment of psychiatric disorders in patients who are not epileptic.

Psychiatric disorder in epilepsy

Psychiatric disorders in the epileptic patient can be intermittent in association with seizure activity or may be more long lasting. Direct results of seizures include, for example, the aura of temporal lobe epilepsy, and automatism Longer-term psychiatric disorders are relatively common, particularly in patients with temporal lobe epilepsy. The commonest disorders are neurotic in nature and apparently secondary to psychosocial difficulties. Psychotic states associated with epilepsy are very varied. Examples are the chronic paranoid-hallucinatory psychosis resembling schizophrenia which occurs particularly in association with temporal lobe epilepsy, and mood disorder. Detailed descriptions of the psychiatric disorders of epilepsy can be found in Neppe and Tucker (1992) and Lishman (1987).

There are several important principles relating to long-term anticonvulsant medication in epileptic patients with associated behavioural or psychiatric disturbances (Reynolds 1982; Neppe and Tucker 1992). Control of epilepsy should be brought about whenever possible by using a single drug. Using several anticonvulsant drugs together will rarely improve seizure control but can have adverse effects upon the mental state. It is often possible to improve the mental state simply by rationalizing anticonvulsant treatment. The single drug which is the most popular in epileptic patients with behavioural or psychiatric disturbance is carbamazepine. This drug has positive psychotropic effects in its own right and causes less cognitive and mood disturbance than some other anticonvulsants such as phenytoin. Carbamazepine is effective for both generalized tonic–clonic seizures and partial seizures such as temporal lobe epilepsy. Treatment with any anticonvulsant needs to be carefully monitored because excessive dosage can lead to loss of seizure control and adverse effects on the mental state. Blood level monitoring is helpful when using carbamazepine. When serious psychiatric disorder persists despite optimal anticonvulsant treatment, it may be necessary to use additional medication such as antipsychotic or antidepressant drugs, though possible interactions between the various medications need to be borne in mind.

The selection of appropriate psychotropic drugs for epileptic patients, and the potential interactions between psychotropic and anticonvulsant drugs, are discussed by Fogel (1988). Both neuroleptics and antidepressants can induce fits in susceptible patients, some drugs more than others. Chlorpromazine and maprotiline are particularly troublesome in this regard. The neuroleptics fluphenazine and thioridazine, and antidepressants of the 'selective serotonin reuptake inhibitor' type such as fluoxetine, appear relatively less likely to provoke seizures (Cooper 1988). A number of interactions between anticonvulsant and psychotropic drugs have been reported (Fogel 1988). Thus, blood levels of haloperidol are reduced by adding carbamazepine, and this may lead to clinical deterioration in schizophrenic patients. Both tricyclic antidepressants and phenothiazines have been reported to increase blood phenytoin levels. Neurotoxic interactions have been reported between lithium and anticonvulsants, particularly carbamazepine. Other possible interactions are recognized. When co-prescribing these drugs, it is necessary first to check the possibility of interactions and to take this into account.

Use of anticonvulsants for psychiatric disorders

Within psychiatry, the mainly therapeutic use for long-term anticonvulsant drugs is in the treatment of manic depressive disorder. The only drug licenced for this use is carbamazepine, though there is research evidence that other anticonvulsants can also be effective.

Lithium is the treatment of choice in manic depressive disorder, but between 20 and 40 per cent of patients do not show an adequate response (Post 1990). An alternative drug treatment is therefore necessary. It has been shown that carbamazepine is as effective as lithium in preventing mood swings in manic depressive patients (Elphick 1989; Coxhead et al. 1992). Furthermore, patients who do not respond adequately to lithium (particularly those whose mood cycles vary rapidly) may show a good response to carbamazepine. For patients who do not respond either to lithium or carbamazepine, the two drugs can be used in combination (Post 1990). Carbamazepine has also been used in other conditions including borderline personality and neuroleptic resistant psychosis (Fogel 1988).

Other anticonvulsant drugs which have been used for long-term prevention in manic depressive patients who have not responded to either lithium or carbamazepine, include valproate (Hayes 1989) and clonazepam (Sachs 1990).

Side effects of anticonvulsants

The side effects of carbamazepine differ considerably from those of lithium. Therefore carbamazepine may be a useful treatment for patients who cannot tolerate lithium. Skin rash is relatively common with carbamazepine,. particularly in psychiatric patients where the incidence has been around 15 per cent in several studies (Elphick 1989). Carbamazepine can also be toxic to the bone marrow with resulting blood disorders (agranulocytosis and aplastic anaemia). It is advised that the blood count should be checked regularly in patients taking carbamazepine. Fatalities are rare, but it is important to be alert to the possibility of a low white cell count if patients taking carbamazepine develop sore throats or other infections. If blood levels of carbamazepine rise too high, signs of toxicity develop which include nausea, dizziness, ataxia and visual symptoms leading to unconsciousness and convulsions if toxicity is severe. Other side effects and drug interactions are reviewed by Elphick (1989).

Valproate is generally well tolerated by psychiatric patients. Some of the more common side effects include gastrointestinal symptoms, tremor, increased appetite and weight gain and, less commonly, rashes. More rarely, liver toxicity may occur. Valproate can damage the foetus during pregnancy, causing abnormalities of the neural tube (McElroy *et al*. 1988). Clonazepam is a benzodiazepine derivative (reviewed by Chouinard 1988). The three most common side effects are ataxia, drowsiness and behavioural changes including disinhibition.

Psychosocial aspects of anti-epileptic treatment

When anticonvulsant drugs are being used to treat psychiatric conditions in patients who are not epileptic, such as those with manic depressive disorder, then the psychosocial management will be the same as for any other patient with that psychiatric disorder.

In patients who do suffer from epilepsy, drug treatment alone is never sufficient and psychosocial aspects must always be considered. The liability to suffer from fits has considerable social repercussions in the areas of education, employment and personal relationships. Supportive counselling will be required, as well as education about epilepsy and the need to take medication regularly. More intensive psychotherapy is seldom indicated. Emotional stress can lead to increased frequency and severity of attacks, so that anxiety management training and other stress management techniques can be helpful. In some patients, behavioural techniques can be used to inhibit or arrest seizures. These are described by Lishman (1987).

Role of the multidisciplinary team

Medication should be presented not as the sole treatment, but as part of a package of care. The relative importance of medication varies according to the condition being treated. Thus, for manic depressive psychosis lithium is the mainstay of treatment and psychosocial measures are primarily supportive, whereas for states of anxiety psychological therapies are paramount and medication has at best a secondary role. Also, the level of involvement of the specialist mental health team will vary. Most patients with schizophrenia or manic depressive disorder will have specialist mental health involvement at some stage, whereas the greater majority of people suffering from anxiety or depression will be treated in a primary care setting, often without the direct involvement of the specialist team. All disciplines are potentially involved. An important and often neglected contribution can come from the pharmacist, whether hospital-based or community-based. Team involvement should occur at all stages of drug treatment.

Decision to use drugs

The long-term management plan for any patient should be devised in a multidisciplinary team setting. This would include discussion as to whether medication should be part of the management package, and details of administration and monitoring medication should be agreed. Team involvement is particularly important when drugs which may be hazardous or which require special monitoring are to be used. These include long-term antipsychotic drugs (particularly in high dosage), lithium therapy, and long-term benzodiazepines.

Once the decision to use medication has been made, then it is the responsibility of the doctor or psychiatrist to ensure that the appropriate drug is chosen and that it is prescribed at the optimum dosage to maximize efficacy and minimize side effects. The pharmacist can offer expert advice on type and dosage of drugs. This may involve a full review of all previous medication, so that patients are not given drugs which have been previously ineffective or poorly tolerated.

Team involvement is also necessary in the decision to discontinue long-term medication. Patients will often register their wish to stop drugs with a non-medical member of the team. It is important to have a full discussion of the possible consequences of discontinuing drugs. The patient and family where appropriate, will need to be fully informed about the potential risks of discontinuing long-term medication such as lithium, neuroleptics or antidepressants. In other cases, for example with benzodiazepines, the pressure to discontinue medication may come from the team rather than from the patient. In all cases, if a decision to discontinue medication is made, it is essential that appropriate support and monitoring procedures are agreed in the high-risk period during and after drug discontinuation. Specific groups such as those for benzodiazepine withdrawal may need to be established. If prescribing is the responsibility of the general practitioner, then psychiatrists and pharmacists will be able to give specific advice regarding withdrawal of benzodiazepines and other medication.

In some cases, patients seen by non-medical team members may benefit from medication. The team members therefore need to have an awareness of the potential benefits of medication and a willingness to seek medical advice, in order to ensure that patients are not deprived of any potentially helpful medical treatment.

Psychosocial treatment

Alternatives and adjuncts to drug treatment should be available from suitably skilled team members. Everybody with a mental health problem will require supportive counselling, and this should be available from any involved staff in either primary care or the specialist mental health team. Counselling in more difficult cases may be provided by practice counsellors, the community psychiatric nurses, or other mental health workers. However, the main function of the specialist team should be to provide specialist therapies which are of proven efficacy. These will include social skills training and family therapy for schizophrenia, cognitive therapy for depression, and psychological treatment for anxiety and insomnia. Team members may be involved in teaching primary care staff the basic skills and concepts involved in some of the simpler therapies, particularly for the management of neurotic disorders.

The relationship between psychosocial treatment and drug treatment will need to be kept under review. For example, it may be possible to reduce the dose of neuroleptic medication when family therapy has been effectively instituted.

Education and health promotion

The specialist mental health team has an important function in educating patients, carers, non-specialist staff and the general public.

Patient education about medication is likely to improve compliance with treatment, ensure that consent is truly informed, and increase the safety of treatment by increasing awareness of side effects and other dangers of medication. It is known that simply handing out information leaflets is of little value in educating patients. It is better to present information in several modalities, including written, verbal and video presentations and possibly including role play to increase medication negotiation skills.

Other family members can sabotage the proper taking of medication if they have not been involved in the education process. Discussions with individual relatives are valuable, and more general presentations to groups such as the National Schizophrenia Fellowship are also helpful.

Primary health care staff can be educated either by working with specialist staff to care for individual clients, or by giving more formal educational sessions to larger groups.

The general public can be educated by health promotion campaigns. The local media can be used for this purpose. For example, one team publicized benzodiazepine dependence in the local newspaper and this led directly to a benzodiazepine withdrawal group being established which was run by ex-addicts. Another example is the 'defeat depression' campaign organized by the Royal College of Psychiatrists. This aims to raise public awareness about depression and its treatment, including the proper use of antidepressants. Items about the campaign have been featured in national and local radio broadcasts, attempting, for example, to dispel the widespread myth that antidepressants are addictive.

Any team member can educate patients about medication, but in many cases team members themselves will require additional training before they would be competent to take on that role.

Administration and monitoring of medication

Discussion of the administration of medication mostly relates to depot antipsychotic drugs. Administration of depot medication can be undertaken either by nursing members of the multidisciplinary mental health team or by primary health care team members. Some centres run depot neuroleptic clinics. These can have the advantage of providing good continuity of care and a focus of contact for both patients and relatives. There is evidence that 'user friendly' clinics will significantly enhance compliance with medication and reduce the use of in-patient facilities (Corrigan *et al.* 1990). However, clinics with an excessively medical pharmacological approach can be detrimental because psychosocial interventions are neglected.

Responsibility for medication ultimately rests with the doctor or psychiatrist who prescribes it. However, members of the multidisciplinary team should have a good awareness of the more important aspects of drug treatment, including the anticipated efficacy and possible side effects, particularly the more severe problems such as tardive dyskinesia, lithium intoxication. and benzodiazepine dependence. Some treatments, particularly depot antipsychotic drugs and lithium, may be suitable for a 'shared care' protocol, in which it is agreed that responsibility will be divided between the specialist and the primary health care teams.

Advocacy

Though it is preferable for patients themselves to learn the skills necessary to negotiate medication, advocacy may be required on behalf of some patients. This is a frequent source of anxiety amongst non-medical team members, who may feel that their patients are being medicated inappropriately, yet they lack the knowledge and confidence to tackle the prescribing doctor who may be antagonistic to their approaches. In such cases, a sound factual knowledge of medication and possibly practice in role play will facilitate the advocacy role.

Summary

Long-term medication is essential for many people who suffer from manic depressive disorder or schizophrenia, and medication is the most commonly used treatment for chronic or recurrent depression. Drugs, when used properly in these conditions, are of proven efficacy but are not 'curative'. Also, side effects are inevitable for some patients, and these vary in severity from trivial to life threatening. Unwanted effects of benzodiazepines have caused such concern that these drugs are no longer recommended for long-term use. It is important that if drugs are used, they should be given in the most skilled way possible, so as to maximize effectiveness whilst minimizing side effects. Drugs should be used as part of an overall treatment package, having due regard to psychological and psychosocial factors. Non-medical members of the multidisciplinary team should be sufficiently knowledgeable about drug treatment to enable full participation in the decision to institute or to discontinue drugs, and they should be able to recognize when drugs are ineffective or causing unacceptable side effects, so that proper medical intervention can be sought. Team members have a particular responsibility to offer alternative effective non-pharmacological treatments and should have the necessary training and expertise to offer these therapies as part of the treatment package. Finally, team members have a wider role with regard to education, health promotion and advocacy in relation to medication.

References

Ashton H (1984). Benzodiazepine withdrawal: an unfinished story. *British Medical Journal*, **288**, 1135–1140.

Ashton C H (1987). Dangers and medico-legal aspects of benzodiazepines. *Journal of the Medical Defence Union*, Summer 1987, 6–8.

Baldessarini R J, Cohen B M and Teicher M H (1988). Significance of neuroleptic dose and plasma level in pharmacological treatment of psychoses. *Archives of General Psychiatry*, **45**, 79–83.

Black D W, Wesner R, Bowers W and Gabel J (1993). A comparison of fluvoxamine, cognitive therapy and placebo in the treatment of depression. *Archives of General Psychiatry*, **50**, 44–50.

Blackburn I M, Eunson K M and Bishop S (1986). A two-year naturalistic follow-up of depressed patients treated with cognitive therapy, pharmacotherapy and a combination of both. *Journal of Affective Disorders*, **10**, 67–75.

Bootzin R R and Perlis M L (1992). Nonpharmacologic treatments of insomnia. *Journal of Clinical Psychiatry*, **53** (suppl.), 37–41.

Bristow M F and Hirsch S R (1993). Pitfalls and problems of the long-term use of neuroleptic drugs in schizophrenia. *Drug Safety*, **8**, 136–148.

Brooker C, Tarrier N, Barrowclough C, Butterworth C and Goldberg D (1992). Training community psychiatric nurses to undertake psychosocial intervention: a pilot study. *British Journal of Psychiatry*, **160**, 836–844.

Brugha T S, Bebbington P E, MacCarthy B, Sturt E and Wykes T (1992). Antidepressants may not assist recovery in practice – a naturalistic prospective study. *Acta Psychiatrica Scandinavica*, **86**, 5–11.

Butler G, Cullington A, Hibbert G, Klimes I and Gelder M (1987). Anxiety management for persistent generalized anxiety. *British Journal of Psychiatry* **151**, 535–542.

Casey D E (1991). Neuropsychiatry of involuntary movement disorders: tardive dyskinesia. *Current Opinion in Psychiatry*, **4**, 86–89.

Catalan J, Gath D, Edmonds G and Ennis J (1984). The effects on non-prescribing anxiolytics in general practice. *British Journal of Psychiatry*, **144**, 593–602.

Catalan J, Gath, D H, Anastasiades P, Bond A K, Day A and Hall L (1991). Evaluation of a brief psychological treatment for emotional disorders in primary care. *Psychological Medicine*, **21**, 1013–1018.

Chouinard G (1988). Clonazepam in the treatment of psychiatric disorders. In: *Use of Anticonvulsants in Psychiatry* (eds. S L M McElroy and H G Pope). Oxford Health Care Inc., Clifton, New York.

Christisen G W, Kirch D G and Wyatt R J (1991). When symptoms persist: choosing among alternative somatic treatments for schizophrenia. *Schizophrenia Bulletin*, **17**, 217–245.

Cohen B M, Benes F M, and Baldessarini R J (1989). Atypical neuroleptics, dose–response relationships, and treatment-resistant psychosis. *Archives of General Psychiatry*, **46**, 381–383.

Coppen A, Noguera R, Bailey J, Burns B H, Swani M S et al. (1971). Prophylactic lithium in affective disorders; controlled trial. *Lancet*, **ii**, 275–279.

Coppen A, Abou-Saleh M, Miln P, Bailey J and Wood K (1983). Decreasing lithium dosage reduces morbidity and side effects during prophylaxis. *Journal of Affective Disorders*, **5**, 353–362.

Coppen A, Standish-Barry H, Bailey J, Houston G, Silcocks P et al. (1991). Does lithium reduce the mortality of recurrent mood disorder? *Journal of Affective Disorders*, **23**, 1–7.

Cooper G L (1988). The safety of fluoxetine – an update. *British Journal of Psychiatry*, **2** (suppl. 3), 77–86.

Corrigan P W, Liberman R P and Engel J D (1990). From noncompliance to collaboration in the treatment of schizophrenia. *Hospital and Community Psychiatry*, **41**, 1203 –1210.

Coxhead N, Silverstone T and Cookson J (1992). Carbamazepine versus lithium in the prophylaxis of bipolar affective disorder. *Acta Psychiatrica Scandinavica*, **85**, 114–118.

Crow T J, MacMillan J F, Johnson A L and Johnstone E (1986). A randomized controlled trial of prophylactic neuroleptic treatment. *British Journal of Psychiatry*, **148**, 120–127.

Davis J M (1975). Overview: maintenance therapy in psychiatry: 1. Schizophrenia. *American Journal of Psychiatry*, **132**, 1237–1245.

Double D B, Warren G C, Evans M and Rowlands M P (1993). Efficacy of maintenance use of anticholinergic agents. *Acta Psychiatrica Scandinavica*, **88**, 381–384.

Drug and Therapeutics Bulletin (1987). Stopping drug treatment in schizophrenia. **25**, 31–32.

Drug and Therapeutics Bulletin (1993*a*). Psychological treatment for anxiety: an alternative to drugs? **31**, 73–75.

Drug and Therapeutics Bulletin (1993*b*). Risperidone and remoxipride for schizophrenia, **31**, 101–102.

Eckman T A, Liberman R P, Phipps C C and Blair K E (1990). Teaching medication management skills to schizophrenic patients. *Journal of Clinical Psychopharmacology*, **10**, 33–38.

Eckman T A, Wirshing W C, Marder S R, Liberman R P, Johnston-Cronk K, Zimmerman K et al. (1992). Technique for training schizophrenic patients in illness self-management: a controlled trial. *American Journal of Psychiatry*, **149**, 1549–1553.

Elkin I, Shea T, Watkins J, Imber S D, Sotsky S M, Collins J F et al. (1989). Treatment of depression collaborative research program I: general effectiveness of treatments. *Archives of General Psychiatry*, **46**, 971–982.

Elphick M (1989). Clinical issues in the use of carbamazepine in psychiatry: a review. *Psychosocial Medicine*, **19**, 591–604.

Evans, M D, Hollon S D. DeRubeis R J, Piaseck J M, Grove W M, Garvey M J et al. (1992). Differential relapse following cognitive therapy and pharmacotherapy for depression. *Archives of General Psychiatry* **49**, 802–808.

Falloon I R H and Brooker C (1992). A critical re-evaluation of social and family interventions in schizophrenia. *Schizophrenia Monitor*, **2**, 1–4.

Falloon I R H, Boyd J L and McGill C W (1984). *Family Care for Schizophrenia: A Problem-Solving Approach to Mental Illness*. Guildford Press, New York.

Falloon I R H, Boyd J L, McGill C W, Williamson M, Razani J, Moss H B et al. (1985). Family management in the prevention of morbidity in schizophrenia. *Archives of General Psychiatry*, **42**, 887–896.

Fieve R R and Peselow E D (1987). The lithium clinic. In *Depression and Mania: Modern Lithium Therapy* (ed. F N Johnson). IRL Press, Oxford, pp. 127–129.

Fogel B S (1988). Combining anticonvulsants with conventional psychopharmacologic agents. In *Use of Anticonvulsants in Psychiatry*, (eds. S L M McElroy and H E Pope). Oxford Health Care Inc., Clifton, New York.

Frank E, Kupfer D J, Perel J M, Jamett, D B, Mallinger A G, Thase M E et al (1990). Three-year outcomes for maintenance therapies in recurrent depression. *Archives* of General Psychiatry, **1**, 1093–1099.

Frank E, Johnson S, and Kupfer D (1992). Psychological treatments in the prevention of relapse. In *Long-Term Treatment of Depression* (eds. S A Montgomery and F Rouillon). John Wiley and Sons, Chichester, UK.

Harvey N S and Peet M (1991). Lithium maintenance: effects of personality and attitude on health information acquisition and compliance. *British Journal of Psychiatry*, **158**, 200–204.

Hayes S G (1989). Long-term use of valproate in primary psychiatric disorders. *Journal of Clinical Psychiatry*, **50** (suppl.) 35–39.

Hogarty G E, Anderson C M, Reiss D J, Kornblith S J, Greenwald D P, Javna C D et al. (1986). Family psychoeducation, social skills training, and maintenance chemotherapy in the aftercare treatment of schizophrenia. One-year effects of a controlled study. *Archives of General Psychiatry*, **43**, 633–642.

Hogarty G E, Anderson C M, Reiss D J, Kornblith S J, Greenwald D P, Ulrigh R F et al. (1991). Family psychoeducation, social skills training, and maintenance chemotherapy in the aftercare treatment of schizophrenia. II. Two-year effects of a controlled study on relapse and adjustment. *Archives of General Psychiatry*, **48**, 340–347.

Hollon S D, DeRubeis R J, Evans M D, Weimer M J, Garvey M J, Grove W M et al. (1992). Cognitive therapy and pharmacotherapy for depression. *Archives of General Psychiatry*, **49**, 774–781.

Hullin R P (1980). Minimum serum lithium levels for effective prophylaxis. In *Handbook of Lithium Therapy* (ed. F N Johnson). MTP Press, Lancaster.

Johnson D (1990). Long-term drug treatment of psychosis: observations on some current issues. *International Review of Psychiatry*, **2**, 341–353.

Johnson D A W, Pasterski G, Ludlow J M, Street K and Taylor R D W (1983). The discontinuance of maintenance neuroleptic therapy in chronic schizophrenic patients: drug and social consequences. *Acta Psychiatrica Scandinavica*, **67**, 339–352.

Johnstone E C, Cunningham Owens D G, Frith C D, McPherson K, Dowie C, Riley G et al. (1980). Neurotic illness and its reponse to anxiolytic and antidepressant treatment. *Psychological Medicine*, **10**, 321–328.

Kane J, Honigfeld G, Singer J and Meltzer H (1988). Clozapine for the treatment-resistant schizophrenic. *Archives of General Psychiatry*, **45**, 789–796.

Kehoe R F and Mander A J (1992). Lithium treatment prescribing and monitoring habits in hospital and general practice. *British Medical Journal*, **304**, 552–554.

Khan R J, McNair D M, Lipman R S, Covi L, Rickels K and Downing R (1986). Imipramine and chlordiazepoxide in depressive and anxiety disorders. Efficacy in anxious outpatients. *Archives of General Psychiatry*, **43**, 79–85.

Kiloh L G, Andrews G and Neilson M (1988). The long-term outcome of depressive illness. *British Journal of Psychiatry*, **153**, 752–757.

Kupfer D J, Frank E, Perel J M, Cornes C, Mallinger A G, Thase M E et al. (1992). Five-year outcome for maintenance therapies in recurrent depression. *Archives of General Psychiatry*, **49**, 769–773.

Lader M (1993). Neuroleptic-induced deficit syndrome (NIDS). *Journal of Clinical Psychiatry*, **54**, 493–500.

Lam D H (1991). Psychosocial family intervention in schizophrenia: a review of empirical studies. *Psychological Medicine*, **21**, 423–441.

Lancet (1987). Treatment of benzodiazepine dependence. Editorial, **1**, 78–79.

Leff J and Vaughn C (1981). The role of maintenance therapy and relatives expressed emotion in relapse of schizophrenia. A two-year follow-up. *British Journal of Psychiatry*, **139**, 102–104.

Lishman W A (1987). *Organic Psychiatry*. Blackwell Scientific Publications, Oxford, pp. 207–276.

McClusky H Y, Milby J B, Switzer P K, Williams V and Wooten V (1991). Efficacy of behavioural versus triazolam treatment in persistent sleep-onset insomnia. *American Journal of Psychiatry*, **148**, 121–126.

McCreadie R G, Robertson L J and Wiles D H (1992). The Nithsdale schizophrenia surveys. IX: Akathisia, parkinsonism, tardive dyskinesia and plasma neuroleptic levels. *British Journal of Psychiatry*, **161**, 793–799.

McElroy S L, Keck P E, Pope H G and Hudson J I (1988). Valproate in primary psychiatric disorders: literature review and clinical experience in a private psychiatric hospital. In *Use of Anticonvulsants in Psychiatry* (eds. S L McElroy and H G Pope). Oxford Health Care Inc., Clifton, New Jersey.

Marks I and O'Sullivan G (1988). Drugs and psychological treatments for agoraphobia/panic and obsessive-compulsive disorders: a review. *British Journal of Psychiatry*, **153**, 650–658.

Marks I M, Swinson R P, Basoglu M, Kuch K, Noshirvani H, O'Sullivan G *et al.* (1993). Alprazolam and exposure alone and combined in panic disorder with agoraphobia. *British Journal of Psychiatry*, **162**, 776–787.

Masterton G, Warner M and Roxburgh B (1988). Supervising lithium. A comparison of a lithium clinic, psychiatric out-patients clinics and general practice. *British Journal of Psychiatry*, **152**, 535–538.

Montgomery S A and Montgomery D B (1992). Prophylactic treatment in recurrent unipolar depression. In: *Long-Term Treatment of Depression* (eds. S Montgomery and F Rouillon). John Wiley and Sons, Chichester.

Montgomery S A, Dufour H, Brion S *et al.* (1988). The prophylactic efficacy of fluoxetine in unipolar depression. *British Journal of Psychiatry*, **3**, 69–76.

Muller-Oerlinghausen B, Volk J, Grof P, Grof E, Schou M *et al.* (1991). Reduced mortality of manic depressive patients in long-term lithium treatment. *Psychiatric Research*, **36**, 329–331.

Myers D H and West T E T (1987). Hormone systems. In *Depression and Mania: Modern Lithium Therapy* (ed. F N Johnson). IRL Press, Oxford, pp. 220–226.

Neppe V M and Tucker C J (1992). Neuropsychiatric aspects of seizure disorders. In *Neuropsychiatry* (eds. S C Yudofsky, and R E Hales). American Psychiatric Press, Washington, pp. 397–426.

Paykel E S and Priest R G (1992). Recognition and management of depression in general practice: consensus statement. *British Medical Journal*, **305**, 1198–1202.

Paykel E S, Mueller P S and De La Vergne P M (1973). Amitriptyline, weight gain and carbohydrate craving: a side-effect. *British Journal of Psychiatry*, **123**, 501–507.

Peet M (1988). The treatment of anxiety with beta-blocking drugs. *Postgraduate Medical Journal*, **64** (suppl. 2), 45–49.

Peet M (1992). The prevention of suicide in patients with recurrent mood disorder. *Journal of Psychopharmacology*, **6** (suppl.), 334–339.

Peet M and Harvey N (1991). Lithium maintenance: 1. A standard education programme for patients. *British Journal of Psychiatry*, **158**, 197–200.

Peet M and Moonie L (1977). Abuse of benzodiazepines. *British Medical Journal*, **1**, 714.

Peet M and Pratt J P (1993). Lithium: current status in psychiatric disorder. *Drugs*, **46**, 7–17.

Petursson H and Lader M H (1981). Withdrawal from long-term benzodiazepine treatment. *British Medical Journal*, **283**, 643–645.

Pollack M H and Rosenbaum J F (1987). Management of antidepressant-induced side effects. *Journal of Clinical Psychiatry*, **48**, 3–8.

Post R M (1990). Non-lithium treatment for bipolar disorder. *Journal of Clinical Psychiatry*, **51** (suppl.), 9–16.

Prien R F and Gelenberg A J (1989). Alternatives to lithium for the preventative treatment of bipolar disorder. *American Journal of Psychiatry*, **146**, 840–848.

Prien R F, Caffey Jr E M and Klett J (1973). Prophylactic efficacy of lithium carbonate in manic-depressive illness. *Archives of General Psychiatry*, **28**, 337–341.

Prien R F, Kupfer D J, Mansky P A, Small J G, Tuason V B *et al*. (1984). Drug therapy in the prevention of recurrences in unipolar and bipolar affective disorders. *Archives of General Psychiatry*, **41**, 1096–1104.

Reynolds E H (1982). The pharmacological management of epilepsy associated with psychological disorders. *British Journal of Psychiatry*, **141**, 549–557.

Rickels K, Downing R, Scwizer E and Hassman H (1993). Antidepressants for the treatment of generalized anxiety disorder. *Archives of General Psychiatry*, **50**, 884–895.

Rifkin A, Quitkin F, Rabiner C J and Klein D F (1977). Fluphenazine decanoate, fluphenazine hydrochloride given orally, and placebo in remitted schizophrenics. *Archives of General Psychiatry*, **34**, 43–47

Rook J A J (1987). Lithium self help groups. In *Depression and Mania: Modern Lithium Therapy* (ed. F N Johnson). IRL Press, Oxford, pp. 129–132,

Rouillon F, Lejoyeux M and Filteau M J (1992). Unwanted effects of long-term treatment. In *Long-Term Treatment of Depression* (eds. S Montgomery and F Rouillon). John Wiley and Sons, Chichester.

Royal College of Psychiatrists (1993). *Consensus Statement on the Use of High Dose Antipsychotic Medication*. Council Report CR26. Royal College of Psychiatrists, London.

Russell J and Lader M (1993). *Guidelines for the Prevention and Treatment of Benzodiazepine Dependence*. Mental Health Foundation, London.

Sachs G S (1990). Use of clonazepam for bipolar affective disorder. *Journal of Clinical Psychiatry*, **51** (suppl.) 31–34.

Schooler N R (1993). Reducing dosage in maintenance treatment of schizophrenia. *British Journal of Psychiatry*, **163** (suppl. 22), 58–65.

Schooler N R, Levine J, Severe J B, Bruzer B, Dimascio A, Klerman G L *et al*. (1980). Prevention of relapse in schizophrenia. An evaluation of fluphenazine decanoate. *Archives of General Psychiatry*, **37**, 16–24.

Schou M. (1988*a*). Effects of long term lithium treatment on kidney function: an overview. *Journal of Psychiatric Research*, **22**, 287–296.

Schou M. (1988*b*). Serum lithium monitoring of prophylactic treatment: critical review and updated recommendations. *Clinical Pharmacokinetics*, **15**, 283–286.

Schou M. (1989). Lithium prophylaxis: myths and realities. *American Journal of Psychiatry*, **146**, 573–576.

Schweizer E, Rickels K, Weiss S and Zanodnick S (1993). Maintenance treatment of panic disorder. Results of a prospective, placebo-controlled comparison of alprazolam and imipramine. *Archives of General Psychiatry*, **50,** 51–60.

Souza F G M and Goodwin G M (1991). Lithium treatment and prophylaxis in unipolar depression; a meta-analysis. *British Journal of Psychiatry*, **158**, 666–667.

Thase M E, Bowler K and Harden T (1991). Cognitive behavior therapy of endogenous depression. *Behaviour Therapy*, **22**, 469–477.

Thomsen K and Schou M (1975). The treatment of lithium poisoning. In *Lithium Research and Therapy* (ed. F N Johnson). Academic Press, London, pp. 519–531.

Tyrer P (1986). *How to Stop Taking Tranquillizers*. Sheldon Press, London.

Tyrer P (1990). Current problems with the benzodiazepines. In *The Anxiolytic Jungle: Where Next?* (ed. D Wheatley). John Wiley, Chichester, pp. 23–36.

Tyrer P, Rutherford D and Huggett T (1981). Benzodiazepine withdrawal symptoms and propranolol. *Lancet* **i**, 520–522.

Tyrer P, Murphy S, Kingdon D, Brothwell J, Gregory S, Seivewright N *et al*. (1988). The Nottingham Study of neurotic disorder: comparison of drug and psychological treatments. *Lancet* **ii** , 235–240.

Tyrer P, Murphy S and Riley P (1990). The benzodiazepine withdrawal symptom questionnaire. *Journal of Affective Disorders*, **19**, 53–61.

Vestergaard P, Poulstrup I and Schou M (1988). Prospective studies on a lithium cohort: tremor, weight gain, diarrhoea, psychological complaints. *Acta Psychiatrica*

Scandinavica, **78**, 434–441.

Van Putten T (1974). Why do schizophrenic patients refuse to take their drugs? *Archives of General Psychiatry*, **31**, 67–72.

Van Putten T, Marder S R and Mintz J (1990). A controlled dose comparison of haloperidol in newly admitted schizophrenic patients. *Archives of General Psychiatry*, **1**, 754–758.

WHO Mental Health Collaborating Centres (1989). Pharmacotherapy of depressive disorders: a consensus statement. *Journal of Affective Disorders*, **17**, 197–198.

15 Daily living skills for clients in the community

D. Hall

Introduction

The purpose of this chapter is to address daily living skills in relation to community mental health care. It will consider what daily living skills mean to different individuals, examine the impact of mental illness upon these skills and discuss the necessity for them. The value of daily living skills as both an assessment and treatment tool will be discussed, together with the importance of the environment within which activities take place. In order to ensure that daily living skills can be developed and maintained throughout an individual's life cycle, the need for flexibility in service provision will be presented and the role of practitioners highlighted.

In the field of mental illness, it is often an alteration or failure in a routine daily life skill which either provokes individuals to seek help or treatment themselves or draws them to the attention of others. This would seem to be the case regardless of age, clinical diagnosis, severity or length of illness. For example, equal concern may be raised over a decline in an individual's ability to maintain the usual levels of personal hygiene whether they be a family member, a neighbour, a work colleague or a person already known to have a diagnosis of mental illness. In each case, the failure in daily living skills is an indication that something has changed or is wrong and as a result some sort of intervention may be required. Thus the area of daily living skills is an important one for community mental health practitioners and their clients.

Terminology

There are several terms which are used in conjunction with daily living skills, the most frequent being activities of daily living (ADL). Others include functional skills and community living skills. Words such as tasks, roles, performance and function are correctly or otherwise associated with these. It is therefore appropriate to begin by looking at semantics to provide the background within which daily living skills can be addressed.

Basic definitions together with some examples which relate to the activity of shopping are presented in Table 15.1. Where it is considered of interest to the reader, the source of a further definition is provided.

A simple conceptualization of the relationship between skills, tasks, activities and function is offered by Unsworth (1993) whereby tasks form activities and skills and activities together make up function. It follows then that one or more skills are necessary to carry out an activity in order to function.

Defining daily living skills and activities

There are many references to daily living skills and activities within mental health literature, much of which has been written by clinicians. Some of them are outlined here.

Table 15.1 Definition of terms used to refer to daily living skills

Skill	A specific ability or integrated set of abilities learnt and practised to a standard for the effective performance of a task (Hagedorn 1992). See also Creek (1990). A skill implies some aptitude or competence, for example the ability to calculate numbers and manage a budget.
Activity	A purposeful behaviour designed to achieve a desired goal – a specific action, function or sphere of action that involves learning or doing by direct experience (Reed and Sanderson 1980). Shopping is such an activity.
Task	A stage or component of an activity (Hagedorn 1992). See also Reed and Sanderson (1980). An example of a task which contributes to the activity of shopping would be handling money.
Role	An identity which directs the individual's social, cultural and occupational behaviour and relationships (Hagedorn 1992). See also Willson (1987). An individual invariably carries out more than one role and these will change throughout their lifetime. For example a secretary may also be (or become) a householder, a customer, a school governor, a parent and a grandparent.
Performance	Accomplishment of the roles that are assumed by individuals in their lives (Hopkins and Smith 1988). See also Kielhofner (1985). Performance is also used as a subjective term relating to the ability with which an individual carried out a task and is sometimes associated with success or failure.
Function	To carry out the tasks that the environment demands of us, requiring our own skills, abilities and knowledge and, sometimes, assistance from others (Mosey 1981).

An early reference to daily living skills was made by Meyer (1917) who described the need for positive structuring of time and development of habits appropriate to daily living. Collis and Ekdawi (1984) present daily living skills as aspects of social adjustment, describing amongst others social behaviour, self-care ability, use of time, attitudes and self-esteem. Shepherd (1983) refers to skills necessary to survive as an independent person in the community, giving examples of basic educational and self-care skills.

A list of eight daily life areas described by clients with a mental health problem is provided by Lehman *et al.* (1982), these being living) situation, family relations, social relations, leisure activities, work, finances, safety and health. Unsworth's work (1993) provides further lists of daily living skills as outlined in functional assessments.

It can be seen from these examples that clinical definitions tend to be fairly prescriptive, providing categories or lists of skills and abilities which form daily living activities. Although useful for the mental health practitioner, these can be restrictive or risk missing vital aspects for some individuals. A more global and flexible framework is provided by Reed and Sanderson (1980). Here, daily living skills are described as 'skill and performance in personal care, maintenance of a self-concept, coping with life situations and participating in the organizational and community environment'. Three key functional areas of self-maintenance, productivity and leisure are highlighted. Each of these comprises activities unique to the individual and in turn demand skills which may be cognitive, motor, sensory, interpersonal and intrapersonal. Using the example of shopping again, in its simplest form this would require budgeting (cognitive), communication (interpersonal) and walking (motor) skills and would contribute to the overall function of self-maintenance.

A completely different approach to looking at daily living is provided by Vorspan (1988) and Deegan (1988). Vorspan describes the skills with which we navigate life and describes daily living activities as 'an expression of humanity, entered into in order for us to engage more fully in the shared ground of daily life'. Deegan, a clinical psychologist who was diagnosed as schizophrenic at a young age, describes daily living simply as 'being able to live, work and love in a community in which one makes a significant contribution'. These concepts are perhaps a more useful foundation for the practitioner because they are open to interpretation according to the lifestyle and background of any individual. Daily living skills and activities are unique to each of us.

Impact of mental illness on daily living skills and activities

The point was raised in the introduction that a decline or failure in daily living skills is likely to bring a person to the attention of the mental health services. This may be directly, as in the case of self-referral, or indirectly, resulting from the concerns and subsequent actions of others, like relatives and neighbours, or bodies such as social services, voluntary organizations and the police. The manifestation of a mental illness can be as wide ranging as a dysfunction in a person's usual practical capabilities or violent intent to self or others. Both cases present a failure to cope in one or more areas of daily life and have consequences for the individual concerned.

Although secondary to the illness itself, an alteration in daily living skill(s) can be equally or more debilitating. Wing and Morris (1981) portray three levels of disability affecting people with mental health problems. They describe primary disabilities as those related to the illness per se, examples of which include lethargy, cognitive impairment, intrusion of unwanted thoughts, disinhibited behaviour and lack of awareness. Secondary disabilities are those which arise from the experience of the illness itself and may be intensified by the length and/or severity of it. These have been described as 'adverse personal reactions' and include factors such as diminished self-esteem and lack of confidence. The tertiary disabilities are referred to as 'social disablements' and stem from society's reaction to mental illness. They include factors such as reduced social contact, unemployment and poverty. Consider the following case scenario.

An individual with a diagnosis of depression has feelings of diminished self-worth and lacks the confidence to attend a regular leisure pursuit in the form of a local bridge club. His attendance is erratic and sometimes he fails to turn up when he has agreed to play in a competition game. On several occasions the club has been unable to keep a commitment with another club and this has caused embarrassment. Unaware of the difficulties the individual is facing, others simply perceive that they have been let down. They view the person as being unreliable and, as such, no longer an appropriate member of the competition team. The group fail to contact him, are anti-social towards him when he does attend and eventually they suggest that he leaves the club altogether. The individual has lost an important team role and source of social contact.

It can be seen from this process that although primary disabilities are warning signs of symptoms which may later indicate a diagnosis of mental illness, secondary and tertiary disabilities have a marked impact on daily living function.

It is often the secondary and tertiary disabilities which will be of initial concern to individuals themselves and the ones that they will be most anxious to overcome. It is likely that people will see themselves failing to fulfil a daily living role or function long before they are aware of an illness which causes this failure. Even when a diagnosis has been made and an individual is presented with an explanation for their failure to cope, they may still consider the ability to cope again the most pressing issue. They may feel humiliated by an apparent inability to carry out what used to be an easy or even 'automatic' task. Deegan (1988) describes the despair experienced by individuals with severe mental illness as being completely overwhelmed at the thought of carrying out a simple activity. This sense of failure can have a devastating effect on someone who is already feeling hopeless or out of control.

The argument against categorizing daily living skills too finely has already been stated. However, it is felt that some discussion is warranted here regarding areas of daily living specifically in relation to mental health and illness. For simplicity, the areas of function outlined by Reed and Sanderson (1980) will be used.

Self-maintenance

Under this heading, Reed and Sanderson (1980) refer to those activities or tasks which are routinely carried out to maintain the individual's health and well-being in the environment. Examples are given of dressing and feeding. A decline in one area of self-maintenance could easily have a knock-on effect on another area of function. This chapter opened with a description of the concerns that may be raised over the decline in an individual's ability to maintain their usual levels of personal hygiene. Not only could this have an effect on the individual's physical and mental health, but it could also impact upon their social life and work situation. Other activities which come under the general heading of self-maintenance include maintaining adequate levels of safety and cleanliness in the living environment, taking regular exercise and adhering to a vital treatment or drugs regimen, as in the case of diabetes.

Productivity

Productivity refers to activities or tasks which are done to enable an individual to provide support to the self, family and society through the production of goods and services to promote health and well-being (Reed and Sanderson 1980). This may be related to fulfilling productive roles such as a secretary, mechanic or homemaker. Such roles provide satisfaction as well as enabling the individual to contribute to the family, community or society. The example given earlier about the bridge player outlined how the role of team member was altered by the effects of an illness. The same illness could prevent that individual from competently fulfilling usual roles and activities within the home and workplace.

The benefits of having a role or purpose which we value are hopefully known to us all. At some time most of us have experienced the consequences of failing, changing, neglecting or losing roles which are of importance to us. For some people, this alteration can be devastating and may further impair their ability to function. In some instances a dramatic, unplanned change of role may be so stressful that it may provoke the onset of a mental illness.

At this point it is useful to consider the subject of work and unemployment and their relationship with mental health and illness.

The sociological effects of unemployment in the wider population have long been reported (Jahoda et al. 1972). Dramatic increases in the level of unemployment, together with concerns over mental health, have provoked further attention in recent years (Feather 1990; Fineman 1990; Smith 1987; Starrin 1989). Additional research has specifically addressed the impact of unemployment on the mentally ill population (Shepherd 1991; Ekdawi 1993). In the same way as reduced socialization can be a symptom of a mental illness or an effect of it, unemployment could result from the impact of symptoms or could be a contributory factor which predisposes an individual to mental illness. Yankowitz (1990) describes the destruction of affective, cognitive, social and other tasks which, unknown to the non-afflicted, create a huge challenge to those mentally ill individuals who seek to obtain and maintain gainful employment.

The benefits of work in the field of mental health have been well documented. Van Weeghel and Zeelan (1991) report that work provides income, autonomy in gaining goods and services, time and space structure, a recognisable societal role and it forces individuals to be active and involved. Shepherd (1984) refers to a sense of personal achievement and mastery and Lehman *et al.* (1982) to the financial and intrinsic rewards of work. Other perspectives are provided by Bachrach (1992), Schwartz (1976) and Ekdawi (1972). Given the central importance of work in the maintenance of function in people with a mental illness and the value they place upon it (Ekdawi 1993), concern is expressed at how little attention this matter receives (Shepherd 1989, 1991).

Leisure

Leisure refers to activities or tasks done for the enjoyment and renewal that the activity or task brings to the person. These may contribute to the promotion of health and well-being (Reed and Sanderson 1980). Football, collecting antiques, knitting, yoga and going to the pub or cinema are all examples of leisure pursuits. They are carried out primarily for enjoyment and relaxation. Some, such as yoga, may fulfil a function of health promotion too and could also be considered under the heading of self-maintenance. Others, such as collecting antiques, could develop into a livelihood and may then be termed productivity. As a general rule though it is important to note that, for most people, leisure only makes sense when compared with productivity or work. It implies 'time off'. Parker (1971) describes leisure time as either an extension of work, the opposite to it or complementary to it. Ravetz (1984) defines leisure time as time left over from work. A poignant reminder of the meaningless of leisure in the absence of work is provided by Vorspan (1988) who states that we do not need leisure time activities if the purpose of leisure is to stand back, unwind or rewind – leisure only makes sense in the context of work. In terms of mental illness, again, disruption to an individual's usual pattern of leisure activities may signify some underlying symptoms. Alternatively, an individual who is in the midst of a mental illness may be forced to spend a considerable amount of time engaged in what others call 'leisure' activities simply because there is nothing else for them to do or because that is all they feel capable of.

In order to maintain the health of an individual, Reed and Sanderson (1980) assert the need for a balance between the functions of self-maintenance, productivity and leisure. The tasks and activities involved are related and some have little or no meaning in the absence of others. For example, some people would see little point in expending time and energy on grooming and appearance if they had nowhere to go once they had done so. Others who live alone have no desire to prepare meals because there is no-one to sit and eat them with. Hence practitioners need to consider the meaning of an activity in relation to each individual's lifestyle and be aware of the fact that a pastime which they regard as, say, leisure may be quite meaningless or fulfil a completely different function for others.

Daily living skills and environment

Environment refers to both human and non-human surroundings and includes objects, people, events, cultural influences, social norms and expectations (Creek 1990). Environments may be diffuse and global such as a whole community or more precisely defined such as a workplace. Reed and Sanderson (1980) outline a useful framework within which daily living skills can be considered here. Their basic premise is that an individual needs to adapt to and with their environment. They stress the fact that, because the environment itself will alter, the daily living skills required of individuals will change. For example, within a workplace the social demands placed on individuals will change when comparing the boardroom to the staff canteen. These demands will alter again on changing the work environment for the home or leisure one.

The community can be discussed under this heading of environment. For every individual, the community in which they live and function presents an ever-changing gamut of people, cultures, norms and expectations. These place demands on individuals which may sometimes be conflicting. Despite a supposed philosophy of community care, for many people with a mental illness the various environments they experience outside organized mental health services remain daunting and, for some, hostile. Turner and Roberts (1992) remind us that, suddenly, two major requirements have been placed on society. These are, first, to 'welcome back' individuals with a mental illness after years of expatriation, and second to regard their continued care and treatment as a priority. Such expectations may be too great. Society may be ill prepared or equipped to deal with these demands and its compliance to the community care ethos cannot be assumed. Consider a recovering individual who is about to be discharged from hospital. The therapeutic community of the psychiatric ward may appear far less threatening than the neighbourhood to which the client is returning. Members of the community, although sympathetic to the individual, may at the same time have misunderstood their illness, be suspicious of them and fearful that their behaviour may threaten public safety (Aviram 1990). The experiences and demands placed upon the individual could alter dramatically between settings and an adaptation of daily living skills will be necessary. Certain individuals may feel drawn to a particular community within which they feel accepted, at ease or with which they have some familiarity. Many 'subcultures' develop within localities which may be beneficial or otherwise. Examples could be a group of ex-employees in, say, a mining fraternity, a group of ex-patients following the closure of a large psychiatric hospital, the homeless 'community' or a group of drug addicts. The wider community varies in its tolerance of such subcultures.

The family can be considered as another aspect of an individual's environment, and discussions continue to take place about the relationship between family life and mental health. Families come in many forms and the numerous personal and sociological influences upon family life ensure no two families function in exactly the same way. What is considered to be normal family life for one family member may appear unusual or disturbing to an outsider, or even another member of the same family.

Research has shown that there is an interaction between certain family processes and the course of established psychiatric conditions. In particular, the disruptive effects of high levels of expressed emotion, criticism, denial or over-involvement within families have been highlighted (Brown 1959; Leff 1978; Kuipers 1979; Shepherd 1984). However, Shepherd (1984) is quick to point out that it does not necessarily follow that family processes cause mental illness. On the positive side, families will often care for, understand and relate to a mentally ill member who has few opportunities for social contact with others and may stand only a limited chance of managing to live independently. Families will often tolerate disturbed and erratic behaviour which others find unmanageable. They may encourage the individual to adopt appropriate roles, providing them with the stability and support they require to live with or overcome their illness. The approval, support and acceptance of a family is sought by most of us and in the case of those who have a mental illness this can prove to be an important factor. For many, attaining or returning to family life provokes thoughts of 'normality' or an environment which they wish to be part of.

The family, then, can have a marked effect on an individual's motivation and ability to function. A family which is over-protective towards a mentally ill relative may inadvertently or otherwise prevent them from developing appropriate skills or roles. Another family may expect such a person to achieve a level of functioning which is beyond him, leaving him with a sense of failure. An individual who is rejected by their family, or perceives this to be so, may be devastated. Alternatively, as has already been stated, the family may be able to assist their relative in developing skills and roles which enable them to live a meaningful and fulfilling existence.

Although many individuals with mental health problems live with their families in the community, it does not automatically follow that this is the most suitable arrangement or one which they would choose. It may result from no alternative being available. It has been suggested that the widely held belief that this is a preferred living arrangement should in itself be a subject for research rather than an accepted assumption (Aviram 1990).

This leads on to another environmental element, that of accommodation. It is not considered relevant here to spend time listing the wide range of living environments in which people with a mental illness live because the practitioner will be aware of these from their own experience. However, it is considered useful to look again at Reed's and Sanderson's (1980) premise of adaptation within the environment and discuss daily living skills in this context. A person who is living independently in a home that they own will require a different set of skills from a person residing in bed and breakfast accommodation. Due to the debilitating effects of mental illness, many individuals may no longer be able to cope with living independently and will be required to adjust to living in some form of supported accommodation. Persons who live in hostel-type accommodation or group homes will be sharing their living space with others and will have to adjust their daily living skills· accordingly. They may be called upon to compromise and tolerate situations and circumstances which would not arise in a family household. The term 'supported' housing should perhaps be viewed with caution. It may reduce the individual's need for competence in certain domestic activities of daily living, but at the same time vastly increase the interpersonal and intrapersonal demands placed upon them. The individual may be motivated and prepared to adapt or develop the necessary skills or could be totally overwhelmed by the prospect. In the event that they do develop skills, these may only be sufficient to cope with that specific living environment and may not prove useful or acceptable elsewhere.

Much has been written on the relationship between the environment and the daily living skills people actually require, develop or lose (Shepherd 1984; Chamberlin 1988; Deegan 1988). Goffman (1961) discusses the impact of an impoverished environment on people suffering from a mental illness. The fact that people were not required to use or develop some of their basic daily living skills meant that over time they eventually lost these skills and the ability to learn new ones. Although Goffman's work related to asylums, the same principle may be applied to any living environment in so much as people may only perform tasks and learn skills relative to the environment they are in. It follows then, that new or adaptive skills are best learned in the environment(s) where they will be required.

Intervention

The various theories and approaches used in assisting individuals to develop daily living skills is discussed under the general heading of intervention.

Rehabilitation is a commonly used term in all fields of health care and disability. Reed and Sanderson (1980) provide a general definition of rehabilitation as being 'the restoration of a person's skills and functions to the fullest physical, mental, social, vocational and economical usefulness of which that person is capable'. Bennett (1978) describes 'the process of helping a physically or psychiatrically disabled person to make the best use of his residual disabilities in order to function at an optimum level in as normal a social context as possible'. Relative to mental health, Wing (1981) describes rehabilitation in terms of its aim – that of social resettlement or adjustment – and Shepherd (1983) views it as an unfolding process culminating from the three stages involved; assessment, treatment and management.

Assessment is summarized by Reed and Sanderson (1980) as 'the process of collecting information, including subjective and objective data, which is relevant to the preparation of an intervention plan.' The purpose of an assessment is to provide an accurate picture of an individual's abilities at a particular time. These will be in relation to the environment they are in and the particular roles and tasks they have to fulfil. The need for accurate assessment is obvious, but the task is a difficult one to achieve. It relies on an objective 'assessor' having the skills, time and opportunity to observe an individual performing all relevant roles and tasks within their normal environment and, in addition, assumes that the individual will carry these out in the usual manner throughout the duration of the assessment. This is a tall order and will not be accomplished lightly. Shepherd (1983) suggests that, in mental health, assessment should be viewed as an ongoing process of accumulating information using interview and discussion as well as direct observation. He stresses the need for assessments to be carried out *in situ* or, failing that, with an as accurate understanding or approximation of the target environment as is possible. Several formal assessment tools have been developed to assist the mental health practitioner in examining an individual's daily living skills and function. Many of these are summarized by Jeffrey (1993) and Unsworth (1993), though Unsworth warns that there may be parallels between these and the criticisms made of some intelligence tests – they may only measure what the tests are designed to measure and this may not be easily translated into the 'real world'.

A thorough assessment of an individual's abilities and difficulties should direct the practitioner or team to aspects of the individual's functioning which may benefit from treatment – the second stage in Shepherd's rehabilitation model (1983). The formulation of a clear statement of an individual's needs and proposed treatment is advocated. This 'treatment plan' will require regular review and modification. Shepherd states that treatment may be by pharmacological and/or psychological means. Again, these would be too numerous to list, but Shepherd emphasizes that practitioners must acknowledge that there is invariably more than one method currently available to treat a specific need and a combination of several approaches may be appropriate. Treatment methods will often require modification to suit different individuals or, indeed, different episodes within a single individual's life cycle. Shepherd goes on to discuss the possibility of an individual not, for whatever reason, responding to the treatment available or offered. In this instance, he presents the concept of 'management' and describes the need for individualized 'packages' of care which address other valid concerns such as the best environment for an individual to experience in the event of treatment being ineffective or untenable.

Bachrach (1992) describes a process of psychosocial rehabilitation, made up of several different approaches to the care of people who suffer from mental illness which 'encourage them to develop their fullest capacities through learning procedures and environmental supports'. It is argued that pharmacological intervention can be, and often is, effective alongside supportive and practical approaches and this combination in fact constitutes a viable intervention method in its own right. Several key concepts are highlighted, including the importance of environmental factors and the fact that it may be as feasible to consider adapting an environment to an individual as it is to help that individual adapt their skills to the environment. Bachrach asserts that rehabilitation has to be orientated to the individual's strengths and they must be actively involved in their own care and the design of intervention protocols. The stated aim of psychosocial rehabilitation is to restore hope to individuals who, by the very nature of their illness, have suffered major setbacks in functional capacity and self-esteem.

Deegan (1988) offers a somewhat different perspective, citing that rehabilitation refers to services and techniques which in turn contribute to an individual's experience of recovery. An individual goes through a process of recovery, not rehabilitation and it is the promotion of this recovery process which should be the chief aim of any intervention. Here, rehabilitation programmes are referred to as being the right sort of environments in which the recovery process can be nurtured and this fits well with the broad definition of environments discussed earlier. Deegan claims that the process of going through daily living skills may offer an individual some feeling of hope and achievement when they have been otherwise devastated by an illness, and thus daily living skills can be regarded as a treatment medium in their own right.

Intervention, then, can be thought of in terms of the different processes, stages or levels involved. Reed and Sanderson (1980) describe five different kinds of intervention which are characterized by the type of input required.

These are preventative, developmental, remedial, environmental, adjustment and maintenance. Needs will fluctuate according to the severity or impact of an individual's mental illness and input aimed at addressing these must adjust accordingly. It can be seen that in the acute episode of a mental illness, or while in a crisis, individuals may require help to maintain basic daily living activities and, if admitted to hospital, possibly environmental adjustment. On recovering from the period of disturbance, the same individuals may respond to remedial input and may later benefit from some preventative work. Each intervention level addresses daily living skills of one sort or another which are relevant to the individuals at the time.

Several important points can be drawn from this discussion on intervention and these are summarized in Table 15.2. The first is the need to tailor interventions to individuals, encompassing their specific needs at the time. There may be a requirement to treat the symptoms of an illness and, at the same time, address the detrimental effects of the symptoms. The symptoms may recede with the prescription of appropriate medication, but in addition the individual may require practical help in developing or adjusting daily living skills. There may be a need to simply support an individual through a crisis, providing no intervention other than daily living skills maintenance until the individual is able to consider and embark upon alternatives. The third point then is the fact that practitioners need to be flexible in the type of interventions they offer, and be prepared to modify these as they go along, reflecting the changing needs of individuals which manifest from their illness. Deegan (1988) explains that, at times, individuals are ruled by the effects of their illness and the timing of intervention is crucial. The value to individuals of being able to dip in and out of treatment programmes as and when their mental state allows should not be underestimated, as this enables them to benefit when they can without experiencing feelings of failure or time wasting. This gives rise to the fourth point that, for interventions to be successful, they must take into account the individual's interests and levels of participation and motivation.

It is possible, of course, that the mental health practitioner could come into contact with clients who are apparently unable to maximize their own independence or have no desire to do so. In such cases it is vital for the practitioner to assess the situation carefully and establish the possible implications of the client's behaviour or inactivity. Wherever possible, this assessment should be carried out in conjunction with the client and relevant family members and carers. Some measure of whether this is a one-off, transient phase or has longer-term implications must be established. The client could be plac-

Table 15.2 Issues to consider during intervention

1 Individuals require tailor-made programmes.
2 Programmes may include practical help in developing or adjusting daily living skills.
3 Interventions need to involve flexible programmes which may require modification in some instances.
4 For interventions to be successful, practitioners must consider individuals' interests, levels of participation and motivation.

ing himself or others at risk, the severity of which may depend upon the illness itself, the circumstances in which he is living, the community around him or other factors. Having established the risk, the practitioner must consider what intervention is necessary to minimize this and whether suitable resources are available locally. In a low-risk situation, it may be possible to address the difficulties with some short-term intensive input or closer supervision. This could be provided by the practitioner, family or friends, statutory or voluntary services. On the other hand, the risk may be considered high and it may not be possible to access the necessary resources to provide the intervention in the community. In this instance, it is vital that the practitioner consults with his colleagues and carefully considers what options are available to alleviate the situation. It may be necessary to remove the client from the community for an episode of in-patient care to ensure that appropriate treatment is implemented. It may also be necessary to consider this course of action if it is felt that the environment in which the client lives will not continue to support or accept him if they are faced with ongoing difficulties. Whatever the outcome and course of action, the practitioner must endeavour to ensure client, family, carers and community are appropriately informed and supported.

Resources

This discussion about intervention leads us to consider resources, as it is often felt that the treatments available to individuals may differ greatly and bear a direct relationship to the local resources – staff and other resources. Given the wide variety and fluctuating nature of community mental health teams, it is not felt appropriate here to discuss the roles and responsibilities of particular professionals, as these will differ between and within localities. Some authorities have developed key worker and case management systems and have a clear brief identified for such individuals (Goldberg 1987; Øvretveit 1992). However, whatever their title, practitioners share some core requirements in skills and knowledge. These are patience, ingenuity and an awareness of the various resources available locally. If resources are viewed purely in terms of statutory services, it becomes very easy for practitioners to get embroiled in the argument to increase them which, although valid and necessary, may distract from the task of day-to-day provision for individuals. The practitioner may be less overawed by this prospect if they can be broadminded and imaginative and actively seek the people and places which provide a resource in their local community.

The families of individuals have already been discussed and reference was made to the fact that many families, given the right support and guidance, will be willing and able to help a relative through the trauma of a mental illness and the adaptation and recovery stages thereafter. Family members may be prepared to become involved with specific intervention techniques and some will value the opportunity of doing something they see as constructive to assist in a relative's recovery. In some instances, it may be appropriate for a practitioner to see as much or more of a relative or carer as the individual themselves. As long as such input is negotiated and reviewed, and the family are not carrying too great a burden of responsibility, this can prove to be a fruitful working arrangement.

The practitioner should be aware of the various voluntary and statutory services in their locality and how to access these resources. Some communities have the benefit of active mental health charities such as MIND or the National Schizophrenia Fellowship which run support groups, lunch clubs, social events and so on. Some run and support low cost or supported housing. Even if local activities are not evident, such organizations may still be worth approaching for volunteer support or with a view to establishing joint ventures. Other non-mental health charities and organizations may be resourced. Many churches run social groups and befriending schemes, for example. Practitioners should not underestimate the help mentally ill individuals can provide for one another and the concept of self-help groups has been advocated by many including Chamberlin (1988), Deegan (1988) and Marks (1992).

In terms of statutory services, the need for practitioners to be aware of current local provision is clear. As well as health and social services, other local authority resources and amenities such as adult education classes and leisure centres should be considered. It may be possible to negotiate preferential rates if these are not already offered.

Given that many health and social services are now arranged on the basis of regularly reviewed contracts, it cannot be assumed that a resource which was available six months ago will be operating on the same basis now. Hence the practitioner must try to keep up to date with changes.

No discussion on resources would be complete without some mention of finance and mental health practitioners will be only too aware of the fact that many individuals exist on a limited or greatly reduced income. Again, the campaign for adequate benefits and user-friendly application procedures is an important one, but the practitioner still has to try and help individuals in the meantime. They must ensure that they are aware of all forms of financial support, allowances and discounts to which they are entitled and should make sure they have access to the necessary information and individuals to enable them to obtain these. On a simpler note, practitioners can assist individuals in developing money management skills and, from their body of local knowledge, provide information on low-cost activities and opportunities.

Conclusion

Daily living skills form part of life itself. Survival in the community, and therefore community care, cannot realistically be achieved without some degree of competence in this area. Practitioners are warned that an absence of psychiatric symptoms does not dictate that an individual can cope in the community (Collis and Ekdawi 1984). This requires skills.

It should not be forgotten that people with a mental illness are no different from any other group of people with special needs – they are the same as us all and have these special needs in addition to the basic needs and aspirations that we all share (Vorspan 1988). As such, they require sensitive and flexible help to enable them to achieve these.

The NHS and Community Care Act (Department of Health 1990) sets the task of providing the right level of intervention and support to enable people to achieve maximum independence and control over their lives (Wheeler 1990). The need for relevant daily living skills is inherent in this philosophy and practitioners are faced with the challenge of enabling individuals to develop them.

References

Aviram U (1990). Community care of the seriously mentally ill: continuing problems and current issues. *Community Mental Health Journal*, **26** (1), 69–88.

Bachrach L L (1992). Psychosocial rehabilitation and psychiatry in the care (of long-term patients. *American Journal of Psychiatry*, **149** (11), 1455–1463.

Bennett D H (1978). Social forms of psychiatric treatment. In *Schizophrenia – Towards a New Synthesis* (ed. J K Wing). Academic Press, London.

Brown G W (1959). Experiences of discharged chronic schizophrenic mental hospital patients in various types of living group. *Millbank Memorial Fund Quarterly*, **37**, 105–134.

Chamberlin J (1988). *On Our Own*. MIND Publications, London.

Collis M and Ekdawi M Y (1984). Social adjustment in rehabilitation. *International Journal of Rehabilitation Research*, **7** (3), 259–272.

Creek J (1990). *Occupational Therapy and Mental Health*, Churchill Livingstone, Edinburgh.

Deegan P E (1988). Recovery: the lived experience of rehabilitation. *Psychosocial Rehabilitation Journal*, **11** (4), 11–19.

Department of Health (1990). *The NHS and Community Care Act*, HMSO, London.

Ekdawi M Y (1972). The Netherne Resettlement Unit: results of ten years. *British Journal of Psychiatry*, **121**, 417–424.

Ekdawi M Y (1993). Work and rehabilitation. *Focus – British Institute of Industrial Therapy*, February, 417–424.

Feather N T (1990). *The Psychological Impact of Unemployment*. Springer-Verlag, New York.

Finemam S (1990). *Supporting the Jobless*. Tavistock/Routledge, London.

Goffman E (1961). *Asylums*. Penguin Books, London.

Goldberg E M (1987). The effectiveness of social care. *British Journal of Social Work*, **17**, 595–614.

Hagedorn R (1992). *Occupational Therapy: Foundations for Practice*. Churchill Livingstone, Edinburgh.

Hopkins H L and Smith H D (eds.) (1988). *Willard and Spackman's Occupational Therapy*, 7th edn. Lippincott, Philadelphia.

Jahoda M *et al.* (1972). *Marienthal, The Sociology of an Unemployed Community*, Tavistock, London.

Jeffrey L I H (1993). Aspects of selecting outcome measures to demonstrate the effectiveness of comprehensive rehabilitation. *British Journal of Occupational Therapy*, **56** (11), 394–400.

Kielhofner G (ed.) (1985). *A Model of Human Occupation*. Williams and Wilkins, Baltimore.

Kuipers E (1979). Schizophrenia and the family. Part 1: the problems of relatives. In *Community Care for the Mentally Disabled* (eds. J K Wing and R Olsen). Oxford University Press, Oxford.

Leff J P (1978). Social and psychological causes of the acute attack. In *Schizophrenia: Towards a New Synthesis* (ed. J K Wing). Academic Press, London.

Lehman A F, Ward A C and Linn L S (1982). Chronic mental patients: the quality of life issue. *American Journal of Psychiatry*, **139** (10), 1271–1276.

Marks I (1992). Innovations in mental health care. *British Journal of Psychiatry*, **160**, 589–597.

Meyer A (1917). The aims and meaning of psychiatric diagnosis. *American Journal of Insanity*, **74**, 163–168.

Mosey A C (1981). *Occupational Therapy – Configuration of a Profession*. Raven Press, New York.

Øvretveit J (1992). Concepts of case management. *British Journal of Occupational Therapy* **55** (6), 225–228.

Parker S (1971). *The Future of Work and Leisure*. Praeger, New York.

Ravetz C (1984). Leisure. In *Occupational Therapy in Short Term Psychiatry* (ed. M Willson). Churchill Livingstone, Edinburgh.

Reed K L and Sanderson S R (1980). *Concepts of Occupational Therapy*. Williams and Wilkins, Baltimore.

Schwartz D B (1976). Expanding a sheltered workshop to replace nonpaying patient jobs. *Hospital and Community Psychiatry*, **27** (2), 98–101.

Shepherd G (1983). Introduction. In *Theory and Practice of Psychiatric Rehabilitation* (eds. F N Watts and D H Bennett). John Wiley and Sons, Chichester.

Shepherd G (1984). *Institutional Care and Rehabilitation*. Longman, London.

Shepherd G (1989). The value of work in the 1980s. *Psychiatric Bulletin*, **13**, 231–233.

Shepherd G (1991).Rehabilitation and the care of the long-term mentally ill. *Current Opinion in Psychiatry*, **4**, 288–294.

Smith R (1987). *Unemployment and Health*. Open University Press, London.

Starrin B (1989). *Unemployment, Poverty and the Quality of Working Life: Some European Experiences*. Germany: Editions Sigma, Berlin.

Turner R and Roberts G (1992). The Worcester Development Project. *British Journal of Psychiatry*, **160**, 103–107.

Unsworth C A (1993). The concept of function. *British Journal of Occupational Therapy*, **56** (8), 287–292.

Van Weeghel J and Zeelan J (1991). *Arbeidsrehabilitatie*. Uitgeverij Lemma BV, Utrecht.

Vorspan R (1988). Activities of daily living in the clubhouse – you can't vacuum in a vacuum. *Psychosocial Rehabilitation Journal*, **12** (2), 15–21.

Wheeler N (1990). 'Working for Patients' and 'Caring for People', the same philosophy? *British Journal of Occupational Therapy*, **53** (10), 409–414.

Willson M (1987). *Occupational Therapy in Long-Term Psychiatry*, 2nd edn. Churchill Livingstone, Edinburgh.

Wing, J K and Morris B (eds.) (1981). *Handbook of Psychiatric Rehabilitation Practice*. Oxford University Press, Oxford.

Yankowitz R B (1990). Employment programmes and psychiatric disabilities. *New Directions for Mental Health Services*, **45** (Spring), 37–48.

16 Support for community psychiatric nurses in multidisciplinary teams: an example

J. Chandler

Introduction

Many of the programmes that offer occupational support seek to address issues of stress and 'burn-out', to counter their corrosive effects on staff morale and performance and limit their impact on turnover. 'Stress' is being discovered in an ever growing number of occupational contexts, including health and social care workers (McCarthy 1985; Handy 1990; Carson *et al.* 1991; Schafer 1992). As discussions of support are commonly adjuncts to and products of studies of stress, there are considerably more studies of its origins than evaluations of the effectiveness of support structures designed to address occupational stressors.

The pervasion of stress and the necessity of support to enhance coping strategies occupies an ideologically unassailable position in the literature on the provision of health and social care. It has strong links with the psychosocial therapeutic models that workers in this field adopt with clients and these models inform their view of themselves and their working relations. Here support is identified as a main contributor to mental health.

Discussion of stressors and support is also allied to human relations management strategies in their efforts to manage a workforce cooperatively and effectively, harness personal commitment and human interest to getting the job done and improve personnel retention. This approach often focuses on the individual and their coping mechanisms, rather than the organization and its work practices. The context of multidisciplinary teamworking makes such an approach less tenable. The reorganization of community services has created opportunities for team bids in care delivery, the introduction of clinical audit, and greater scope for the evaluation of team performance. Furthermore, for Øvretveit, the maintenance of effective and supportive networks is indicative of the quality of client care. He comments that it 'is a striking observation that teams which practise co-service and partnership, also work hard at creating and maintaining open and participatory relationships within the team' (1993, pp. 175–6). Good support for team members then becomes not an optional extra, but an essential process of team functioning.

This chapter will identify the importance of support for those working in multidisciplinary teams, how it can be provided and the importance and difficulties of assessing the value of support structures. The development of multidisciplinary teams has been particularly influential in shaping the working relations of community psychiatric workers and throughout this chapter they will be used as an exemplar in the discussion of the provision of occupational support for those involved in the provision of health and social care.

The context of support

The professional context of psychiatric nursing has changed dramatically in the last 20 years. As the care of mental health patients moves from hospital to community the practice of the relatively recent profession of community psychiatric nurse (CPN) has been ever dynamic. The structure of teams, the bases from which teams operate, and lines of professional and managerial accountability have been subject to organizational flux.

The current pattern of CPN work and its recent developments is evident in White's national survey of community psychiatric nursing (1990a). In the last decade the network for referrals for many CPNs has widened with almost as many referrals coming from GPs as psychiatrists and there has developed a closer identification with primary care. Schafer (1992) also found that hospital referrals had increased in recent years while referrals from the community had continued to rise.

In this context Handy (1990) argues that the stress of CPN work has been heightened by their own professional ambition and expansionist philosophy. The desire to escape from the medical superordinancy of psychiatrists has encouraged the widening base of referrals and participation in primary health care teams. These moves have been welcomed by GPs who see them as an opportunity to pass over more difficult and time-consuming clients. This has improved the status of CPNs as independent practitioners but has created new problems for caseload management and new sources of professional insecurity. There is the risk that CPNs are 'captured' by primary health care and psychosocial models of health care. Here 'intransigent psychiatrists' are seen as a threat to the smooth functioning of multidisciplinary teams. But it also changes the bases of potential conflict moving it from a debate between CPN and psychiatrist to debates between psychiatrists and GPs about what CPNs should properly be doing.

However, White (1993) suggests that the Department of Health circular, *Care Programme Approach,* may halt or even reverse this trend. It reasserts the primacy of the psychiatrist in interprofessional mental health care and re-emphasizes the importance of providing long-term support to those leaving mental hospitals. Furthermore two in five CPNs report themselves as specializing with a particular client group, the bulk of whom are the elderly, a group who are demographically set to rise and who are targeted as major recipients of community care. CPNs are working in different types of teams which require mixtures of specialist and generic skills and the ability to work with different client groups. This has implications for training and the balance between uni-professional expertise and multiskilling.

The recent history of community psychiatric care has also been characterized by physical dispersion. It is clearer where CPNs have moved from rather than where they have moved to. Nearly a quarter claim to have no main base and for many the move to new office accommodation has been driven by opportunism rather than rational planning. Locus is important to professional functioning and to team participation. These organizational features inform the support structures that are necessary to sustain professional practice and personal commitment.

In a review of support in multidisciplinary teams it is important to recognize the variability of team organization and the conceptual problems of identifying 'support' and its consequences. The concept of the team identifies an occupational structure and a style of working where individuals operate within a prescribed network, share the same objectives and adopt more egalitarian work practices. Operationally teams differ; some function to provide services to a particular client, others are loose networks and yet more are formally constituted teams. Each type of team differs in its level of permanence, the degree of interdisciplinary cooperation required and in the nature of the support CPNs may need.

Any discussion of the nature and effectiveness of team support must be grounded in the nature of the team itself. Here Simmons (1988) suggests that there are two main ways in which CPNs find themselves working in multidisciplinary teams. The first way is through attachment to primary health care teams or community care groups, an attachment which may or may not be coupled with a second base within a CPN team. On the positive side, Skidmore and Friend (1984) have suggested that the majority of CPNs prefer a dual base and this preference may be seen as indicative of the extent to which they need single disciplinary support to be effective in multidisciplinary contexts. Such support may override any tugs of loyalty and responsibility that this duality engenders. Second, they may be working within a community mental health team which incorporates other disciplinary groups in the provision of a district psychiatric service.

These different types of teams provide different contexts for the implementation of support systems although the need for support remains much the same. However, before the forms that this might take are assessed it is important to examine some of the reasons why CPNs are seen to need support and the organizational and professional context for such support.

The need for support

The sources of stress and the objectives for support for CPNs are many and varied. In broad terms the problems include lack of clarity and boundaries in their occupational role, the breadth of their referral base and the pressure this brings to caseloads, the personally demanding nature of their client group, and the new demands of teamworking. Many of these issues are residual problems for the CPN but their experience of them is influenced by their participation in multidisciplinary teams (Simmons and Brooker 1986).

Relationships with clients

Pollock (1989) has argued that the goals of community psychiatric nursing are vague both to health care planners and to CPNs themselves. The breadth of their occupational role makes it hard for them to identify which problems are suitable for clinical intervention and which are not. The scope for professional judgment and uncertainty is greater in the community where the boundaries of psychopathology are less obvious and the goals of care more diffuse. The changing locus of work has implications for the model of care used but the move towards psychosocial models both reflects and exacerbates boundary problems. Problems of living and personal distress are endemic in wider society and the CPN may have difficulty and require support in identifying what falls within and outside of their professional remit. The desire to have frequent personal contact with the client is the motivation for the job but its daily reality is also a key source of stress. Their ambivalence to the client group is noted by Handy (1990) as clients are regarded as both commodities in and consumers of the health service.

Much of the work of CPNs scores highly on the dimension of emotional labour. This is a drain on their own psychological resources and may threaten their own mental health. The discourse of care may incline CPNs towards self-sacrifice and hence it is part of all forms of support to delimit the job and to ensure that it is realistic and its goals are achievable. The nature of the job is personally wearing and in the past it has been suggested that community psychiatric nursing was so demanding that it could only be done on a part-time basis (Maisey 1975). CPNs who identify their therapeutic skills with their capacity to forge good interpersonal relations are more vulnerable to the dangers of over-involvement, the swamping of compassion and the problems of containing disappointment with non-responsive clients. Both Pollock (1989) and Handy (1990) describe the difficulties of CPNs in sustaining therapeutic relationships with patients who are difficult and demanding and the ways in which patients with whom CPNs have become over-involved eventually suffer by being rejected. As both GPs and psychiatrists refer the most difficult cases to CPNs, they need clear guidance about who to accept and how to manage their caseload.

The shape of support should reflect the nature of the client group. Handy's research contrasts the working lives of CPNs in an acute team with those who specialize in care of the elderly. Those in the acute team found their jobs both more stressful and more rewarding as this reflected the greater scope for improvement and disappointment in the care of this client group. In the delivery of care there was ambivalence about how patient care and client rights should be tempered by their supervisory responsibilities. Also their work brought them into daily contact with carers and families and involved them in the dynamic tensions that surrounded the question of 'who is my client?'

Those suffering mental illness remain social actors in the world, with power to influence the lives of others. Here the multidisciplinary team provides great scope for the manipulation of staff by patients, the progressive involvement of more professionals and the opportunity to exploit inconsistencies and divergences in their therapeutic strategies. The actions of some clients may light the touch paper if not fan the flames of interprofessional rivalry. The cohesiveness of the team may not always work to the benefit of clients. The jointness of responsibility may lead to the passing on of difficult clients and inconclusive case conferences in which decisions are slow to emerge. Also one must not also assume that collective views are always best. Close-knit teams provide an environment for the sharing of client information and the confirmation and circulation of pejorative labels. The looser-knit frameworks of care may create more social space within which clients can operate. Effective support should enable CPNs to sustain therapeutic relationships with clients and to be reflexive about the impact of team care.

Team leadership and coordination

The moving of services has led to greater involvement with primary health care teams and to work with other health professionals, paramedics, social workers and voluntary groups. These teams are multidisciplinary rather than interdisciplinary, blending specific areas of expertise rather than spawning new breeds of generic workers, although this may happen in the future. Here professional line management may be at variance with team demands and the CPN may find themselves caught at the crossroads where line and team management intersect.

Multidisciplinary teamwork may enhance rather than diminish a sense of professional isolation. The team widens the group who may be considered as colleagues but it is not always easy to be collegiate with others whose practice is informed by different disciplinary assumptions. Here Fox's analysis of primary health care teams (1991) describes a mental handicap nurse who finds that a multidisciplinary team does not compensate for the support they previously obtained from other mental handicap nurses. The same could be true for CPNs.

The concept of teamwork is a metaphor for cooperation and joint decision-making in work practice. Teamwork both demands higher levels of cooperation and coordination and creates more scope for cross-disciplinary rivalry and here conflicts with social workers have proved the most likely. As community psychiatric work moves from biomedical to psychosocial models the differences in therapeutic stance may diminish and their capacity to obviously complement one another may shrink. This is the basis for heightened professional competition where the lack of equivalent legal powers for CPNs remains a further source of resentment.

The theory of teamwork assumes that different members of the team have complementary models of the client and clear views about their particular professional input. However Pollock's research (1989) has demonstrated that CPNs work eclectically and this has some merit in permitting flexibility in relation to clients and the professional input of other key workers. However, in reality, there may be wide discrepancies in team members' perceptions of other members' roles and members may be quite literally unable to see the other workers' point of view (Brunning and Huffington 1985) or engage with other occupational cultures and languages. Effective liaison may demand specific disciplinary practice to be set within a more generic framework.

In an analysis of the perceptions of professional differences in a primary care team, Young (1991) found that members had great difficulty in describing either their or others' roles with one clear exception – they could all identify the role of medical practitioners. She also found that commitment to and involvement in the team was variable as medical professionals, either GPs or psychiatrists, have more power to opt out of team accountability. Young (1991) describes the ways in which GPs distance themselves from primary health care teams and White (1990*b*) similarly argues that psychiatrists are unwilling to be involved in the daily workings of the mental health multidisciplinary team. This was confirmed in Pollock's analysis of multi-disciplinary team functioning where members' practice was geared to medical authority (1989). When challenged they responded by closing ranks and involving the consultant. This creates some variability in who is a colleague and what is the team.

The constituent members of the team are variable. White (1990a) found that almost half the teams in which CPNs functioned included contributions from social services, a quarter of teams contained psychologists and a quarter of teams contained general managers. Psychiatrists were contributing to 86 per cent of teams but the extent of their contribution was very variable and only 29 per cent of psychiatrists were reported by local services managers as sympathetic to the professional remits of the community psychiatric service. Harrigan *et al.* (1993) found that team contacts were more extensive for CPNs working with clients suffering from psychotic or organic disorders rather than those with neurotic or other complaints. Here CPNs worked in a more independent way.

There are also practical issues in sustaining support and improving coordination. As Øvretveit points out, in the multidisciplinary context, no one person 'owns' the problem of coordination as it is an issue which is at once everyone's and no one's concern. Here the barriers to effective teamwork are also the barriers to support, in the lack of time to develop and sustain team links, the use of part-time and sessional staff, the use of different information systems and rules about access to client information. Obstacles to the smooth flow of information and the functioning of teams generate frustration, inhibit team effectiveness and strain systems of support.

Resource issues

Øvretveit argues that the purpose of community-based teams is 'to get the best and quickest "match" between a person's needs and resources available' (1993, p. 53). With the closure of hospitals and the movement towards trust status, the problems of matching the needs of the client population with community resources is more acute. In a recent questionnaire survey, which attempted to identify stressors for CPNs, the issue of 'not having enough facilities in the community to refer my client to' generated the highest scores (Carson *et al.* 1991).

Discussion on support needs suggests that support systems must have both personal and organizational dimensions if they are to be effective. Effective systems of support must also recognize how services are organized locally – the extent to which they are accountable to consultant psychiatrists, managed by nurses and sectorized to blend with local social services. The changing nature and context of community psychiatric nursing has raised new demands and new foci for support. These will be discussed in the next section.

Forms of support

The need for support has an emotional appeal and there is more call for its development than scrutiny of the effectiveness of different support systems.

One problem is that the concept of support, like that of care, is slippery and hard to define. Both are used descriptively and evaluatively. In any group there may be dispute about what counts as support and argument about whether individuals should receive 'support' whether they like it or not. It has a strong ideological and moral tinge (Pines and Maslach 1978). This is particularly evident in contemporary discussions of 'personality hardiness' (Boyle *et al.* 1991) and where psychiatric staff may judge colleagues who attended stress management workshops as personally weak (Kunkler and Whittick 1991). These findings demonstrate the lingering importance of traditional approaches to 'character' in nursing and these may be antithetic to the establishment of support systems.

There is a need to say what the support is, who should give it and to whom. Support may take many forms and its constituent elements are examined below. Any solutions that are taken must also reflect local conditions, and systems emerging in direct response to local problem solving.

Training

A major and continuing problem for CPNs is the level of training that most practitioners have received to facilitate their work in the community and within multidisciplinary teams. Training has been slow in adjusting to organization change. Although the community element in basic training has been expanding since the 1960s, it was only in 1974 that the first clinical course for CPNs, with the express aim of preparing mental health nurses to work in multidisciplinary teams, was established. But, as White notes, the main struggle has not been about educational objectives, but to secure and protect finance and secure secondment. Although the recent survey of CPNs demonstrated that more have completed CPN courses, the majority (62.5 per cent) have not been trained specifically to work in the community or in multidisciplinary contexts (White 1990*a*). This occurred at a time when one in five places on CPN courses remained empty (Rushford 1990), a product of insufficient funds rather than insufficient applicants.

There have been developments in the field of open learning and the pooling of training resources in health authority consortia. But some nationally regarded courses have closed recently (White 1993) and the movement to trusts is likely further to fragment training initiatives. Post-basic training for CPNs is inevitably shaped by the development of Project 2000. The changing structure of basic training is intended to create a broader knowledge base for mental health nurses as all will be trained to work both in hospital and community settings. These developments were a continuation of the 1982 registered mental nurse (RMN) curricula and grounded in the gathering pace of hospital closure.

Such developments undermine free-standing post-basic courses. However, White (1993) found that a quarter of those who had undertaken the 1982 RMN syllabus had already gone on to complete the CPN course. This says much about practitioners' desire to extend their skills and the pressure to achieve higher levels of accredited learning. Here the closer links with higher education being forged by nurse education are leading to the academic accreditation of a wide range of post-basic courses. CPN courses are likely to be included in the changes which are moving all practitioners to membership of a diplomate and graduate profession. This is a widespread trend among all nursing and paramedical groups and it is important that CPNs are included, as this will enhance their status as members of multidisciplinary teams and may facilitate the development of new relationships with other community nurses.

White (1990b) has argued that the real consumers of courses are managers and feared that CPN training is more likely to become increasingly instrumental, subject to budgetary limitations and contract training. However, in the future, when part of a broader and often modularized educational programme within higher education and located in the English National Board Higher Award, such courses may be less vulnerable and more central to a national strategy for the delivery of community care.

There is no systematic evaluation of CPN courses at a national level. Training can seem to offer the complete answer to groups who are denied access to extended professional training. It is unrealistic and perhaps dangerous to assume that training will equip participants to 'solve' patient problems. Also evaluations of courses suggest that careful consideration is needed in how to blend life experience and expert knowledge. But how far course content will be orientated towards the multidisciplinary teams in which CPNs will find themselves functioning depends on the course planners and the accrediting bodies.

Related to this, there have been suggestions that professions should change their methods of training, to include more elements of joint and interdisciplinary education (Hutt 1986; Gomes 1985) and to further multi-skilling. But most educational programmes focus on the development of single-discipline expertise with sessions on working with others. Any change would blur professional identity and may not be popular with the accreditation bodies who police professional boundaries. Training programmes should also specifically address a range of issues in relation to support. All training needs to balance the acquisition of distinct practitioner skills and shared management skills, to value others in the team, to have a clear view of where their expertise fits and to participate effectively in team networks and team meetings.

In the community context, contacts with clients are less open to routine professional support and are located in the client's web of relationships. Hence training must reflect settings of families and neighbourhoods, the wide variety of living arrangements and a therapeutic context where patients have more power. Here the job is less routine and the individual CPN has to be more resourceful. Where care is shared, individualized treatment models of therapist and client are often less appropriate.

Working with clients in natural settings makes those who became violent or threatening potentially more difficult and dangerous. Whitfield and Shelley (1991) found that 9 per cent of CPNs surveyed had sustained a physical injury and 24 per cent had been threatened with physical violence in the previous 12 months. Their work also identifies the poor guidelines and policies operative at local level and the deficit of training in this area. This is a key training issue for all members of the multidisciplinary team; it provides opportunities for shared training and is a issue that recurs in discussions of peer support.

One area where training links into peer support is in participation in stress-management workshops. Kunkler and Whittick have assessed their value for psychiatric nurses. In their study they describe the positive evaluation such workshops received from those who participated in the programme, but also note the problems of achieving regular attendance. This was attributed to staff resistance and more particularly the lack of managerial support to attend workshop sessions. One conclusion from their work is that stress-management must be seen as a part of the work programme, not an additional activity for 'Once stressed, staff are less likely to want to participate in any new initiatives which may lead to a temporary increase in stress levels' (1991, pp. 175–6). When staff feel overloaded, the stress-management workshop becomes another task to be fitted into their busy schedules. There is also scope for 'positive re-framing' where the pace and unpredictability of work is viewed as adding spice rather than stress to the job (Finch and Krantz 1991).

However, training is not only about courses that give once and for all qualifications. It should be a continuous process. The newly-qualified are to receive continuing support as preceptors and established practitioners are to obtain regular updates in study days within the post-registration education for practice programme. Here supervision becomes an adjunct to training as it seeks to develop professional skills.

Supervision

In management literature, supervision is seen as a positive process in professional development and guidance, but it is not always seen as supportive by its recipients (Hill 1989). Platt-Loch (1986) found psychiatric nurses suspicious of the role of supervisors and their capacity to control and evaluate their work. However, more recent research by Major (1993) found very positive attitudes to supervision among CPNs and their managers. Here supportive supervision is aimed at limiting and assessing CPN activity, to ensure the quality of clinical intervention, provide advice and monitor caseloads. It aims to safeguard against burn-out, improve morale and reduce absenteeism. Supervision is especially important in giving direction, especially for new and for part-time members of staff.

Although much of the literature points out the benefits of supervision, there is some debate about the form that it should take. Simmons and Brooker (1986) suggest that supervision may be either individual or group. Group sessions may encourage nurses to learn more from each other and increase the visibility of their work. But this can be threatening and demands good relations with peer and supervisor to be effective. It is unclear whether this should be undertaken by another psychiatric nurse or by another senior member of the team. If it is undertaken by someone from a different disciplinary background, models of care must still be shared. Finally there is comment on the effectiveness and supportiveness of different supervisory styles. Major (1993) notes the dilemma; more egalitarian styles may be experienced as more emotionally supportive but may do little to extend clinical skills and self-evaluation, whereas a more managerial approach may help CPNs to meet team targets, but are more stressful.

But the onus is not only on the CPN to accept and use supervision, but also on supervisors to manage realistically, to act as a buffer between policy-makers and practitioners, to evaluate current caseloads and interpersonal difficulties with individuals in the client group. Supervisors need training and should be mindful not only of their own management hierarchy but the place of the CPN in the team, where professionals may feel relatively isolated and unsupported in their disciplinary area. Multidisciplinary teams both challenge and necessitate the continuance of systems of supervision within a nursing framework. Here Simmons argues that 'only when a professional group has security in its professional identity can that group contribute fully to a team made up of other professions' (Simmons 1988, p. 17).

In the swings and roundabouts of supervision Fineman (1985) suggests that there were more supervisory difficulties when supervisors were also managers. But when they are managers they are more empowered to alter working conditions, review caseloads, allocate resources and offer career development. There needs to be some clarity about what is meant by supervisory support and how it relates both to line management and team working. Where health services have been subject to the processes of continuous reorganization, the quality of supervision and leadership available to CPNs has often suffered.

There is considerable variability and lack of clarity in how counselling relates to support and management. Counselling as an adjunct to supervision can be seen as the first line of disciplinary action (King 1989). Here there are organizational penalties for those seen to lack coping skills and this type of counselling is likely to generate reserve amongst staff in acknowledging and confessing that they have problems. Handy argues that counselling could do more than combat occupational stress among CPNs; it could facilitate more contextually and socially aware reflection 'by introducing them to alternative theoretical frameworks for examining the ways in which they conceptualize and respond to the demands of their working environment' (1990, p. 210). Many organizations now employ the services of a psychologist or trained counsellor – but there is probably too much unacceptable irony in a psychiatric service embarking on such a venture.

Supervision is an area where there are many claims and little evaluation of the system in operation and where the training of supervisors themselves could be improved. However, at the other end of the supervisory spectrum, there is obvious scope for peer support and co-counselling and it is to this that the chapter now turns.

Peer support and counselling

Good collegiate relationships both reflect and enhance morale. At one level collegiality relates to the informal relationships amongst team members and this is always as important as the formal organization. Thompson (1986) argues that this is especially true for multidisciplinary teams. Personal knowledge smoothes the pathways of referral and Thompson found that effective teams were characterized by a more comfortable atmosphere amongst members who knew and liked each other. Furthermore, White (1986) found that GPs were keener to refer patients to CPNs whom they knew. It may be hard to orchestrate, but the message is that team support is easier where attention is paid to the affective and informal aspects of teamwork. However, although informal work groups may be more satisfying to the members, organizational research has long suggested that their objectives may not always match official objectives of the organization. This may be avoided where peer support and supervision are integrated into a single system.

The work of Marcelissen and colleagues (1988) adds critical comment to the discussion of peer support. They suggest that it cannot compensate for the strains of the job. They found that, as stress levels rose, co-worker support declined and, as perceived stress fell, so support increased. They emphasize the importance of greater sensitivity to the complex interpersonal environment in which support is exchanged, as support systems are ineffective in the over-stressed environment. Their research demonstrates that vocalized stress and the experience of co-worker support cannot be easily identified as separate phenomena that can be placed in a causal relationship to one another. The rhetoric of stress is a safe grievance, a useful cipher in the workplace as it identifies a problem without blaming individuals.

A peer support programme may have a more specific focus, such as that described by Dawson and his colleagues (1988). This was designed specifically to support staff after a patient assault and, although established within an acute setting, what it identifies as good practice could be easily transferred to the community context. The support project identified the problem of excessive self-blame and its corrosive effects on professional confidence as common in the aftermath of an assault and it used the 'buddy system' to provide immediate and purposeful support. The programme was evaluated well by its participants and its implementation coincided with a fall in staff turnover. Although the research team argued that it was hard to demonstrate that this resulted directly from the scheme, the establishment of the programme had other benefits in that it provided a focus for training days and consultation. These findings contrast with those of Whitfield and Shelley (1991), where despite widespread membership of informal and formal support networks, these were seen to provide little help to staff who had experienced violence or its threat.

Most examples of team support are less specific and fall more into the category of team-building.

Team-building and communication

The establishment of teams is commonly accompanied by team-building exercises and these have both formal and informal objectives. On the formal side joint seminars are useful to facilitate understanding of professional roles and responsibilities and to ease communication. Young (1991) described these as a feature only of the initiation of the community care groups she surveyed. Once established the sessions stopped and there was little or no further discussion of members' roles. Team-building exercises were a product of innovation and change, of heightened commitment and enthusiasm, as evidenced in these comments of a CPN:

It was time of okay, let's get together and let's do something ... let's move forward. It was a very enthusiastic time, very stimulating. (Fox 1991)

However, team-working that relies on enthusiasm alone is vulnerable and Fox describes how, since the inception of a primary care group, attendance at formal meetings had declined. The formal support system atrophied as those attending felt that what was being discussed had little relevance for themselves and they had become doubtful about the value of continuing participation. Ironically, the failures of formal meetings to team build were matched by the establishment of an informal support group. Perhaps the word 'group' is misleading, as what individuals most frequently developed and relied upon was a particular relationship with a single individual.

Øvretveit (1993) emphasizes that team-building is not a once and for all activity. As new members join and others leave the team objectives need reaffirmation. Team-building and team maintenance should be constant and routine activities and this takes time. He notes that time pressures threaten team functioning, as members become more inclined to miss meetings and resent those they feel they must attend. For team-working to be supportive to individuals, Øvretveit argues that members must understand the importance and effectiveness of cooperation, invest time in network maintenance, hold others who don't use team mechanisms accountable for their laxity and ensure that team meetings are well organized and give value for time spent.

Team support depends on the flow of information. Young (1991) found that nurses were the principal communicators in primary health care teams. They acted as the go-between for paramedical workers and doctors and were the most committed to teamwork. Location was also important and much of the success of the team functioning in the context of primary health care was associated with its geography, as this influenced the frequency and opportunity for formal and informal contact.

The increasing use of computers may enhance teamwork as they facilitate the accessibility of notes to all members of the team and provide a genuine network of information. Computerized notes may assist genuine networking where information flows across disciplines rather than just from top to bottom. For Øvretveit (1993) smooth information flow is an essential aspect of team support and a measure of effectiveness and cohesion, but raises issues about the commonality and confidentiality of client records. However, computerization has not always been viewed positively as input facilities may not be easily accessible and its introduction appears initially merely to increase the work burden.

Team leadership

The management of teams is less clear than professional line management. Some teams may function by straddling the cracks between line management while others may attempt to lessen disciplinary rivalry by constructing themselves as leaderless networks. Teams require active management for them to orchestrate productive meetings, to avoid purposeless discussion (Pollock 1989) and to ensure that what is discussed in general meetings is of widespread interest (Young 1991). This is a residual problem of team organization. Here the skills required are those of coordination, of agenda setting and chairing. Fox describes how the introduction of group managers has altered this, bringing more accountability to the use of resources and equipment.

The effectiveness of teams and their leadership are influenced by their resourcing. In the delivery of health care, power follows resources and the creation of community resource teams in the wake of the Griffiths Report means the move to local social-services-based teams and their empowerment. Financial support is a key to their successful operation and teamwork can never resolve resource issues. This is a constant pressure of the job and a key item for team discussion and occupational support.

Conclusion

Support is an adjunct to good management in clarifying professional responsibilities, managing caseloads, acting as sounding-boards when professional problems are encountered, the resourcing of practice and the backing of staff decision-making when reasonable risk has gone wrong. It is also indicative of general team functioning.

Support is also an important buzz-word in modern management circles and in the delivery of health and social care. However, there is a need to critically and unsentimentally appraise the structures and processes identified as supportive. It is an important part of team leadership and team review. Handy's critical account of occupational stress among CPNs is a model for subsequent research with other professional groups contributing to multidisciplinary teams. She presents a case for good qualitative research that probes the ways in which individuals and organizations function rather than an overall reliance on quantitative techniques which attempt empirically to gauge the ways in which 'surface stressors cluster together'. The latter may provide a useful thermometer of job satisfaction but is not helpful in fully understanding the ways in which different professional groups work within multidisciplinary teams. It is also probably easier to assess what support structures and processes are trying to achieve than enter the academic minefield of researching stress and its many manifestations with its 'lack of conceptual clarity, disagreement on definitions and divergent operationalizations' (Marcelissen *et al.* 1988).

Research is needed to examine how those involved in different multidisciplinary teams deliver care and manage their professional interface with other team members. Such research would benefit from an improved ethnography of health and social care workers as well as the testing of skills within support systems. Multidisciplinary teams are largely the product of local and ad hoc responses to policy changes and there is no evidence that any future planning will contain more rationality than planning to date. But such localism also provides opportunities for building support mechanisms that truly reflect local need. Part of such research would be a review of the role of support in individual and team performance and it would examine not only the activities of individual workers but also identify ways of supporting the supporters.

References

Boyle A, Grap M J, Younger J and Thornby D (1991). Personality hardiness, ways of coping, social support and burnout in critical care nurses, *Journal of Advanced Nursing*, **16**, 850–857.
Brunning H and Huffington C (1985). Altered images. *Nursing Times*, **81** (31), 24–27.
Carson J, Barlett H and Croucher P (1991). Stress in community psychiatric nursing: a preliminary investigation. *Community Psychiatric Nursing Journal*, **11** (April), 8–17.

Dawson J, Johnston M, Kehiayan N, Kyanko S and Martinez R (1988). Response to patient assault. A peer support program for nurses. *Journal of Psychosocial Nursing*, **26** (2), 1–12.

Finch E S and Krantz S R (1991). Low burnout in a high stress setting: a study of staff at Fountain House. *Psychosocial Rehabilitation Journal*, **14** (Jan), 15–26.

Fineman S (1985). *Social Work Stress and Intervention*. Gower, Aldershot.

Fox J M (1991). Working in a community care group: factors influencing professional views. A paper presented at the Medical Sociology Conference, University of York, September.

Gomes J (1985). Cooperation through core courses, *Nursing Times*, 31 January, 5.

Handy J (1990). *Occupational Stress in a Caring Profession: the Social Context of Psychiatric Nursing*. Avebury, Aldershot.

Harrigan P, Sorensen J and Ryder S (1993). Clinical audit and CPN services. In *Community Psychiatric Nursing. A Research Perspective*, Vol. 2 (eds. C Brooker and E White). Chapman and Hall, London.

Hill J (1989). Supervision in the caring professions: a literature review. *Community Psychiatric Nursing Journal*, **9** (Oct), 9–15.

Hutt A (1986). What exactly is the team approach? *Midwife. Health Visitor and Community Nurse*, **22** (10), 340, 342, 350.

King C (1989). Staff counselling. *Community Psychiatry: its Practice and Management*. **2** (2), 25–26.

Kunkler J and Whittick J (1991). Stress-management workshops for nurses: practical problems and possible solutions. *Journal of Advanced Nursing*, **16**, 172–176.

Maisey M (1975). Hospital based psychiatric nursing in the community. *Nursing Times*, **71** (9), 354–355.

Major S (1993). Attitudes towards supervision: a comparison of CPNs and managers. In *Community Psychiatric Nursing. A Research Perspective*, vol. 2 (eds. C Brooker and E White). Chapman and Hall, London.

Marcelissen F H G, Winnubst J A M, Buunk B and de Wolff C J (1988). Social support and occupational stress: a causal analysis. *Social Science and Medicine*, **26** (3), 365–373.

McCarthy P (1985). Burnout in psychiatric nursing. *Journal of Advanced Nursing*, **10**, 305–310.

Øvretveit J (1993). *Coordinating Community Care. Multidisciplinary Teams and Care Management*. Open University Press, Buckingham.

Pines A and Maslach C (1978). Characteristics of staff burn-out in mental health settings. *Hospital and Community Psychiatry*, **29**, 233–237.

Platt-Loch L M (1986). Clinical supervision for psychiatric nurses. *Journal of Psychiatric Nursing*, **26** (1), 7–15.

Pollock L C (1989). *Community Psychiatric Nursing: Myth and Reality*. RCN Research Series, Scutari Press, London.

Rushford D (1990). Recruitment to post-basic certificate courses in the United Kingdom for 1989–90. *Community Psychiatric Journal*. **10** (Feb), 17–20.

Schafer T (1992). CPN stress and occupational change. *Community Psychiatric Nursing Journal*, **12** (Feb), 16–24.

Simmons S and Brooker C (1986). *Community Psychiatric Nursing: A Social Perspective*. Heinemann, London.

Simmons S (1988). Community psychiatric nurses and multidisciplinary working. *Community Psychiatric Nursing Journal*, **8** (Sept), 14–18.

Skidmore D and Friend W (1984). Should CPNs be in the primary health care team? *Nursing Times*, 19 September, 310–312.

Thompson T L (1986). *Communication for Health Professionals: a Relational Perspective*. Harper and Rowe, New York.

White E (1986). Factors influencing general practitioners to refer patients to community psychiatric nurses. In *Psychiatric Nursing Research* (ed. C Brooker) Wiley, Chichester.

White E (1990*a*). *Community Psychiatric Nursing: The 1990 National Survey*. CPNA, Nuneaton.

White E (1990*b*). Psychiatrists' influence on the development of community psychiatric nursing services. *Community Psychiatric Nursing. A Research Perspective* (ed. C Brooker). Chapman and Hall, London.

White E (1993). Community psychiatric nursing 1980 to 1990: a review of organization, education and practice. *Community Psychiatric Nursing. A Research Perspective*, vol. 2 (eds. C Brooker and E White). Chapman and Hall, London.

Whitfield W and Shelley P (1991). Violence and the CPN: a survey. *Community Psychiatric Journal*, **11** (April), 13–17.

Young K (1991). Multi-disciplinary teamwork in the community. A paper presented at the Medical Sociology Conference, University of York, September.

Acknowledgement

I would like to thank Tim Hardwick for his helpful comments during the preparation of this chapter.

17 Principles of evaluation

B. Thomas

Introduction

In recent years evaluation has become increasingly important in the effective delivery of community mental health care. Stemming initially from general financial problems which created controversy about the NHS in the late 1980s, evaluation of community services has developed not in a planned and systematic manner but more haphazardly resulting from a number of disparate strands coming together. These include the lack of efficacy found with traditional psychiatric hospital treatment and the government's major prioritizing of community care. The Audit Commission (delegated by the government to monitor value for money in the public sector) reported in 1986 on the poor coordination and fragmentation of funding sources for community care. This resulted in the White Paper *Caring for People* (Department of Health 1989) and the introduction of the 1990 NHS and Community Care Act which established the concepts of purchaser and provider, trusts and the close working relationships between health and local authorities.

In addition there is a new professional attention to quality in the public services, increasing involvement of users and carers in service planning and delivery. There is a growth of the user movement, campaigning for more accountability on the part of service providers, increased public awareness and a shift in attitudes towards higher expectations of health care. The government's drive for effective, efficient and economic use of resources adds impetus for the identification of appropriate evaluation processes and a widening search for outcome measures particularly in relation to symptom reduction, health gain, social functioning and quality of life. Evaluation of community mental health services incorporates a wide range of methods and represents various interests and perspectives. Despite its gradual development unifying principles are now emerging for community mental health care evaluation and a body of knowledge is growing.

This chapter is not intended to present a comprehensive survey of existing research. Rather it examines some of the principles that underpin the evaluation of community mental health services and highlights some of developments that have occurred in this area. Community mental health services are changing rapidly. Evaluation cannot be seen in isolation. Recording and disseminating information about the impact of mental health services on the quality of life for those who depend on them is necessarily political, particularly when there is a shortfall in provision and a growing public unease about the problem. Evaluative research is throwing some light on the type of community services that work for service users. It is imperative that these results should influence practice and thereby improve future service provision and generate further evaluation. Community mental health services are multifaceted and therefore one of the basic principles involves ensuring that the evaluation is wide enough to incorporate the concerns of the different stakeholders.

Systematic evaluation is called for as a way of demonstrating greater accountability on the part of health service providers, particularly in an era of increasing demand and severe financial constraints. Community mental health services, like all health care provision, are cash limited. The government's clamp-down on public spending means that every aspect of expenditure is placed under rigorous scrutiny (Bottomley 1993). Health programmes are expected to produce evidence that they work and that they are cost effective. As rationing and prioritizing become commonly accepted in discussions of choice between different patients, psychiatric treatments and mental health services evaluation data will be all the more important in influencing the decision-making process. These decisions will only be as good as the information on which they are based. This in turn depends on the quality of the evaluation carried out. Increasing pressures on available resources mean that one of the major principles of health service evaluation is the inclusion of an economic perspective. Although not all health service evaluation studies have been concerned with the efficient use of resources, there is vast and increasing literature on economic evaluation in relation to health care.

Economic evaluation

Economic evaluation refers to the systematic appraisal of the costs and benefits of a service, treatment programme or project. It is usually carried out to determine the relative economic efficiency of a service. Efficiency is about getting the most out of available resources. In health care it is essential to identify efficient ways of using limited resources since any decision to provide a particular service uses resources which could have been used in other ways. This section highlights some of the main issues incorporating economics into evaluation studies. For those who wish to pursue the topic in more detail, Mooney *et al.* (1986), McGuire *et al.* (1992) and Drummond (1990) are highly recommended. Economists define two concepts of efficiency. The first accepts a particular end as given and is concerned with how to achieve this at least cost. This is called technical efficiency. For example, if it is accepted that treating people with schizophrenia in the community is worthwhile then the question of efficiency relates to how to treat people at least cost. The technique used to address this 'how' question is cost effectiveness analysis (CEA). The second approach considers maximizing the benefit obtained from available resources. This is known as allocative efficiency. Allocative efficiency is approached by using the technique of cost benefit analysis (CBA). The costs and benefits of competing ways of using resources are assessed in monetary terms. For example, if a community programme has to be compared with an in-patient facility, then the question is whether it is more beneficial to use resources in one programme or the other.

Both of these techniques are problematic in their application to community care and indeed to health care generally, since it is rarely appropriate that the outcome of community care is one-dimensional. For example, if managers compare community care with in-patient care using cost effectiveness analysis (CEA) it may be assumed that patients' satisfaction is the same for all treatments. However, in treating people with schizophrenia, both community and in-patient programmes may use pharmacological treatments which reduce core symptoms but patients' levels of satisfaction may be very different for each programme (Muijen *et al.* 1992). In using cost benefit analysis (CBA) to determine whether community care or in-patient treatment is most beneficial in relation to the money spent we are limited to measuring the benefits only in monetary terms.

To compensate for this deficit, health economists have devised a multidimensional approach known as cost-utility analysis (CUA). This approach uses a combined quantity of life gained with quality of life measure, generally called the QALYs or quality adjusted life years. Without denying the importance of measuring the health outputs, QALYs is restrictive if there is anything else that patients want from their treatment and care. For example, many users of mental services have financial and social problems. These deficits have led some critics to want to abandon QALYs altogether. However, others are more favourable towards their potential for development. A more detailed discussion of QALYs follows under the heading 'Quality of life'.

The reduction of hospital beds and in-patient facilities is based on the premise that community care will provide more beneficial treatments, with increased choice, less personal restriction and greater consumer responsiveness, all at a lower cost, at least for low-dependency groups. It is now acknowledged that community care may cost more for some groups of patients. For example, Goldberg (1991), in his review of cost effectiveness in the treatment of schizophrenia, emphasizes that although care in the community is generally cheaper than care in a hospital there are individuals who can be cared for more cheaply in hospitals. As hospitals empty of their easy-to-discharge patients the more severely mentally ill will remain The essential elements of community services include needs-based assessment and planning, care management, domicilary, day and respite services, and better support for carers and for patients in their own homes. In addition in-patient facilities are required for assessment and short-term treatment. The *Health of the Nation: Key Area Handbook, Mental Illness* (DoH 1992) lists nineteen service settings for the delivery of mental health care.

O'Donnell *et al.* (1992) suggest that, so far, major policy changes towards hospital closures and the development of community services are being implemented with little systematic evaluation of costs or their benefits to patients and carers. In this review, O'Donnell found only eight UK studies of costs and outcomes of mental health care alternatives. Goldberg (1991) suggests that although several carefully conducted cost studies have indicated that care in the community is generally cheaper than care in a hospital, none of the studies indicate that it is better. In his review Goldberg presents data which show that more expensive treatment may sometimes be cheaper for society. However, this is not a general rule and some methods of providing care are more expensive and less effective.

There is a need for more evaluation studies examining the efficacy of community services and their comparative costs if the best use is to be made of scarce resources. Economic evaluation will need to be considered in controlled studies and will need to involve the measurement of a number of outcomes since mental health care is multidimensional. Knapp *et al.* (1990) found that care in the community was less expensive for patients discharged from the Claybury and Friern hospitals in North London. The lower cost of care in the community does not appear to be at the expense of effectiveness since on average patients preferred community care to hospitalization. Such studies are becoming more and more sophisticated. For example, Strathdee and Thornicroft (1992) are currently carrying out a comprehensive evaluation study of a sectorized psychiatric service in Camberwell, South London. In addition to developing a comprehensive, innovative psychiatric service the researchers intend to rigorously evaluate the service including the development and dissemination of a comprehensive set of computerized clinical and research measures of needs and outcomes including family burden. Satisfaction with care and an interagency care assessment instrument. The study also includes a comprehensive cost effectiveness evaluation of experimental and control sector services.

With health economics becoming a stronger driving force in strategic planning and policy formulation for mental health services there is an expectation that more evaluation studies will be carefully controlled and directed around financially led considerations. From the mid-1970s in the United States there has been rapidly growing interest in the methods of economic analysis as a means of developing policy solutions for the problems facing the delivery of mental health services, (Frank and Manning 1992). Karluk and Astrachan (1993) suggest that research is growing impressively in this field. However, efficiency is not the only criterion that needs to be considered when evaluating community care. Karluk and Astrachan (1993) warn that current policies may lead to a fragmentation of services which are multitiered and lack equity. Equity is the degree to which a distribution is judged to be 'fair'. Bartlett and Le Grand (1993) suggest that equity is a concept of many interpretations which is rarely made explicit in today's policy objectives, probably because they are being driven by a government for which equity considerations are not necessarily a high priority. However, in the delivery of community services for the mentally ill notions of equity are becoming more prominent, for example, equal access for all client groups, particularly black and minority racial groups (DoH 1993*b*). Bartlett and Le Grand define equity in relation to need. An equitable service is one which is determined primarily by need and not by irrelevant factors such as income, socioeconomic status, gender or ethnic origin.

The argument relating to equity is elaborated by Knapp (1990). He suggests that economics is not confined to economy, effectiveness and efficiency but that these have to be accompanied by an equity enquiry. Knapp is opposed to grand generalizations about the benefits of community care. He suggests that evaluation studies should be focused on individuals, their needs and consequences for their carers. He argues that few evaluation studies of mental health services have analysed or presented their findings below the aggregate level. Good community care is not necessarily cheaper than hospital provision but it may be more cost effective. However, for some people community care may not be cost effective. Knapp suggests that we need to establish who and under what circumstances community care is more cost effective than hospital treatment. This issue has now been acknowledged by the government and is emphasized in its *Research for Health* document (DoH 1993*3c*).

To illustrate his argument Knapp quotes Hafner (1987) who found that the total costs of complementary care in psychiatric homes and group homes in Mannheim amount to an average of only 43 per cent of the costs of continuous in-patient hospital care for 145 patients with schizophrenia admitted to hospital. But for eight of the 145 patients the complementary care was more expensive than continuous hospital treatment. From these results Hafner suggested that certain patients require such intensive care that it is more cost effective to treat them in hospital than in the community.

Appropriateness and acceptability

Without denying the need for economic appraisal there are a number of other important principles which should form the basis of any evaluation programme. These include appraising the social acceptability of services (Doll 1973). Regardless of the economic viability of a service, if it is not acceptable to the people it is aimed at then it will not succeed, since users will either ignore what is provided or find alternative forms of help. Finding out whether or not patients use a service seems like a fairly easy task. Until 1987 the hospital activity analysis (HAA) was the major source of infommation processing for hospitals. This information was used for planning and for evaluation. Unfortunately, psychiatric services were generally excluded. The collection of such routine data within the NHS for evaluation purposes has been so problematic that a Royal Commission on the NHS was particularly critical of timeliness and questioned its accuracy. This led to a DHSS review into the existing health service information systems and a proposal for changes. Following the recommendations of the Korner Committee a new form of routine data collection came into operation in 1987. Community services were covered in the fifth Korner Report and a separate classification system set up for mental illness services. Clinical data included initial contact, location of contact, source of referral, client's age and sex. St Leger *et al.* (1992) suggest that the NHS infommation system which has developed out of the Korner reports will enable activity to be linked with resources more effectively and for more reliable costing of procedures to be carried out.

Since the introduction of the NHS and Community Care Act (1992) provider units need to be much more timely and accurate about their recording of patient information including numbers of referrals, service uptake and activity levels. Purchasers are becoming more astute in monitoring performance and comparing statistics between provider units, including planned and actual patient episodes, average length of stay, suicide rates, untoward incidents and other indices which provide information relating to cost, volume and quality.

Due to the increasing volume and complexity of data to be collected, stored, analysed and retrieved most health services now use some form of computerized information system. In mental health services computerized patient information systems are less developed than in general medicine and so far the data collected is fragmented and variable. For example, it is difficult to show relationships between the care and treatment delivered, the costs incurred and patient outcomes. Greater technical sophistication will improve the accuracy and integration of the data obtained, linking cost, volume and quality. As far as psychiatry is concerned Shepherd (1989) suggests that at a technical level the best tool for service evaluation is the case register. Such a system records the individual's contacts with the service and is used for a given population of a geographical area. Most of the present patient-recording systems do not include such comprehensive data and are not suitable for storage of longitudinal histories of patient care. Case registers can monitor specific kinds of service usage (e.g. Sturt *et al.* 1982) and different types of contacts can be cross-referenced, etc. (Wooff *et al.* 1983). A good example is provided by the Worcester Psychiatric Case Register which contains a computerized record of all patients in the psychiatric services from 1973 until 1987. From the case register it has been possible to determine the average number of service days delivered per year, to demonstrate that there has been a trend towards patients using more services and an increase in the contribution of local authority social services (Hassall 1991).

Health outcome measures

Case registers have provided a large amount of important evaluative and epidemiological data. However, they are difficult and expensive to set up and despite their revived popularity they cannot provide information about the quality of a service or anything significant about health outcomes. At the heart of health service evaluation is the assessment of outcomes or the impact of treatment and care on a given population. Despite the controversy surrounding measurement of health outcomes, attempts are being made to move away from negative conceptualizations of health to more positive measures of well-being. A full review of these developments can be found in Bowling (1990). Health outcomes are usually dependent on technical appraisal and are described in terms of the effectiveness of treatments and caring services. Shepherd (1988) suggests that outcome indices should reflect what happens to people as a result of their being involved in the service. However, it is necessary not only to decide according to certain criteria but also according to whom. This not only includes the judgments of the professional staff but must be extended to include users and, where appropriate, relatives and the wider community.

Until recently the process of evaluation in health care concentrated on structure and process despite continued pressure and interest in outcome determination. Many of the changes introduced to mental health services in the NHS and Community Care Act can be seen as creating an environment which facilitates a focus on outcomes. The context of health outcomes is usually defined in terms of the achievement of, or failure to achieve, desired goals. In psychiatry the measurement of outcomes is particularly difficult. Outcomes relate to the impact of the community mental health service on individuals and families and on communities and society as a whole. The analysis of a causal relationship between the service and an assumed outcome requires consideration of intervening variables and exclusion of other competing factors. St Leger *et al.* (1992) remind us that intervention studies are the most powerful means of evaluation. The most rigorous approach to intervention studies is the randomized controlled trial (RCT). Although used frequently in the evaluation of clinical procedures, particularly drug trials, it can in principle be applied to service provision in general. A full discussion on outcome measures and RCTs is beyond the scope of this chapter. For further details see Cochrane (1972) and Pocock (1987).

According to Weiss (1972) the evaluation of outcomes is determined by measuring the effects of a programme against its goals. Whilst agreeing that this is an essential requirement, Milne (1987) points out some of the difficulties that can arise when goals are not stated clearly and the problems of real-life situations when priorities change and programmes are modified. At a general level there is agreement about the main goals of community mental health care, for example, the *Health of the Nation, Key Area Handbook* on mental illness suggests that care outside the institutional setting of large mental hospitals can improve health outcomes for the mentally ill (DoH 1993). One of the primary targets set out in *Health of the Nation* is to improve significantly the health and social functioning of mentally ill people. However, such general goals have to be broken down into measurable objectives otherwise it is impossible to assess their effectiveness (Rossi *et al.* 1985). Explicitly defined objectives, seem to be less common in community mental health care than in more acute specialities.

Community mental health care programmes are dynamic and complex by nature involving a number of practitioners, who for the most part do not remain constant. They apply various kinds of interventions, which are prone to change, and sometimes they work towards different outcomes and have different priorities. This is not to mention other intervening variables such as other agencies who may be involved, including voluntary organizations and similar informal sources. To determine plausible conclusions in relation to outcomes careful consideration must be given to the design of any evaluation study. The control and exclusion of other explanations are particularly important. Milne (1987) discusses a number of threats to the internal validity of evaluation studies and the difficulties of teasing out the effects of a programme from other factors affecting the client's well-being. The classic design for the elimination of the influence of intervening variables in causal analysis of outcome is the experiment. Newcombe (1988) suggests that the randomized controlled trial (RCT) be adopted as the norm in all studies of mental health care but, as Milne points out, while this is a relatively straightforward matter in a laboratory it is unattainable as an ideal in mental health services.

Hafner and an der Heiden (1989*b*) suggest that there are three prerequisites for a sensible evaluation of any type of care programme:

- A standardized intervention programme with the active components identified. If for some reason this is not possible then the treatment programme must be reproducible by describing all its active component parts.
- The active components of the programme must be administered when indicated.

- Differences in outcome must not be accounted for by other factors, for example readmission rates are not influenced solely by the patient's mental state but by financial resources and bed availability.

A full description of experimental, quasi-experimental and naturalistic approaches to mental health service evaluation in relation to causal analyses of effectiveness is provided by Hafner and an der Heiden in *Evaluating Effectiveness and Cost of Community Care for Schizophrenic Patients* (1991). The choice of research design will depend on a number of factors including practical considerations, the objectives requiring evaluation and the selection of appropriate outcome measures. In addition to cost effectiveness, clinical efficacy and quantitative data relating to service use, there are a number of other outcome measures which are increasingly important in evaluating the impact of community mental health services. Quality of life has become one such variable and measures for it are regarded as central to any evaluation of the impact of community mental health care.

Quality of life

Prior (1993) suggests that with the advent of community psychiatry a new range of outcome measures has emerged, including independence, social support and quality of life. Quality of life has become one of the explicit goals for community mental health care. In a review of the literature Goodinson and Singleton (1989) suggest that the concept is discussed in two major contexts: first in the context of treatment selection and therapeutic approaches, and second to develop a new concept, that of the quality adjusted life years (QALY) (Kind *et al.* 1982). Referring to the latter context, QALY has been developed from an economic perspective to provide a basis for allocating resources to those treatments judged to be most effective and those individuals who have the potential to maximize benefit, i.e. the number of quality adjusted life years. Gudex and Kind (1990) suggest that the ability to adjust for quality of life is an important advance which allows comparisons to be made between specific forms of intervention and between competing programmes. QALYs are a powerful addition to the range of evaluative techniques for use in assessing the impact of health care. However, QALYs have been criticized from a number of perspectives and these arguments are summarized in Mooney (1992). Despite their limitations in the current economic climate it seems likely that interest in their ability and application to mental health care will increase. A study by Wilkinson *et al.* (1992) in community care for the mentally ill suggests that the QALYs methodology may require the adoption of multidimensional measures of health to fulfil its role in comparing medical and mental health programmes.

In relation to treatment selection and therapeutic approaches Goodinson and Singleton (1989) suggest that early studies of quality of life most commonly used to evaluate treatment were rates of cure, survival response and duration of response. Realization that many treatments have the potential to cause unpleasant side effects brought into question survival in terms of the personal cost of receiving these and their effect on a person's quality of life. However, problems of measurement and lack of consensus of definition prevented widespread assessment in many evaluative studies. Barry *et al.* (1993) propose that quality of life is defined as referring to a sense of well-being and satisfaction experienced by people under their current life conditions. Similarly Young and Longman (1983) define quality of life as the degree of satisfaction with perceived present life circumstances.

Quality of life is usually accepted as adequacy of material circumstances and people's feelings about these. However, as McDowell and Newell (1987) point out, changing social circumstances tend to bring about changes in definitions and there has been a clear evolution in definitions of quality of life, from viewing it in material terms of income, career success and possessions, towards emphasizing spiritual rewards such as satisfaction, personal development and subjective well-being. Current methods of obtaining judgments of quality of life tend to rely on self-report measures of both objective and subjective indicators of well-being.

Barry *et al.* (1993) suggest that the objective of improved quality of life is of particular relevance for those clients who experience long-term chronic mental health problems. They argue that the extent to which mental health services can have a positive impact on the lifestyle of the long-term clients and maximize their quality of life is an important test for any new service. A multidimensional construct such as quality of life is a good outcome measure against which to evaluate the success of a programme of care, offering a useful means of incorporating the client's perspective into the evaluation process. Renshaw (1985) identifies seven components of quality of life which are relevant in evaluating the benefits of care for the long-term mentally ill. These are symptoms, behaviour and social functioning; morale and satisfaction; engagement in activity; social contracts, friends and outings, significant events and personal presentation. Measuring quality of life usually fall into two main categories (Kind 1990). First, rather than measuring quality of life directly, an indicator which seems closely linked to it is used as a measure. For example, Feinstein *et al.* (1986), in a review of the literature, found 43 widely used indices that focus in whole or in part on activities of daily living. Social support, social functioning and measures of psychological well-being are also used as indicators of quality of life. Kind (1990) is critical of such measurements since the linkage between these variables and quality of life is often a matter of conjecture.

The second approach to the measure of quality of life uses instruments specifically developed for this purpose. These have either been developed as generic measures or for a particular client group, for example Spitzer *et al.*'s (1981) quality of life index for patients with cancer. A number of quality of life instruments have now been developed for use with the long-term mentally ill, for example, the 'satisfaction with life domains scale' (Baker and Integliata 1982) and the 'quality of life interview' (Lehman 1988).

In a longitudinal study, Barry *et al.* used a wide range of evaluation measures to determine quality of life in a group of 62 patients who were being discharged from long-term care and resettled in the community. Included were Lehman's 'quality of life interview' which was adapted for use with the present subjects. A number of open-ended questions were added to explore individual perceptions of significant life events and experiences, aspirations and attitude to discharge. In addition to this a list of questions concerning the objective indicators of life quality for each of the residents was also completed by a member of the care staff. In their conclusion they confirm that the quality of life schedule used in their study provided valuable information on the life situation and subjective perceptions of patients whose views may be rarely represented in the care planning process. They again raise the issue of imposing an external value system on subjects, ignoring their own values and preferences. To prevent this from happening they suggest the use of more exploratory methods of data collection, rather than relying solely on satisfaction ratings to tap subjective perceptions and feelings. One approach would be the use of qualitative approaches in conjunction with structured interview schedules.

Users' views

The last few years has seen a gradual increase in the interest in obtaining the views of patients using mental health services, to the extent that no decent evaluation study would fail to include the experiences and perceptions of service users. However, Rogers *et al.* (1993), citing a review on patient satisfaction literature by Hall and Dorrian (1988), argue that obtaining the views and levels of satisfaction from psychiatric patients has seriously lagged behind other client groups. This has resulted mostly from the widely held belief that psychiatric patients are incapable of providing a rational and valid opinion about the services they are receiving. Rogers *et al.* suggest that this view is shared by mental health research funding bodies. To highlight this point they give the example of the Medical Research Council who, in their recommendations regarding future research, placed evaluation of services to patients in eighth position out of ten priorities and did not make any mention of user evaluation of services.

Dissatisfaction with mental health services has given rise to a user movement which challenges the paternalistic style of the NHS in which patients were previously passive recipients of care complying with prescribed treatment. Today mental health service users are demanding information about their diagnoses, treatment and care. They are also requiring information about alternative treatments in order that they can make informed choices. Users want to maintain as much control over their lives as possible by being treated as equal partners. They want to have influence over decisions affecting them and whenever possible contribute to service planning and evaluation.

Many of these rights and standards are embodied in the Patient's Charter (DoH 1991) which seeks to make services more patient-orientated and more responsive. Seeking users' views is, therefore, essential if services are to be 'user-friendly'. There are many different methods which can be used to obtain users' 'views including the use of advocacy services, community health councils, user groups, focus groups, suggestion boxes, informal and formal interviews, telephone follow-up and complaints. The most popular way of recording users' views is through written user surveys. Popularly known as patient satisfaction surveys. Fitzpatrick (1992) suggests that there are three reasons besides external pressures from government why health professionals should include satisfaction as a measurement. First, many evaluation studies now include user satisfaction as an outcome measure, e.g. Thomas *et al.* (1990).

Second, patient satisfaction is useful in assessing consultations and patterns of communication, particularly information giving, and including the user in decisions about their care. Third, user feedback can be used systematically to make choices regarding different ways of organizing or providing health care, for example, arranging to see psychiatrists or community psychiatric nurses at health centres as opposed to traditional out-patient departments.

Assessing users' satisfaction with the service they receive is assuming greater importance and a wealth of information has developed in this area, including methodological challenges. A number of reviews on this subject have been carried out, for example, Fitzpatrick (1992). Frequency in the use of satisfaction surveys has led many service evaluators to use standard rating scales based on aspects of care defined and regarded as relevant by professionals. However, such use has been severely criticized. For example, Carr-Hill *et al.* (1989) argue that responses other than those stated are restricted, the uni-dimensionality of the concept is assumed and also there is a risk of response-set bias. Hansson *et al.* (1993) suggests that most studies have used interviews or questionnaires developed by professionals that contain characteristics and variables of attitude and satisfaction which reflect the service provider and staff conception of what patients should base their evaluations on. This is in spite of all the research which shows differences between staff and perception of the importance of different treatment characteristics.

To evaluate services truly from a user perspective it is necessary to see the world from the user's point of view. Hansson *et al.* (1993) adopted a qualitative methodology to determine a user's perspective about service provision. Although their work relates to in-patient care, the methodology could just as easily be applied to users receiving community care. Barham and Hayward (1991) suggest that, in order to capture users' experience, a shift in research style is required from the quantitative to the qualitative in which the profession of expertise cedes to a more collaborative way of working with the subjects of research. In their own work they used semi-structured interviews with 24 patients who had been discharged from psychiatric hospitals, to explore their experiences of trying to live outside hospital. Such an approach, they argue, teaches us something about the difficulties we have put in the way of people with mental illness and the cause of their demoralization and shows us how we might think and act more helpfully.

Rogers *et al.* (1993) suggest that there needs to be more of an attempt to involve users themselves in research. Health and social services involved in evaluation research need to take into account a user perspective, perhaps by employing researchers who have been on the receiving end of psychiatry to do field work. At the very least, considering that all mental health services have access to clients, there is no reason why a user perspective could not be built into all mental health research, particularly when evaluating service provision. Donabedian (1987) suggests that users are indispensable sources of information in judging the quality of care. It is generally accepted that future evaluations of community services will involve more user input. In preparation for this some services are beginning to run training seminars for users who wish to have more say in mental health policy and service provision. Norsigien (1989) suggests that better informed users can ask more relevant questions and can help care-givers be more effective.

Quality of care

Recent years have seen an increasing interest in providing a quality health service. The two government White Papers *Working for Patients* and *Caring for People* have led to demands for NHS staff to improve the quality of their services to users and generally raise the standards of care provision overall. However, quality has many interpretations and is a difficult concept to define. Donabedian (1988) defines quality as the ability to achieve desirable objectives using legitimate means. The British Standard 4778 (1987) defines quality as: 'The totality of features and characteristics of a product or service that bear on its ability to satisfy stated or implied needs'.

In the USA the Joint Commission on Accreditation of Healthcare Organizations identify accessibility, appropriateness, continuity, effectiveness, efficacy, efficiency, incorporation of the patient perspective, safety and timeliness as necessary components of quality care. These are outlined in Table 17.1.

Many initiatives have been introduced within community mental health services to bring about quality improvement. These include standard setting, measuring performance and changing practice and procedures. Reviews of such activities are provided by Carr-Hill and Dailey (1990) and Shaw (1993). While it is clear that there are a wide range of quality initiatives taking place, these are often uncoordinated and do not form part of any quality strategy or overall programme. Without such a strategy or programme it is difficult to demonstrate quality assurance activities leading to actual improvement in the quality of care, since quality assurance programmes are aimed at improv-

Table 17.1 The Joint Commission on Accreditation of Healthcare Organizations: components of quality care

Components of quality that indicators may assess
1 *Accessibility of care*: the ease with which patients can obtain the care they need when they need it.
2 *Appropriateness of care*: the degree to which the correct care is provided, given the current state of the art.
3 *Continuity of care*: the degree to which the care needed by patients is coordinated among the practitioners and across organizations and time.
4 *Effectiveness of care*: the degree to which care is provided in the correct manner, given the current state of the art.
5 *Efficacy of care*: the degree to which service has the potential to meet the need for which it is used.
6 *Efficiency of care*: the degree to which the care received has the desired effect, with a minimum of effort, expense or waste.
7 *Patient perspective issues*: the degree to which patients and their families are involved in the decision-making processes in matters pertaining to health, and the degree to which they are satisfied with patient care.
8 *Safety of the care environment*: the degree to which the environment is free from hazard or danger.
9 *Timeliness of care*: the degree to which care is provided to patients when it is needed.

ing deficiencies in care through a feedback loop which often involves educating service providers. Wells and Brook (1988) suggest that, unfortunately, there is little empirical data to guide mental health service providers in their selection of a quality assurance programme. In a literature review they only found one study that evaluated the effectiveness of quality assurance activities using a control group and a prospective design (Sinclair and Frankel 1982). These authors evaluated the process of care of community mental health treatment teams that either had or did not have a quality assurance programme. The programme involved peer review and the education of clinical supervisors and case workers in delivering high-quality care. One year after implementing the programme significant improvements were found in the process of care for the experimental groups but not the control groups. Wells and Brook (1988) suggest that this study is consistent with other studies that report positive effects of quality assurance programmes in community mental health services where peer review, clinical supervision and continuing education is combined in a supportive professional environment.

There are a few British studies which have demonstrated the impact of quality assurance on the improvement of clinical practice and patient care. One of the rare exceptions is the work of Perkins *et al.* (1992) who describe how the process of quality assurance and audit have been effective in changing care practices on a rehabilitation unit. The system not only offers criteria by which to assess performance in a long-term and rehabilitation setting, but also provides a method for evaluating the multidisciplinary team's performance.

Wells and Brook (1988) suggest that the hallmark of evaluations of the quality of care is the establishment of standards of care. A standard is a desired and achievable level (or range) of performance corresponding to a criterion against which actual performance is compared. In mental health services, standards of practice and instruments for objectively measuring practice have been slow to develop. Wells and Brook suggest that disagreement over the definition of mental health problems and treatments and concerns about confidentiality have made it difficult to establish standards of care for mental health care services. They propose that it should be a high priority of all professional groups to develop and empirically test standards for specific conditions including diagnostic groups or client problems.

Work is well under way in developing standards particularly in nursing. For example, the Bethlem Royal Hospital and the Maudsley Hospital have developed eleven key mental health nursing standards based on the dynamic standard setting system (DySSSy) using Donabedian's interrelated concepts of structure process and outcome (Kitson 1988). The standards and criteria provide a tool to measure and evaluate the quality of nursing care. whilst uni-professional standard setting will continue to be important, community mental health services depend on the combined work of a number of professionals. Standard setting therefore needs to reflect this approach. The development of clinical standards and clinical protocols for diagnosis, care and treatment has recently begun to take place. The trend towards multidisciplinary teams means that quality of care can be audited by comparing the actual delivery of the service against those standards set by all the professionals concerned.

A coordinated approach

The numerous aspects to be considered and included in any evaluation programme matched to the purpose of the study demonstrates the importance
of a coordinated and comprehensive approach. A number of frameworks
and methods for evaluating community mental health services have now
evolved. For example, Raeburn and Seymour (1977) suggest a systems
approach to planning and evaluating community care. The systems model is
particularly useful for the inclusion of the three classic components of quality care formulated by Donabedian (1966, 1969, 1980) in his review of the
evaluation of medical care. These are structure, process and outcome.

Structure refers to support facilities. Included in this are organizational
arrangements, financial resources, and personnel and administrative procedures which underpin the delivery of the service. Staffing levels, the availability of facilities and environmental factors are also included. Shaw (1992)
suggests that structural details are far removed from the outcome of treatment and are at best a very indirect measure. However, usually resources
can be easily measured and information is accessible. Due to this conve-
nience dependence on measuring structural details has developed but it
should not be assumed that quality environments and facilities always equate
with good care.

Process refers to the transactions between health care staff and patients
during episodes of care. Although this is probably the most difficult approach
to carry out it is the most telling in judging whether or not good care is being
carried out (Donabedian 1969). In measuring process, a value judgment by
clinical experts is required. It is often differences of opinion which make this
approach less objective than the others.

Outcomes according to Donabedian means what is achieved, i.e. an
improvement in health status, attitudes, knowledge or behaviour conducive
to future health. As previously discussed outcome measurement in mental
health is in its infancy. However, outcome research is gaining in momentum,
for example Shapiro (1989).

Smeltzer (1992) identifies ten steps in the evaluation process:

Step 1   State the goal or purpose of the evaluation study.
Step 2   Describe the information that is needed to achieve the stated goal.
Step 3   Identify available information to answer the questions formulated
           in Step 2.
Step 4   Describe the methodology to collect the information
Step 5   Select or construct the information-gathering data instrument.
Step 6   Operationalize the evaluation plan.
Step 7   Record and analyse the information collected.
Step 8   Formulate value judgments after the data analysis.
Step 9   Make decisions concerning future programme development.
Step 10 Summarize and report the evaluation results.

McCollam and White (1993) provide a guide on evaluation methods and the
practical issues to be considered when carrying out evaluation in mental health
care. Their sequence of the different stages involved is shown in
Fig. 17.1. McCollam and White emphasize that the stages do not necessaily
follow on in a linear fashion; for example, applying the results and dissemi-

nation can take place simultaneously. The important consideration is the purpose of the evaluation. The authors suggest that it is no good just collecting information and then deciding what to do with it. The key to good evaluation is to set out with a clear purpose.

In the United States the Evaluation Society (Rossi 1982) has developed standards for programme evaluation for the various models. These standards consist of six components:

- formulation and negotiation
- structure and design
- data collection and preparation
- data analysis and interpretation
- communication and disclosure
- utilization.

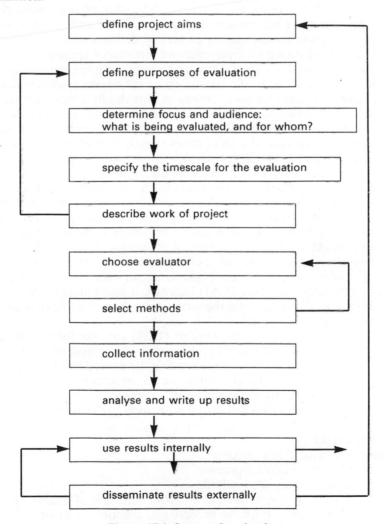

Figure 17.1 Stages of evaluation

Principles of evaluation

Evaluation, research and audit

Confusion often exists over the similarities and differences between evaluation, research and audit. Similarities between evaluation and research include their systematic processes, their need for resources and support to undertake the activities and their purpose in seeking to improve health care. However, so far the direct relationship between much scientific investigation and its value in improving health care has been difficult to identify since many academic pursuits seem to have little relevance to clinical practice. Moreover, when research has major relevance there is often a gap between potential and actual use of findings.

Differences between evaluation, audit and research include the goals of each. The purpose of evaluation is to provide feedback about a service or programme in order to make decisions about the allocation of resources, to plan services and make improvements. Similarly, audit aims to analyse systematically and critically the quality of service delivery in terms of use of resources and the outcomes for patients and introduces appropriate change in response to that analysis. Health service managers require answers quickly and are therefore likely to be the consumers of evaluation studies and audit. Research, however, takes longer to complete. It is chiefly concerned with the generation of new knowledge for the purpose of refining relevant theories. Research is designed to ensure that it can be replicated and that its results are able to be generalized. The chief characteristic of evaluation is its focus on making a judgment. The World Health Organization defines evaluation as 'the systematic and scientific process of determining the extent to which an action or set of actions was successful in the achievement of predetermined objectives' (Shaw 1992). Evaluation involves judging the worthwhileness of some activity. This element of judgment is certainly consistent with the general usage of the term and should obviously serve as a foundation for assessing whether an activity is indeed evaluative in nature. Evaluation is used to determine the effectiveness, efficiency and quality of a specific programme. The objectives of the programme are an essential prerequisite to any evaluation study. As Milne (1987) suggests, it is meaningless to ask the basic evaluative question (e.g. did the programme work?) without some predetermined objective in mind.

The publication of *Working for Patients* (1989) saw the formal introduction of clinical audit. Clinical audit is defined as the systematic and critical analysis of the quality of clinical care, including the procedures used for diagnosis, treatment and care, the associated use of resources and the resulting outcome and quality of life for the patient.

The fundamental principles associated with audit are that it should (DoH 1993*a*):

- be professionally led
- be seen as an educational process
- form part of routine clinical practice
- be based on the setting of standards
- generate results that can be used to improve outcome of quality of care
- involve management in both the process and outcome of audit
- be confidential at the individual/clinician level
- be informed by the views of patients/clients.

Clinical audit provides opportunities for service evaluation to be carried out by clinical staff directly involved in providing care. Firth-Cozens (1993) suggests that audit is specific and local to particular patient groups. Shaw (1992) suggests that since most methods of clinical audit rely heavily on the assumption that good care produces good outcomes, audit and evaluation are thus complementary. Similarly, only by using objective research methods can specified patterns of clinical management be related to their effect on clinical outcome.

Although there is a good track record of health service research in the UK, most of this has been scientifically driven and despite being highly productive, inevitably the effort has placed emphasis on areas of high scientific interest to the neglect of less scientifically attractive yet important problems facing the health service (DoH 1993c). There is a less enviable history of collaboration between researchers and managers in the process of shaping the research agenda. It is important to acknowledge that the two groups may have different interests and objectives. For example, researchers may need to undertake studies that ensure reproducibility and academic credibility in order to advance academic careers. This may limit the type of research in which they are prepared to become involved. Managers on the other hand, may need quick answers to pressing problems. The Department of Health's research and development strategy is intended to cut across these divides and places collective responsibility on academic researchers, clinicians, managers and other health service staff to maximize the contribution of research and development to the nation's health and quality of life, as well as to the efficient and effective use of public funds. The research community has a new opportunity to work closely with NHS managers and clinicians to identify the obstacles caused by lack of information and to identify existing knowledge or new research which can directly help the service (DoH 1993c).

In the same ways as audit and evaluation are complementary, evaluation and research are often integrated into one activity. This consists of the application of the principles of research to the process of evaluation. Many writers have been at pains to identify the distinctions between evaluation and research and more recently those of audit. Combining the work of Popham (1975) and Suchman (1967), Milne identifies eleven distinctions between basic and evaluative research, as shown in Table 17.2 (Milne 1987).

Lang (1982) suggests that although the development of standardized instruments for use in audit exercises and selected controlled studies should be viewed as relevant research activity, they are not usually perceived as rigid highly controlled studies. Rather these activities are part of routine organizational and professional functions. In nursing particularly, most studies are categorized either as evaluation or research with little integration of the two processes. Lang suggests that the challenge facing nursing is to develop an interrelationship between quality, audit and the domain of research as well as integrating the processes of evaluation and research. This type of integration is now being encouraged, through the contracting process between providers and purchasers where it is essential to provide reliable information about audit procedures designed to evaluate service quality, and research results and activities which must be integrated in daily practice. The role of the purchaser in supporting the evolution of clinical audit is set

Table 17.2 Distinction between basic and evaluative research (after Milne 1987)

Factor	Basic research	'Evaluative' research
1 Purpose of research	To build theories and improve understanding	To make decisions and improve programmes
2 Applicability of findings	Widely applicable	Results only directly relevant to same programme and setting
3 Value of research	To establish 'truth'	To improve worth of programme
4 Measurement	Standardized instruments; rigorous control; scientific standards essential (e.g randomization)	Ragbag of measuring tools; control very difficult to achieve; scientific standards desirable
5 Topics	Anything	Socially important phenomena
6 Judgment	Eschewed	Integral
7 Research consumers	Secondary, not identified	Primary
8 Politics	An improper consideration	A necessary and important consideration
9 Replicability	Important hallmark	Neither important nor possible
10 Setting	Not treated as significant: highly controlled	Essential aspect; control very limited
11 Publication	Major academic goal of research	Uncommon and secondary

out in Annex B of EL(93)34. This shows the legitimate role of purchaser in negotiating topics for audit.

Purchasing and providing mental health care

Under new legislation the key means of delivering community mental health services will be through the development of effective purchasing. Purchasers and providers are encouraged to develop strategies for a five-year period and contracts are expected to reflect longer-term arrangements as well as providing flexibility to meet shorter-term needs. The contracting arrangements between purchasers and providers of community mental health care have identified the need for more and better information. Longer-term strategies particularly need to be underpinned by information about good practice and evidence of the effectiveness of different treatment programmes and interventions. The inclusion of research-based information into purchase and provider contracts will ensure that these needs are met, that scarce resources are used efficiently and that achievable health targets are set.

Similarly audit results are expected to influence the purchasing process. At present contracts specify quality requirements, the mechanisms by which standards are to be monitored and the remedies available if a provider fails to meet the terms of the contract. However, this is a prescriptive approach by purchasers and a reactive process for providers. In future providers need to be much more proactive. They need to negotiate with purchasers areas for improvement and develop rolling programmes for developments in service provision and quality initiatives.

The government identifies the seven hallmarks of successful purchasing as:

- a strategic approach
- well informed decision-making
- responsiveness to local people
- local alliances
- working closely with providers
- improving quality and value for money
- organizational fitness for purchasing.

The implementation of many of these will depend on good evaluation data.

Conclusion

Evaluation is a goal that requires commitment, objectivity, critical and analytical abilities, a systematic approach, creativity and above all an openness to change. Evaluation of community mental health services has developed since the mid-1980s as a result of government policy initiatives, from a professional concern with accountability, from a desire to improve standards of service delivery and from users who want to be more informed, consulted and involved in decision-making and planning about their treatment and care. This is not an isolated endeavour but must be an integral part of health care delivery. This chapter has examined the principles upon which evaluation studies have so far been developed in pursuit of this goal. These principles are not absolutes but rather contemporary requirements which are needed in enhancing evaluations of community mental health services, given the state of current knowledge.

Community mental health care is provided by a complex delivery system involving many agencies. Quality evaluation, therefore, depends on collaboration amongst these agencies and among clinicians, economists, statisticians and administrative agencies. The process of evaluation involves deciding what to evaluate and carrying out the evaluation. The methodology chosen should be appropriate to the question(s) under review. The purpose of the evaluation and its context should determine the most suitable methods. In addition to determining technical considerations, there will be resource implications and it is important that economic appraisal is included at the planning stage of an evaluation. Evaluating the efficiency and effectiveness of a mental health service is problematic if that very process distracts staff from their work or prevents patients from receiving the care they require. Finally, evaluation involves using the information acquired. Evaluation should ultimately lead to the improvement of services. Evaluation will provide feedback on performance and aid decision-making about future developments of a service. Evaluation will help prioritize expenditure and promote changes that will improve the quality of patient care. As Finkelman (1992) suggests, the delivery of health care without an evaluation system is frightening to imagine.

References

Baker F and Integliata J (1982). Quality of life in the evaluation of community support systems. *Evaluation and Programme Planning*, **5**, 69–79.

Barham P and Hayward R (1991). *From the Mental Patient to the Person*. Routledge, London.

Barry M M, Crosby C and Bogg J (1993). Methodological issues in evaluating the quality of life of long-stay psychiatric patients. *Journal of Mental Health* **2**, 43–56.

Bartlett W and Le Grand J (1993). The theory of quasi-markets. *Quasi-Markets and Social Policy* (eds. J Le Grand and W Bartlett). Macmillan, London.

Bottomley V (1993). Measuring the quality of care. *Guardian*, Wednesday, 16 June 1993.

Bowling A (1990). *Measuring Health: A Review of Quality of Life Measurement Scales*. Open University Press, Milton Keynes.

Carr-Hill R, McIver S and Dixon P (1989). *The NHS and its Customs*. Centre for Health Economics, University of York.

Carr-Hill R and Dailey G (1990). Question of quality. *The Health Service Journal*, 2 August, 1146–1147.

Cochrane A L (1972). *Effectiveness and Efficiency: Random Reflections on Health Services*. Nuffield Provincial Hospitals Trust, London.

Department of Health (1989). *Caring for People: Community Care in the Next Decade and Beyond*. HMSO, London.

Department of Health (1989). *Working for Patients*. Medical Audit Working Paper no. 6. HMSO, London.

Department of Health (1990). *NHS and Community Care Act*. HMSO, London.

Department of Health (1993a). *Clinical Audit: Meeting and Improving Standards in Health Care*. NHS Management, London.

Department of Health (1993b). *The Health of the Nation: Key Area Handbook Mental Illness*. HMSO, London.

Department of Health (1993c). *Research for Health*. HMSO, London.

Doll R (1973). Monitoring the National Health Service. *Proceedings of the Royal Society of Medicine*, **66**, 729–740.

Donabedian A (1966). Evaluating the quality of medical care. *Millbank Memorial Federation of Quality*, **44**, 166–208.

Donabedian A (1969). *A Guide to Medical Care Administration, Medical Care Appraisal*. American Public Health Association, New York.

Donabedian A (1980). *Explorations in Quality Assessment and Monitoring: The Definition of Quality and Approaches to its Assessment*. Health Administration Press, Ann Arbor, Mich.

Donabedian A (1987). Commentary on some studies of the quality of care. *Health Care Financing Review* (annual supplement), 75–85.

Donabedian A (1988). The quality of care. *Journal of the American Medical Association*, **260**, 1743–1748.

Drummond M F (1990). *Principles of Economic Appraisal in Health Care*. Oxford Medical Publications, Oxford.

Feinstein A R, Joseph B R and Wells C K (1986). Scientific and clinical problems in indexes of functional disability. *Annals of International Medicine*, **105**, 413–420.

Finkelman A W (1992). *Quality Assurance for Psychiatric Nursing.* Aspen, Md.

Firth-Cozens J (1993). *Audit in Mental Health Services.* Lawrence Erlbaum Associates, Hove.

Fitzpatrick R (1992). Surveys of patient satisfaction: I – important general considerations. In *Audit in Action* (ed. R Smith), British Medical Journal, London.

Frank R G and Manning W G (1992). *Economics and Mental Health,* Johns Hopkins University Press, Baltimore, Md.

Goldberg D (1991). Cost-effectiveness studies in the treatment of schizophrenia: a review. *Schizophrenia Bulletin,* **17** (3), 453–460.

Goodinson S M and Singleton J (1989). Quality of life: a critical review of current concepts, measures and their clinical implications. *International Journal of Nursing Studies,* **26** (4), 327–341.

Gudex C and Kind P (1990). *The QALY Tool Kit.* Discussion Paper 38, Centre for Health Economics: University of York.

Hafner H (1987). Do we still need beds for psychiatric patients? *Acta Psychiatrica Scandinavica,* **75**, 113–126.

Hafner H and an der Heiden W (1989). Evaluation of care for the disabled mentally ill: Theoretical issues. *European Archives of Psychiatry and Neurological Sciences,* **238**, 179–184.

Hafner H and an der Heiden W (1991). Evaluating effectiveness and cost of community care for schizophrenic patients. *Schizophrenia Bulletin,* **17**, 441–451.

Hall J and Dornan M (1988). What patients like about their medical care and how often they are asked: A Meta-Analysis of the Satisfaction Literature. *Social Science and Medicine,* **27**, 935–939.

Hansson L, Bjorkman T and Berglund I (1993). What is important in psychiatric inpatient care? Quality of care from the patient's perspective. *Quality Assurance in Health Care,* **5** (1) 41–47.

Hassall C (1991). The Worcester Psychiatric Case Register In *The Closure of Mental Hospitals* (eds. P Hall and I F Brockington). Gaskell, London.

Karluk M and Astrachan B (1993). Economics and mental health care. *Current Opinion in Psychiatry,* **6** (2), 263–268.

Kind P, Rosser R and Williams A (1982). Valuation of quality of life: some psychometric evidence. In *The Value of Life and Strategy* (ed. M W Jones-Lee). Elsevier, Amsterdam.

Kind P (1990). *The Design and Construction of Quality of Life Measures.* Discussion Paper 43, Centre for Health Economics, University of York.

Kitson A (1988). Raising the standards ... providing care of a consistently high standard. Dynamic Standard Setting System. *Nursing Times,* **84**, 28–32.

Knapp M (1990). Economic barriers to innovation in mental health care: community care in the United Kingdom. In *Mental Health Care Delivery* (eds. I Marks and R Scott). Cambridge University Press, Cambridge.

Knapp M, Beecham J, Anderson J, Dayson D, Leff J, Margolius O, O'Driscoll C and Willis W (1990). The TAPS Project predicting the community costs of closing psychiatric hospitals. *British Journal of Psychiatry,* **157**, 661–670.

Lang N M (1982). Introduction: trends and issues in nursing quality assurance. *Quality Review Bulletin,* **Spring**, 2.

Lavender A (1987). Improving the quality of care on psychiatric hospital rehabilitation wards: a controlled evaluation. *British Journal of Psychiatry,* **150**, 476–481.

Lehman A F (1988). A quality of life interview for the chronically mentally ill. *Evaluation and Programme Planning,* **11**, 51–62.

Lehman A F. Ward N C and Lynn L S (1982). Chronic mental patients: The quality of life issue. *American Journal of Psychiatry,* **139**, 1271–1276.

McCollam A and White J (1993). *Building on Experience: Evaluation and Mental Health Projects.* Scottish Association for Mental Health, Edinburgh.

McDowell I and Newell C (1987). *Measuring Health: A Guide to Rating Scales and*

Questionnaires. Oxford University Press, New York.

McGuire A, Henderson J and Mooney G (1992). *The Economics of Health Care*, Routledge, London.

Milne D (ed.) (1987). *Evaluating Mental Health Practice: Methods and Applications*. Croom Helm, London

Mooney G H (1992). *Economics Medicine and Health Care*. Harvester Wheatsheaf, London, 2nd edn.

Mooney G H, Russell M and Weir R D (1986). *Choices for Health Care: A Practical Introduction to the Economics of Health Provision*. Macmillan, London.

Muijen M, Marks I, Connolly J and Audini B (1992). The 3 months' outcome of the Daily Living Program: A randomised controlled study evaluating home care versus hospital care. *British Medical Journal*, **304**, 749–754.

Newcombe R G (1988). Evaluation of treatment effectiveness in psychiatric research. *British Journal of Psychiatry*, **152**, 696–697.

Norsigian J (1989). Informed consumers are key. *Health Management Quarterly*, **11** (4), 22–23.

O'Donnell O, Maynard A and Wright K (1992). Evaluating mental health care: the role of economics. *Journal of Mental Health*, **1**, 39–51.

Perkins R, Hollyman J and Serracino M (1992). Do we measure up? The development of multidisciplinary quality assurance and audit systems in a psychiatric rehabilitation setting. *Health Trends*, **14** (2), 56–59.

Pocock S J (1987). *Clinical Trials: A Practical Approach*. John Wiley, Chichester.

Popham W J (1975). *Education Evaluation*. Prentice-Hall, Englewood Cliffs, N.J.

Prior L (1993). *The Social Organisation of Mental Illness*. Sage Publications, London.

Raeburn J M and Seymour F W (1977). Planning and evaluating community health and related projects; a systems approach. *New Zealand Medical Journal*, **86**, 188–190.

Renshaw J, Hampson R, Thomason C, Darton R, Judge K and Knapp M (1988). *Care in the Community: The First Steps*. Gower, Aldershot.

Rogers A, Pilgrim D and Lacey R (1993). *Experiencing Psychiatry: Users' Views of Services*. Macmillan in association with MIND Publications, London.

Rossi P H and Freeman H E (1985). *Evaluation: a systematic approach*. Sage, Beverly Hills, CA, 3rd edn.

Shapiro D A (1989). Outcome research in behavioural and mental health research. In *A Handbook of Skills and Methods* (eds. G Parry and A R Rodriguez). Lawrence Erlbaum Associates Publishers, Hove.

Sinclair C and Frankel M (1982).The effect of quality assurance activities on the quality of mental health services. *Quality Review Bulletin*, **8** (7), 7–15.

Shaw C D (1992). The background. In *Audit in Action* (ed. R Smith). British Medical Journal, London.

Shaw C D (1993). Quality assurance in the United Kingdom. *Quality Assurance in Health Care*, **5** (2), 107–118.

Shepherd G (1989). Research in service planning and evaluation. In *Behavioural and Mental Health Research: A Handbook of Skills and Methods* (eds. G Parry and F N Watts). Lawrence Erlbaum Associates, Hove.

Shepherd G (1988). Evaluation and service planning. In *Community Care in Practice: Services for the Continuing Care Client* (eds. A Lavender and F Holloway). Wiley, Chichester.

Smeltzer C H (1992). Evaluating quality assurance program effectiveness. In *Improving Quality: A Guide to Effective Programs* (ed. C G Meisenheimer). Aspen, Md.

Spitzer W O (1987). State of science 1986: Quality of life and functional status as target variables for research. *Journal of Chronic Diseases*, **40**, 465–471.

Spitzer W O, Dobson A J, Hall J, Chesterman E and Levi J (1981). Measuring the quality of life of cancer patients. *Journal of Chronic Diseases*, **34**, 585–597.

St Leger A S, Schneiden H and Walsworth-Bell J P (1992). *Evaluating Health Service Effectiveness*. Open University Press, Milton Keynes.

Strathdee G and Thornicroft G (1992). Community sectors for needs-led mental health services. In *Measuring Mental Health Needs* (eds. G Thornicroft, C R Brewin and J Wing). Gaskell, Royal College of Psychiatrists, London.

Stricker G and Rodriguez A R (1988). *Handbook of Quality Assurance in Mental Health*. Plenum Press, New York.

Sturt E, Wykes T and Creer C (1982). Demographic, social and clinical characteristics of the sample: In *Long-term Community Care: Experience in a London Borough* (ed. J K Wing). Psychological Monograph Supplement 2, Cambridge University Press, Cambridge.

Suchman E A (1967). *Evaluative Research*. Russell Sage, New York.

Thomas B, Muijen M F and Brooking J I (1991). Community psychiatry: reactions to a new service. *Nursing*, **9**, 9–11.

Weiss C H (1972). *Evaluation Research*. Prentice-Hall, Englewood Cliffs, N.J.

Wells K and Brook R H (1988). Historical trends in quality assurance for mental health services. In *Handbook of Quality Assurance in Mental Health* (eds. G Stricker and A R Rodriguez). Plenum Press, New York.

Wilkinson G, Williams B, Krekorian H, McLees S and Falloon I (1992). QALYs in mental health: a case study. *Psychological Medicine*, **22**, 725–731.

Wing J K and Hasiley A (1972). *Evaluating, a Community Service. The Camberwell Register 1964–1971*. Oxford University Press, London.

Wooff K, Freeman H L and Fryers T (1983). Psychiatric service use in Salford: a comparison of point-prevalence ratios, 1968 and 1978. *British Journal of Psychiatry*, **142**, 588–597.

Young K J and Longman A J (1983). Quality of life and persons with melanoma: a pilot study. *Cancer Nursing*, **6**, 219–225.

18 Evaluating community services

S. Ramon

The objectives and desirability of evaluating community services seem to be straightforward, providing answers to the following questions:

- Are services delivering what they have set out to deliver? If not, why not?
- Is the service provided useful in terms of leading to an improvement in clients' lives?
- Is the service delivered in a way which meets clients' and carers' needs and their wishes?
- Is the service delivered in a way which is respectful of clients, including members of ethnic minorities and women?
- Is the service effective in the way it is run and in the use made of resources? How does it compare in cost effectiveness with other services?
- What are the main gaps in the services on offer?

However, those who have attempted an evaluation of community services have quickly become aware of the complexity of the exercise, and its potentially conflictual nature.

In part, both the complexity and the conflictual nature relate to the large number of stakeholders interested in evaluation. Stakeholders include clients and carers, service providers, service purchasers, local and central government, professional associations and the general public.

The high visibility of community services in comparison with the lower visibility of psychiatric hospitals, the relative newness of their existence and the controversy which has accompanied their establishment add an edge of tension to any such evaluation. Thus a major additional objective is that of comparison with non-community-based services, and of services before and after a restructuring has taken place.

Although service evaluation has been around for a long time, it is still perceived as an external imposition on a service, by either management or researchers. So far, the demand for evaluation has not come from service providers, users or carers. A somewhat hostile reaction to being evaluated can often be detected, with service providers feeling imposed upon and passive. The value of research to everyday practice is often negated by practitioners, most of whom are not updated in their knowledge of relevant research findings. It is rare to find a service which has generated its own means of evaluation. In these rare cases the initiative was likely to have come because of the innovatory nature of the service, which providers wish to assess and promote. If the evaluation highlights the positive aspects of the service, then attempts at dissemination will follow. If, however, the data indicates negative aspects, the responsibility for the implications of these findings is likely to be deflected elsewhere.

The attitude of service providers to evaluation reflects an assumption that evaluation is aimed at fault-finding, at attempts to cut resources allocated to the service, and that criticism can never be constructive. Furthermore, practitioners tend to assume that researchers neither understand, nor are interested to learn about, the complexity of the work situation, the life circumstances of clients, and the layers of bureaucracy – all of which affect the service, and therefore it is a waste of time to ensure that researchers will be better informed. Consequently they feel that there is no need to listen to researchers or to be updated in research-led information.

This chapter will focus on evaluating mental health services for adult continuing care clients. This will include public sector services (health and social services) and the voluntary and the commercial sectors. It will focus on psychiatric hospital closure and resettlement, community mental health centres, day care, housing, care management and multidisciplinary work.

Continuing care clients are defined here as such by their length of contact with a service and the duration of their problems as people who have been using mental health services for more than two years, rather than by psychiatric diagnosis. In the literature, however, most continuing care clients are attached a diagnosis of psychosis (Lavender and Holloway 1988). However, as services in the community are not designed for the carriers of diagnostic labels, and as diagnostic categories do not tell us much about the relationships between a service and a client, or even about the client's needs, abilities, disabilities or circumstances, they are not useful for the purpose of evaluating services.

Examples will be taken mainly from Britain, but also from American and Italian experiences. The text is not going to focus on clients' outcomes, even though these are the ultimate objective of a service, and therefore provide an indication of the service performance by definition. Changes in clients' outcomes are influenced by factors other than the contribution of the service, hence a lack of improvement in a client's outcome does not necessarily reflect the service activity, nor does a positive outcome necessarily reflect on the service contribution. When looking at clients' outcomes as an indicator in community services evaluation, it is important to separate out those outcomes which have been directly influenced by the service, and those which have not. In principle this separation is clear and straightforward; in everyday reality it is much more difficult to maintain.

Clients' outcomes will be reported as one indicator of service performance, attempting to relate them to specific service activities. A good knowledge of the clients' strengths and weaknesses, life circumstances and mental distress is a necessary prerequisite to constructing services, as is an assessment of their needs and wishes.

Issues of cost will be dealt with under the specific service evaluation. Due to lack of systematic evaluation, services for ethnic minorities by ethnic minority providers, for women by women providers only, and user-run services will not be looked at in this chapter. The existing evidence relating to these three types of services demonstrates that they meet clients' needs by attracting people who would not otherwise use mainstream mental health services, or who have been frustrated by those services (Fernando 1991; Chamberlin 1988).

Methodology

The aim of this section is:

- to provide an overview of the methodologies used in evaluating community services
- to highlight the connections between the questions asked and the answers which can be obtained by specific methodologies
- to indicate the limitations which methodology puts on what can be asked and the type of information to be gathered and made sense of.

Most evaluation of community services is empirical, and quantitative in focus. This is hardly surprising, as the main issue is that of judging a specific empirical phenomenon, namely a service.

The tendency towards quantitative measurements, as opposed to qualitative indicators, reflects the assumption that figures are perceived as more objective and hence scientific than non-numerical statements, and that everyone understands figures better than statements. Thus the focus on quantitative measures expresses the bias towards natural science methodology and a positivistic research framework.

Within such a framework it is assumed that experimental designs, in which some variables are manipulated and other variables remain untouched by the same manipulation ('controlled variables') are the best methodology with which to test out the efficacy of a new way of working. In turn, this assumption too is based on the wish for approximation to the natural sciences. Indeed, medicine sees itself as part of the natural sciences, and those psychiatrists who see no difference between their focus and that of other doctors would see it as self-evident that the methodology used in the natural sciences should apply to psychiatry too.

There are three major problems with this perspective. First, the social world influences the natural world. Medicine provides us with many instances of such influences, be it in terms of access to services mediated by age, class, gender and race or psychological and social responses to illness and disability which influence both the availability and the response to medical interventions (Tuckett 1984). Second, the psychosocial components of mental illness are even more difficult to deny than in the case of physical illness. There is sufficient evidence to suggest that in a number of mental distress conditions there are major psychological, rather than physical, components at work. Social factors play a continuous part in the way psychiatric symptoms are interpreted by individuals, families and social groups (Warner 1985; Pilgrim and Rogers 1993). Third, decisions concerning interventions and ways of organizing professional responses to people suffering from mental illness are heavily influenced by social considerations, notably governments' policy decisions, as well as the type of training which professional groups receive (Ramon 1985). The training too is influenced in turn by social attitudes, while it also plays a part in shaping these attitudes. Therefore, the application of social sciences methodologies is more justified than the application of natural science methodology in the evaluation of community mental health services.

Evaluative strategies include the following designs:

- experimental design
- quasi-experimental design
- cross-institutional design
- single case study
- longitudinal study
- users' perspective
- pluralistic evaluation.

As outlined above, in an experimental design it is attempted to change either the quantity, or the form, or the content of one factor only, while leaving the others constant. In relation to service evaluation, this could entail the introduction of a new service/discipline/intervention to which one group of people will be allocated, while another group – with the same characteristics – will continue to receive the old service (Gibbons 1981). The problem with this 'pure' design is that it bears little relation to reality, in which people are different from each other even if they suffer from the same mental distress, in which things change in their lives during the trial period, and in which service providers are not the same even when they work in the same service. An additional critical issue which requires careful attention in this strategy is that of the ethics of providing a service to one group, but denying it another.

The quasi-experimental design aims at remedying some of these flaws, by imposing an experimental design on a change in intervention which has taken place anyhow. This often implies that a comparison group, rather than a control group is used for the purpose of evaluating the usefulness of the change which took place in one (called 'experimental'), but not the other, group. An example is provided by a study evaluating health and social work input into the homes of elderly clients, where the specific intervention was compared through outcome measures of a group which received the targeted intervention, and one which did not. The group was similar in age, length of stay in hospital and diagnosis. To minimize the ethical issue of some clients not being offered a service, the comparison group was drawn from another area, where such a service did not operate (Simic *et al.* 1992).

Cross-institutional design simply implies comparison of the same service, or intervention, across different sites – especially useful for evaluating a new policy. However, the impact of variables such as teamwork and home atmosphere would need to be taken into account, side by side with the effect of the intervention on clients (assuming that differences in clients' characteristics had been considered and controlled for (Thornicroft 1991).

Case studies are useful for the purpose of understanding processes and outcomes where the subject is compared with herself at different stages. This strategy also fits in with the way practitioners operate. A range of case study designs and methods exist (Yin 1989), and a number of studies in mental health use this strategy. However, only a few of these studies focus on service evaluation, such as Vasconcelos's study (1991) of the development of community mental health services in one Brazilian state, Bel Horizonte. In this study the researcher interviewed professionals, relatives and service users, observed a number of service provision encounters and studied the documentation available concerning the state policy and media coverage of mental health issues during a ten-year period.

Longitudinal studies can be a variation of a case study over a longer period of time, or of a group (cohort) of people participating in a change process, where they are studied at specific points in time (time-sampling) within the process. This is especially useful for the evaluation of structural changes, such as hospital closure and resettlement in the community (Segal and Kotler 1991; TAPS 1990; Fetch 1992). The problematic issue of extrapolating from what has happened to individuals to the effectiveness of the service remains unresolved with this method too.

As far as direct and indirect users' perspectives are concerned, in terms of service evaluation consumers' views are an indispensable indicator of the usefulness of a service. They have become fashionable now, as part of the focus on quality assurance. Such studies may be conducted through questionnaires, individual and group interviews, and self-reporting (McIvor 1991). Their problematic aspects include:

• the difficulty of ensuring representation from the different subgroups of users of a service
• the usually low rate of participation due to lack of involvement of users in decision-making
• their unsurprisingly suspicious attitude when suddenly asked for their views
• the tendency to rate positively a service because you do not wish to antagonize those who have power over you
• the alienation felt when confronted by questionnaires and researchers.

Despite all of these difficulties, there is a lot to be learned from the process of eliciting users' and carers' views and from what they have to say (Rogers *et al.* 1992; Lieper and Field 1993).

Pluralistic evaluation, or triangulation, is based on the logical assumption that, given the complexity of a service and the incompleteness of any given evaluation measure, it would be necessary to use more than one method of evaluation (Smith and Cantley 1985). Yet it remains doubtful whether the combination of different methods results in a coherent whole, and whether even triangulation can adequately cover the complexity. Triangulation can be seen as an insurance policy device, based on the inherent weaknesses of the available repertoire of evaluation methods.

Action research is often left unmentioned as an evaluation strategy, though it is a strategy designed a priori to include an in-built evaluation of a proposed course of action (Friere 1970; Room 1993). In some projects the research team has been a separate group from the action team, while in others the same people were initiating the action and the evaluation. This raises the issue of whether evaluating one's own activities can be sufficiently unbiased to render results which may highlight doubtful or negative aspects of the project, incorporating the vexing issue of mental health workers' self-critical abilities. As a model of practice, there is no substitute for the ability to examine one's own actions and for a group to evaluate its activities. An outside researcher may be less biased but is also further removed from what is taking place, tends to care less, and is only there for a short period of time. Therefore, the issue should not be whether it is appropriate for workers to evaluate their own service, but how to ensure that this happens regularly, in conjunction with systematic evaluation by service users and the agency. Involving service providers systematically in evaluation and allowing them to own it will only enhance the accountability of the service, and ensure that evaluation is not a one-off, distanced activity (Ramon 1993).

Community mental health service evaluation: main findings

Hospital closure and resettlement

Elsewhere I have argued that services in the community reflect the type of hospital closure which has taken place, leading up to the establishment of such services, or in conjunction with their establishment (Ramon 1992). Furthermore, as most hospital closure programmes include a substantial component of resettlement in the community, it is logical to include hospital closure and resettlement as part of the evaluation of community services.

In evaluating hospital closure and resettlement there are a number of central issues which require to be addressed:

- evaluating the effectiveness of the different stages of the closure and resettlement process
- evaluating the effectiveness of the contribution of the different actors in the process
- evaluating both the outcomes of the closure, and the process by which it was carried out, including the different types of costs
- ensuring that the major participants in the process contribute to the evaluation.

Although American psychiatric hospitals were the first to be closed, no evaluation of the process of closure and its stages took place. Thus we are left with British and Italian findings. On the whole, the Italian findings tended to describe the process and the outcomes, rather than to have an in-built measured evaluation. Plenty of documentary evidence exists, including videos and verbatim transcripts of staff and patients' meetings in which decisions concerning the closure were taken (Basaglia 1968). Since the establishment of community mental health centres evaluation is taking place more systematically. With few exceptions, British research tends to focus on outcomes, especially clients' outcomes, rather than on processes.

The planning and implementation process

The effectiveness of the different stages depends on the definition of the objectives of the closure and hence of the stages. While planning seems a neutral enough activity, decisions as to who participates in the planning, the pace, and what should be the end results, determine to a large extent what will in fact take place.

British planning was led and controlled by health service planners, who approached the closure objectives in terms of 'what would the resettled patients need in the community', and how to translate these identified needs into concrete, quantitative, outcomes: such as housing (often more than one type), day care and leisure activities. A few planners identified a need for employment training programmes for a small number of resettled clients. Other planners saw the need to develop advocacy schemes and resource/ information centres.

In addition it seems to have been self-evident that there would be a need for general hospital units for acute admissions and for people with 'special needs' (i.e. those the staff in hospital have found too difficult to handle, self-harming or potentially a threat to others). Alternative approaches to asylum facilities in the community were usually not even discussed, despite the fact that a number of users' surveys highlight their wish for non-medical asylum facilities in the community, and the existence of several such alternatives within mainstream services in the US (Rogers *et al.* 1992; Warner 1991).

There were no plans to involve carers, or their organizations, in the process. In some places with active community health councils or local MIND branches a degree of public consultation took place in meetings. This often felt like the planners going through the motions of consultation, but no more than that. While representatives of social services were invited to participate in the planning meetings, it was made clear to them that they were not equal partners in terms of access to finance and other resources, and in a number of instances they walked out of the planning processes.

There were no consultations with groups of workers in the hospitals, or the unions. In response to unions' threats to boycott the whole process, assurances were given that people would be redeployed, though it took a long time to sort out the process of redeployment. From the beginning it was assumed that resettlement teams would be brought from the outside, based on the belief that the workers inside were overworked, or would not want or be able to carry out the new type of work. No consideration was given to the alternative view that bringing a team from the outside would demoralize and de-motivate the insiders.

Tomlinson (1992), following Korman and Glennerster's study (1985) of the process of closing of Darenth Park, a hospital for people with learning difficulties, has applied the concept of 'organisational culture' to the closure process. He suggests that authorities differed in the degree to which they were closer to one of five types: the controlled (rigidly following government's instructions), guided (product champions), autarchic (the market competition-led authority), decentralized (allowing other organizations to have a major say) and Athenian (democratic and participatory) authority. Tomlinson's analysis of the closure process of two large British psychiatric hospitals would lend support to the view that planning and decision-making depended on the personalities involved as much as on objective conditions, or pressure that could be exerted by groups external to a planning authority. This conclusion is important for understanding the planning processes which go beyond hospital closure, into the planning of community services.

A comparison of mental health development work in five districts undertaken by the King's Fund in the last two years has also highlighted that the change process does not follow the formula laid down in management books. The principal development officer has observed that the existence of a vision does not necessarily lead to change. Interpersonal interaction focused on shared interests and views, the formation of a number of interest and pressure groups, and the existence of people ready to assume leadership are some of the dimensions more likely to facilitate change, whereas the vision develops as part of the process. A further observation is that the attempt to impose a particular view of desirable services by outsiders is likely to backfire, unless the insiders come to see this particular perspective as their own (Echlin 1993).

Echlin's observations also highlight that the pace of developing active user participation in planning services is slower than that of professionals and administrators. This is hardly surprising, given the long lasting experience of disempowerment that users have often gone through. Furthermore, the more participatory a process is, the longer it takes, as has been demonstrated in community development and action research programmes (Lees and Smith 1975).

Clients' outcomes as an indicator of the effectiveness of hospital closure and resettlement

So far, outcomes studies of resettled ex-patients in the community, defined a priori as 'the long long stay', indicate that most of them have been able to lead a better quality of life outside the hospital, have improved their level of social functioning but have not necessarily reduced their levels of symptomatology, and that they are satisfied with their current way of living (McCourt Perring 1993; Segal and Kotler 1991; TAPS 1990). These outcomes would indicate that the resettlement process has been relatively successful and that the services in the community have offered useful personal and social support. The British findings are similar to the American and Italian outcomes (Tansella *et al.* 1987; Mosher and Burti 1989), even though on the whole the Italian group homes have a lower level of staff cover.

Clients' outcomes as an indicator for the hospital vs. home as the predominant treatment setting

By now there are a number of British home treatment schemes, as well as American and Italian services where this is the main delivery method. They all demonstrate that the need to be removed from home for the purpose of hospitalization is greatly reduced when home treatment becomes the main form of service delivery (Tansella 1987; Stein and Test 1980; Burns *et al.* 1993). Some British evaluations of such schemes highlight that, apart from the considerable reduction in hospitalization, there are no other significant differences in clients' outcomes between hospital and home treatment (Burns *et al.* 1993; Simpson *et al.* 1993). This should hardly be surprising, as the content of the interventions has not changed in the move from hospital to clients' homes in these schemes. On the whole, the intervention in the British projects continues to be medication-focused. Where the focus has changed to include not only medication but, for example, a family education programme (Falloon *et al.* 1992) or a comprehensive service (Test and Stein 1980), the outcomes for those worked with in the community demonstrate a significantly more positive overall outcome. Even the reduction in the need to use hospitalization signifies reduced financial cost, reduced stigmatization and institutionalization.

Workers' responses

Studies focused on the responses of workers to the closure, and its implications for professional identity and knowledge, are even more rare than studies on the planning and the implementation processes. The lack of such research highlights the difficulty which politicians, planners and researchers have in recognizing the centrality of grassroots workers in implementing changes such as hospital closure, and the ease with which they fall into the trap of believing that workers simply follow any decision imposed on them. This strange omission highlights that planners and politicians are unaware of the lessons learned in business and large industries of the importance of workers' motivation and their active involvement in change and innovation.

The one British study on the reactions of grassroots workers to the closure of a psychiatric hospital focused on three teams of social workers located within one large hospital, working for three similar inner city social services departments. The study covered two major stages, the middle phase and the final phase of a ten-year closure process. The issues looked at were views about closure and whether these changed as closure became a reality, changes in the roles, tasks and knowledge required, as perceived by the workers, and changes in professional identity. The methodology included six-monthly individual interviews of the workers, interviewing key workers from other professions and management, observation of staff meetings and observation of some workers in practice (Ramon 1992; Shears 1994). The findings highlight that a more immediate concern with the perceived inferior power position of the workers vs. the multidisciplinary team in the hospital and the social services hierarchy outside the hospital occupied the workers much more than the closure. Furthermore, while the workers welcomed the closure and were committed to securing community living for their clients, they were sceptical of central government's policies, and of the ability of both health and social services to deliver what had been promised. Changes in roles and tasks took place, and social workers became more involved in supporting new resettlement projects at the management level and later in everyday practice, but this had not led to perceived changes in professional identity or to the identification of gaps in knowledge. The social workers did not feel themselves to be wanted partners in a process of change, but more a doubly marginalized group within the hospital and in their own social services departments. Consequently although intelligent and resourceful and committed to community care ideals, the three teams initiated little by way of innovation, though they responded well to the initiatives of trusted line managers.

Studies focused on the stresses and satisfactions experienced by nurses in a psychiatric hospital and in the community have recently been carried out by Carson, Bartlett, Brown and Fagin (1990 1993). The initial study highlighted that while levels of stress for the community psychiatric nurses (CPNs) in the community were higher than in hospital, so was the level of satisfaction. The second study indicated that the differences are smaller in relation to both stress and satisfaction. As this study is still in the process of analysing its data, it is too early to conclude what has led to this finding, though the possibility of the contribution of a constant process of organizational change in the NHS and of each working place requires to be considered.

Only one study has looked at the issues faced by the largely unqualified care staff in group homes (McCourt Perring 1993). This qualitative study has highlighted the dilemmas coming out of the continuing power of the medical approach to mental illness, and the application of a 'family-like' living model for people who are not part of one family and where the 'children' are much older than the parent substitutes. It also addresses the lack of sufficient psychosocial knowledge and skills, and the relative isolation felt by the staff.

Community mental health centres

Such centres are a recent addition to British mental health services. A survey by Sayce *et al.* (1991) highlighted the pace of their development (from 25 in 1985 to 150 in 1989), the differences in organizational affiliation (health, health and social services, social services, voluntary organizations), the variety of client groups served (some serve only continung care clients, others offer services predominately to people with mild mental health problems), and the range of intervention methods (medication focus, and/or individual counselling, family work, psychotherapy, group work, day care/activities, occupational therapy, housing, welfare advice, support workers in people's homes, home treatment, advocacy, self-advocacy, establishing user-run services).

Sayce suggests four broad types of such centres:

- a local comprehensive mental health service
- a low key sessional service
- a day care model
- a community development model.

The types seem to reflect the preferences of the key local professionals involved in setting up the centres. Often centres are set up despite the opposition of such key figures, notably consultant psychiatrists, even if there is a formal acceptance of the role to be played by such a centre (Goldie *et al.* 1989).

Further in-depth evaluation of six such centres (Patmore and Weaver 1991) has highlighted the lack of comprehensive cover for different groups of clients in four out of the six centres, and the shortfall in providing a range of services. The two teams which were willing and able to provide a comprehensive service to continuing care clients were based in social services, were designated as working with vulnerable clients, and had a smaller caseload than the others. The study illustrates relatives' appreciation of the service provided by these teams, especially having access to services on a 24-hour basis and the focus on practical needs. The two teams also provided a reaching-out model. Such an approach marks a departure from a medical and health-needs model to that of social and personal care. This is further illustrated by the wide-ranging background of the support workers, most of whom did not come from mental health work.

By demonstrating the demand from both people with mild and severe mental distress for the new mental health centres, the findings highlight indirectly the inadequacy of the services provided by traditional out-patient clinics. If the latter were adequate, then the demand from these two groups would not have been so high, especially not the demand from those with milder problems. The findings indicate that four of the teams were not attracted to working with continuing care clients, but were working with people suffering from milder difficulties, a finding reflecting similar studies from American mental health centres, but not from those in Italy (Mosher and Burti 1989). The Italian context is characterized by the relative absence of private counselling and psychotherapy outside of the large cities, and by a restructuring of mental health services coming from the perspective of the positive rediscovery of the continuing care client as a person with potential for dignified living. If anything, Italian mental health centres tend to focus on, and attract, continuing care clients more than those with mild difficulties. Most of the workers establishing such centres would come out of psychiatric hospitals literally together with their long-term clients. The community mental health service was constructed with the view to providing a comprehensive service, including 24-hour cover.

All of these features, plus the informality of the worker–client relationships, have enabled them to work more closely with the young new long-stay (Dell'Acqua and Mezzina 1990). Unlike their British counterparts they did not feel the need to establish subteams, or separate out support work and home treatment from the mainstream of the community mental health centres. Yet their caseloads are on the smaller side, like those of the British support teams (Savio 1993).

The relative newness of community mental health centres in Britain means that they are under-researched. The tendency not to have in-built evaluation beyond the collation of basic statistics is apparent in these centres already. Those centres which have established mechanisms of user involvement benefit from having an in-built quality assurance and evacuation device through the periodic feedback of users' views.

An interesting perspective concerning community mental health centres is highlighted in the study carried out by Handyside and Heyman (1989) on clients' outcomes and satisfaction in a comparison between those who were connected to a centre run by a voluntary organization, in addition to being treated by a multidisciplinary team in the community, and those treated only by the latter. The findings indicate no significant difference in clients' outcomes, as both groups improved greatly. The people connected to the voluntary organization were less satisfied with the service provided within the public sector and would have liked to have been seen only in the voluntary organization service. Contact with CPNs and social workers was preferred to contact with other professional figures. The latter finding differs from that found in the large-scale survey of 500 people reported by Rogers *et al.* (1992), where contact with the GP was perceived as the most satisfactory.

Day care

Day care has developed slowly since the 1950s, first as an adjacent facility to hospital ('day hospital') and later in the form of day centres in the community. The section below focuses on the second type, within which there are a number of subtypes, such as centres aimed at work-related activities, structured psychotherapeutic activities, and drop-in club-like centres, which may also offer counselling and welfare advice. Most of the day centres in the community are run by social services or a voluntary organization (usually MIND), and provide a purposely non-medicalized environment.

Only a few evaluations of day centres exist, even though a major survey of day centres took place in the late 1970s (Carter 1981). It would seem that there is no significant difference in the characteristics of people using day centres from those in day hospitals (Holloway 1989), despite the differences in objectives and staff background. However, centres more orientated towards verbal activities have the more articulate clients.

The open-ended nature of attending most day centres and the lack of clear-cut individualized objectives periodically reviewed, make it quite difficult to evaluate them in terms of clients' outcomes. There have been attempts to look at quality of life indicators for clients attending day care, but these have been one-offs rather than involving a before and after assessment, taking stock of changes in quality of life (Holloway 1989).

Users' views on the value of a particular day centre seem to have replaced other aspects of evaluation. Methodologically these range from a ticking-off questionnaire to individual interviews and group discussion. Conceptually a different range exists, from a maintenance perspective, through a rehabilitation angle to the position taken by the normalization, or social role valorization (SRV) approach. The conceptual choice dictates the methodology to a great extent. In the study conducted by Wainwright *et al.* (1988) the two latter approaches are used for comparative purposes within the same inner city day centre. In the first, users' views were requested to evaluate satisfaction with specific activities and to correlate their views with those of the staff in relation to their level of functioning and degree of mental health symptomatology. Following the second approach, users and staff were asked to rate the centre and its activities in terms of its competence-enhancing and image-enhancing success. The results were much less favourable to the centre when judged by the criteria of the SRV approach, and the staff felt bad about them.

Even more important than the difference revealed by following a different conceptual approach is perhaps the following statement made by the researchers, one of whom was a worker there for a long time: 'the evaluation of the day service as a whole revealed a paradoxical situation. There was considerable unmet need for treatment and care within day settings where significant numbers of users also required less treatment and care of the kind that they were receiving' (p. 242). This relates in part to the multiplicity of services offered by the day centre, but also to the lack of a sufficient degree of catering for individual needs and wishes.

Day care is presently undergoing considerable changes, in part due to continuous cuts in the budgets of social services and the view that day services are not as essential as housing or hospitalization. Yet some of the changes have come in response to users' views and the critique voiced above, namely of offering an inappropriate service too much of the time, and not enough of the individualized service which clients want. Many residential establishments are constructing their own day activities, a number of which take place in ordinary facilities in the community; some day centres offer more of the specific activities for shorter periods of time, and still others are restructured to cater for the needs and wishes of a specific subgroup of clients.

Clients have indicated in each study that they value nonmedicalized settings which offer them opportunities to socialize, as well as work opportunities, access to counselling, and welfare advice (Mangen 1990; Rogers *et al.* 1992). They have also indicated that many of the traditional activities of day centres are not to their liking, voting with their feet. In those few settings where clients have a considerable say in the decision-making concerning a centre's activities, most of them are able to make decisions and conduct a number of these activities (Hennelly 1990).

Housing

Developments in housing for continuing care clients have been central to the shift of services from a hospital to a community base. They have also mirrored changes not only in community care and normalization policies but in preferences concerning funding. These changes include the funding of public, voluntary and private sector services and services for ethnic minorities, public opinion concerning the visibility of people with mental illness, and the general shortage of low-cost housing. The evaluation of housing services has been about comparative cost across service sectors, catering for the assumed differentiated needs of subgroups, the provision of 'a home away from home', and reducing/reversing hopelessness.

The government's insistence on privatization of health and social services is more pronounced in housing than in any other mental health service, and provides an example of how government financial support and/or penalty can change not only the ownership of a service, but its focus. Cost depends on ownership; private housing seems to be consistently cheaper for any subgroup (Oliver and Mohammed 1992; Petch 1992). However, the focus on investigating cost sometimes comes at the expense of looking at what, apart from a roof over one's head, is on offer. Furthermore, it is necessary to compare housing across the sectors for the same subgroup, i.e. clients with a similar degree not only of mental distress and level of personal and social functioning, but also of abilities, years of institutionalized life, social network, and degree of supporting services.

The housing solutions for clients with a similar profile would then need to be compared as to the range of services which they offer (e.g. level of physical comfort, privacy and cleanliness; attention to physical health; nutrition and catering for residents' preferences in food; access to day activities and their quality; pastoral skills of the staff; degree of residents' involvement in caring for themselves and in looking after the house; extent of involvement in making decisions; degree of ties and connections with the local community and the resident's family and friends; the impact of registration and inspection legislation on care standards).

Studies have rarely incorporated all of these dimensions. Pre-1985

American and British studies are summarized by Garety (1988). These have focused on the 'new long stay' and people coming out of acute admissions, rather than on the 'long long stay'. In contrast a number of the post-1985 studies concentrate on the resettled 'long long stay' in the community. The most revealing studies are those in which qualitative and participatory methods have been used. Three such studies stand out as valuable examples of evaluative research (McCourt Perring 1993; Youll and McCourt Perring 1993; Smith and Kurriesh 1993). The findings illustrate:

- the relative lack of choice which residents had in where and with whom they were going to live
- the high level of satisfaction from current housing in comparison with hospital life in terms of degree of privacy, choice and freedom in everyday life and links to non-mentally ill people
- the ability of residents to contribute to the management and quality control of the houses
- the continuing high level of care staff power over the residents
- the high level of tension within the staff group
- the need to question the validity of applying a family-like model to this group of people.

All studies report high levels of satisfaction and low levels of relapse into acute mental illness as long as people continue to live in the supported housing scheme. They also record the relatively low level of meaningful contacts with the community of the resettled people.

Although there are projects focused on homeless people suffering from mental illness, a subgroup with a high public visibility, there are very few evaluation studies of these services (Onyett *et al.* 1990; Bachrach 1992). These highlight the usefulness of early intervention, provided trust has been established between the client and the worker. Achieving such trust requires persistence and readiness to reach out, and a high degree of disregard of the prevalent prejudices against homeless people suffering from mental illness.

Professional responses

Care management

Care management is a method of working which has operated in the United States since the 1970s (Berkowitz 1992; Holloway 1991), and has been hailed in Britain as the way forward to improved efficiency, effectiveness, meeting of client's needs and involving them and their carers. Onyett (1992) has provided us with a good summary of the range of care management forms in the Anglo-Saxon mental health services.

Despite being in existence for twenty years, the number of thorough evaluation studies is small. Existing evaluation studies, such as those carried out in Madison, Wisconsin and Australia, illustrate better client outcomes in terms of reduction of hospitalization episodes, days spent in hospital, days spent in employment, and the size and depth of users' social networks. This was true for most of the group which received an intensive and assertive/aggressive reaching-out service, in comparison with a group of people with a similar degree of mental health difficulties who used the ordinary service. Overall costs were lower for the experimental group, though only marginally so. This in-depth evaluation of the Madison project also highlighted the need for continuous support in the community (Stein and Test 1980; Test and Stein 1980). Similar findings were reported for an Australian scheme influenced by the American model (Hoult 1986). However, the findings from a British project based on the Madison model demonstrated less successful outcomes (Muijen *et al.* 1992).

In both the American and the Australian schemes the workers came from a mixed background, but tended to be professionally qualified providers. In the most researched British example, which focused on older people with a variety of difficulties, including mental distress but not mental illness, the care managers were not professionally qualified (Chalis and Davies 1986). Positive client outcomes and considerably lower costs of care were reported for that programme. A number of American programmes are now training ex-service users to become care managers, paying them much less than a professionally qualified care manager would be paid. Thus the evaluation of care management raises the uncomfortable issue of who is the best care manager and what are the qualities of such a provider.

Brokerage schemes usually get a footnote in the literature on care management, but deserve a closer look and evaluation, as they are based on the principle of giving the client a much greater degree of control over the services she wants, and over who will deliver the service, starting with appointing the broker (Brandon and Towe 1989; Ellis 1993).

The systematic evaluation of British pilot care management schemes in five areas is yet to be completed by the Research and Development in Psychiatry team which has overseen the projects. So far the evidence illustrates a reasonable level of client satisfaction (Conlan 1992), a high level of worker satisfaction (which may be related to the enthusiasm generated by participating in a pilot project) and the generation of a much higher level of information about clients (raising the question of standards of required information and how information is used) (RDP 1992).

Multidisciplinary work

Of necessity mental health work requires collaboration between health and social services, to cater for the health and social needs of clients. Such collaboration has taken place in a number of forms, either by disciplines working separately but collaborating over individual cases, or by being placed in the same team. Every textbook tells us that multidisciplinary work is a good thing, yet this issue has not been the subject of much evaluation research in mental health, or in health and social care in general. The lack of such an evaluation reflects in part the ease with which we are ready to accept new ideologies of intervention, and in part the difficulty of separating out multidisciplinary work from all other service factors within a research design. This gap in our knowledge also reflects the low priority given to evaluating the way we organize our work in comparison to the evaluation of direct work with clients.

Existing evidence relates mainly to the views and feelings which professionals have about multidisciplinary work, and indirect evidence of the impact of the specific format of such work on ways of working. In the two-phased study which looked at the responses of social workers to the closure of a psychiatric hospital, mentioned above in the section on hospital closure (Ramon 1992; Shears 1994), it was found that frustration with multidisciplinary work within the hospital was the main feature attributed to such work. The social workers stated that one of the major attractions of going to work in a psychiatric setting was the wish to engage in what they termed 'genuine multidisciplinary work', by which they meant that respect towards the contribution of each discipline should have been demonstrated. The frustration, which was deeply felt, was about being treated as providing a contribution inferior to that of psychiatrists, and a lack of understanding of what social work was by nurses. The views expressed by key informants from psychiatry and management who were interviewed as part of the research project reinforce the social workers' belief. The message from the key informants was that either social workers were not doing what they should be doing, or that they were not an indispensable part of the multidisciplinary team.

Social workers spoke of lack of respect of, and care for, clients by psychiatrists, but did not suggest that mental health services need not employ psychiatrists. However, some of them concluded that they preferred to work in uni-disciplinary teams rather than in a multidisciplinary team.

A comparative study of the development of community psychiatric nurses in Britain and Italy illustrated that the meaning of multidisciplinary work differs. Whereas British nurses worked in CPN-only teams and did not wish to work in a proper multidisciplinary team, Italian nurses worked only in the latter and did not consider the alternative as viable. Multidisciplinarity in the Italian context meant a lot more overlap and joint working among the different disciplines than would be the case in a British setting, accompanied by a much greater degree of informality in the relationships with clients and with colleagues (Savio 1992, 1993).

Comparative studies of the contribution of different disciplines, in which the focus was on a specific method of intervention, are also rare. Wooff *et al.* (1988) have highlighted the fact that social workers are better than nurses in providing counselling. This is hardly surprising, as nurses' training focuses less on counselling than social work training has. There is no evidence to suggest that once trained to do so, nurses are less effective than social workers.

Concluding comments

This review of evaluative research on community mental health services has highlighted the following:

- There are considerable gaps in our current knowledge. Some of these gaps are a reflection of recent and rapid developments, while some others come out of lack of recognition of the importance of a specific aspect. Other lacunae relate to methodological difficulties, and/or the limitations of any one given methodology as an effective evaluation tool.
- Evaluation is valuable in re-thinking the contribution of existing services, both in terms of service organization and content,

- It is useful to include users, carers and grassroots workers' views as an integral part of service evaluation.
- Factors external to community mental health services have an impact on the ways services are organized and the content of interventions. A number of non-mental health disciplines have a significant contribution to make to the evaluation of mental health services, such as anthropology, economics, social policy and sociology.
- The major restructuring which has taken place so far in British mental health services, namely the closure of psychiatric hospitals and the resettlement of long-stay patients in the community, has had reasonably positive outcomes. The outcomes related to the established services in the community are less clear-cut.
- Some strategies of interventions are not put into everyday practice despite consistent existing evidence concerning their effectivness vs. more traditional forms of intervention. Home treatment is one such example; crisis facilities in the community provide another. It would seem that the barriers to adopting a service innovation need to be better understood and worked with.

As we are in the midst of a fundamental restructuring of the British mental health services, it needs to be remembered that evaluation studies cannot replace the systematic evaluation of one's own work, or of a team's work. Yet such studies can provide community mental health teams with some of the useful tools required for the evaluation of their work. Other tools, and working out the framework for in-service evaluation, may come from action research models and from the original solutions which specific teams and their clientele will come up with.

References

Bachrach L (1992). The urban environment and mental health. *International Journal of Social Psychiatry*, **38**, 1.

Basaglia F (ed.) (1968). *L'istituzione negata*. Einaudi, Milan.

Berkowitz N (1992). Care management in American health settings. In: *Care Management: Implications for Training* (ed. S Ramon). ATSWE (Association of Teachers in Social Work Education) Publication, Sheffield University.

Brandon D and Towe N (1989). *Free to Choose: An Introduction to Brokerage*. Good Impressions, London.

Burns T, Beadsmoore A, Bhat AV, Oliver A and Mathers C (1993). A controlled trial of home-based acute psychiatric services: I: clinical and social outcomes. *British Journal of Psychiatry*, **162**, 239–243. II: treatment patterns and costs. *British Journal of Psychiatry*, **162**, 55–61.

Carsons J and Bartlett H (1990). Care in the Community – Are the Staff as Stressed by the Changes as the Patients? TAPS Annual Conference, London 5 July.

Carsons J, Bartlett H, Brown D and Fagin L (1993). Stress at Work for Psychiatric Hospital Nurses and Community Psychiatric Nurses, Paper given at the International Congress on Psychiatric Nursing, Manchester, 21 September.

Carter J (1981). *Day Services for Adults.*, Allen and Unwin, London.

Challis D and Davies B (1986). *Case Management in Community Care*. Gower, Aldershot.

Chamberlin J (1988). *On Our Own*. MIND Publications, London.

Conlan E (1992). Users' Views on Care Management. Presentation given at the study day on Care Management in Mental Health, Research and Development in Psychiatry, 11 March, London.

Dell'Acqua G and Mezzina R (1990). Approaching mental distress. In *Psychiatry in Transition* (ed. S Ramon). Pluto Press, London, pp. 60–71.

Echlin R (1993). Changing Large Scale Systems. Seminar given for the Diploma in Innovation in Mental Health Work, The London School of Economics, 30 September.

Ellis K (1993). *Squaring the Circle: User and Carer Participation.* Joseph Rowntree Foundation, York.

Falloon I R H, Laporta M, Fadden G and Graham-Hole V (1992). *Managing Stress in Families: Cognitive and Behavioural Strategies for Enhancing Coping Skills.* Routledge, London.

Fernando S (1991). *Mental Health, Race and Culture.* MIND in collaboration with Macmillan, Basingstoke.

Friere P (1970). *The Pedagogy of the Oppressed.* Herder and Herder, New York.

Garety P (1988). Housing. In *Community Care in Practice: Services for the Continuing Care Client* (eds. A Lavender and F Holloway). Wiley, Chichester, pp. 143–160.

Gibbons J (1981). An evaluation of the effectiveness of social work intervention using task-centred methods after deliberate self-posioning. In *Evaluative Research in Social Care* (eds. E M Goldberg and N Connelly). Heinemann, London.

Goldie N, Pilgrim D and Rogers A (1989). *Community Mental Health Centres: Policy and Practice.* Good Practices in Mental Health, London.

Handyside L and Heyman B (1989). Community mental health care: clients' perceptions of services and an evaluation of a voluntary agency support scheme. *International Journal of Social Psychiatry,* **36** (4), 280–290.

Hennelly R (1990). Mental health resource centres. In *Psychiatry in Transition* (ed. S Ramon). Pluto Press, London, pp. 208–218.

Holloway F (1989). Psychiatric day care: the users' perspective, *International Journal of Social Psychiatry,* **35** (3), 252–264.

Holloway F (1991). Case management for the mentally ill: looking at the evidence, *International Journal of Social Psychiatry,* **37** (1), 2–13.

Hoult J (1986). Community care of the acutely mentally ill. *British Journal of Psychiatry,* **149**, 137–144.

Korman N and Glennerster H (1985). *Closing A Hospital: The Darenth Park Project,* Bedford Square Press, London.

Lavender A and Holloway F (eds.) (1988). *Community Care in Practice: Services for the Continuing Care Client.* Wiley, Chichester, pp. 3–8.

Lees R and Smith G (eds.) (1975). *Action Research in Community Development,* Routledge, London.

Leiper R and Field V (eds.). (1993). *Counting for Something in Mental Health Services: Effective User Feedback.* Avebury, Aldershot.

Mangan S (1990). Dependency or autonomy. In *Psychiatry in Transition* (ed. S Ramon). Pluto Press, London, pp. 72–81.

McCourt Perring C (1993). *The Experience of Psychiatric Hospital Closure,* Avebury, Aldershot.

McIver S (1991). *Obtaining the Views of Users of Mental Health Services.* King's Fund Centre, London.

Mosher L and Burti L (1989). *Community Mental Health: Principles and Practice,* Norton, New York.

Muijen M, Marks I and Connolly J (1992). The daily living programme: preliminary comparison of community vs. hospital-based treatment for the seriously mentally ill facing emergency admission, *British Journal of Psychiatry,* **159**.

Oliver J and Mohamad H (1992). The quality of life of the chronically mentally ill: a comparison of public, private and voluntary residential provisions, *British Journal of Social Work*, **22** (4), 391–404.

Onyett S, Tyrer P and Connolly J (1990). The early intervention service: the first 18 months of an inner London demonstration project. *Psychiatric Bulletin*, **14**, 267–269.

Onyett S (1992). *Case Management in Mental Health*. Chapman Hall, London.

Patmore C and Weaver T (1991). *Community Mental Health Teams: Lessons for Planners and Managers*. Good Practice in Mental Health, London.

Petch A (1992). *At Home in the Community*. Avebury, Aldershot.

Pilgrim D and Rogers A (1993). *A Sociology of Mental Illness*. The Open University Press, Milton Keynes.

Ramon S (1985). *Psychiatry in Britain: Meaning and Policy*. Croom Helm, London.

Ramon S (1992). The workers' perspective: living with ambiguity and ambivalence. In *Psychiatric Hospital Closure: Myths and Realities* (eds. S Ramon). Chapman and Hall, London.

Ramon S (1993). Educating and training professionals for innovation in mental health services. In *Joint Strategies for Community Care Training* (eds. S Ramon and C Ward). ATSWE Papers No. 1, University of Sheffield.

RDP (Research and Development in Psychiatry) (1992). Partnership in Care Management. Study Day, 11 March.

Rogers A, Pilgrim D and Lacey R (1992). *Experiencing Psychiatry: Users' Views of Services*. MIND in collaboration with Macmillan, Basingstoke.

Room G (ed.) (1993). Anti-Poverty Action – Research in Europe. School for Advanced Urban Studies, University of Bristol.

Savio M (1992). Psychiatric nursing in Italy: An extinguished profession or an emerging professionalism? *International Journal of Social Psychiatry*, **37** (4), 293–299.

Savio M (1993). Pathway to Professionalism: The Development of Community Psychiatric Nursing in Britain and Italy. Unpublished Ph.D. thesis, The London School of Economics.

Sayce L, Graig T and Boardman A (1991). The development of community mental health centres in the UK. *Social Psychiatry and Psychiatric Epidemiology*, **26**.

Segal S and Kotler P (1991). *Sheltered-Care Residence and Personal Outcomes Ten Years Later*. Mental Health and Social Welfare Group, School of Social Welfare, University of California at Berkeley.

Shears J (1994). Social Work Teams' Responses to the Closure of a Psychiatric Hospital. Unpublished Ph.D. thesis, The London School of Economics.

Simic P, Gilfillan S and O'Donnell O (1992). *A Study of the Rehabilitation and Discharge of Long Term Psychiatric Patients from the Royal Edinburgh Hospital*, Scottish Office, Edinburgh.

Simpson C J, Seager C P and Robertson J A (1993). Home-based care and standard hospital care for patients with severe mental illness: a randomized controlled trial. *British Journal of Psychiatry*, **162**, 239–243.

Smith G and Cantley C (1985). *Assessing Health Care*. Open University Press, Milton Keynes.

Smith H and Kerruish A (1993). *Quality for People – Working in Partnership*. Longman, London.

Stein L and Test M A (1980). Alternative to mental hospital treatment, I. *Archives of General Psychiatry*, **37**, 392–397.

Tansella M, De Salvia D and Williams P (1987). The Italian psychiatric reform: Some quantitative evidence. *Social Psychiatry*, **22**, 37–48.

TAPS (Team for the assessment of psychiatric services) (1990). Moving Long Stay Patients into the Community: First Results. TAPS Fourth Annual Conference, London, North East Thames Regional Health Authority.

Test M A and Stein L (1980). Alternative to mental hospital treatment III: Social cost. *Archives of General Psychiatry*, **37**, 409–412.

Thornicroft G (1991). The concept of case management for long-term mental illness.

International Review of Psychiatry, **3**, 125–132.

Tomlinson D (1992). *Utopia, Community Care and the Retreat from the Asylums.* Open University Press, Milton Keynes.

Tuckett D (1984). *Introduction to Medical Sociology*, Tavistock, London.

Vasconcelos E (1991). Alienists of the Poor: The Development of Community Mental Health in Bel Horizonte. Unpublished Ph.D. thesis, The London School of Economics.

Yin R K (1989). *Case Study Research.* Sage, London.

Youll P and McCourt Perring C (1993). *Raising Voices: Changing Practices in Residential Care.* HMSO, London.

Wainwright T, Holloway F and Brugha T (1988). Day care in an inner city. In *Community Care in Practice: Services for the Continuing Care Client* (eds. A Lavender and F Holloway). Wiley, Chichester, pp. 231–257.

Warner R (1985). *Recovery from Schizophrenia.* Routledge, London.

Warner R (1991). Creative programming. In *Beyond Community Care: Normalization and Integration Work* (ed. S Ramon). MIND in collaboration with Macmillan, Basingstoke.

Wooff K, Goldberg D and Fryers T (1988). The practice of community psychiatric nursing and mental health social work in Salford. *British Journal of Psychiatry*, **152**, 783–792.

19 Multidisciplinary care in the community for clients with mental health problems: guidelines for the future

J. Lucas

Introduction: the power to treat and the will to care

Historically the psychiatric professions have held most of the power in mental health services. This power is derived from years of history, any number of accidental associations and personalities and is entrenched in daily, and often unquestioned, routine. The psychiatric professions have had the power to define illnesses and who is diagnosed as having them, to determine their treatments, to treat people against their will in hospital, to organize services within the NHS, to spend the vast budgets that are tied up in the old asylums, to influence public opinion, and to select those that are to be endowed with or deprived of these powers. This power was supported by the general perception of the medical profession as a benign force and the complete unwillingness of many other parts of society to take any interest in people affected by mental health problems as well as earlier legislation.

This history is that of all public institutions. Prisons and private schools share a very similar course of development with the consequent wide range of traditions and abuses. The worst outcome was that all sorts of perverse and oppressive abuses of that power developed behind closed doors, in institutions that were far away from society, in the name of psychiatric medicine. This power was not just legal power and technical competence but was also expressed as brute physical force. The 'treatments' forced on people in the Victorian asylums bear witness to that expression. Also, whole populations of individuals were forgotten and ignored, including both the staff and the patients, and they became thoroughly institutionalized and accepted very low standards of care and lifestyle.

This power and the force of entrenched routine are now being challenged, and this challenge is sometimes initiated from within psychiatry, by the growth of other interest groups in mental health, notably users themselves, and slowly changing professional and public expectations. These have been altered slightly, and also legitimized by, the Mental Health Act 1983 and the NHS and Community Care Act 1991.

Understanding mental distress

Different models

A recent influence on this history is the belief that mental distress is not a disease or an illness. Rather it is a manifestation of social and psychological factors. If mental distress is purely social and psychological in origin then community care needs to be responding to those issues alone and hospital beds will have a minimal role. This does not take away the need for asylum – for somewhere for people to go when they are in crisis and in need of some support, but it does change the criteria for providing it and the resources available within it.

A more generally held view is that the causes of mental distress are multiple and complex and that, given the current levels of understanding, all the professions now involved in the services have something to offer. Indeed, to be able to offer people a wide choice, the medical response should remain one of the elements of community care along with other very different forms of service.

Implications for community care

These different models or belief systems have profound implications for the sorts of services that are offered, the understanding on which they are based and the training of the professionals involved in them. The contribution of the medical professions within this model is the diagnosis and treatment of genuinely organic and physical problems and the offering of medication for short-term symptom relief.

Racism in mental health services

There is no doubt, however, that British psychiatric services are based on a eurocentric model. This model does not acknowledge the validity of some of the older and more traditional ways of responding to mental health problems and it alienates many British citizens who come from other communities. Suman Fernando in 'Roots of racism' notes that:

> Psychiatry depends on identifying 'illness', but it has neither an objective means of measuring nor a precise culture-free classiffcation, of illness. At best psychiatry is a body of knowledge built on a framework of hypotheses and information. It has always been 'permeable to the social and political norms of the time'. (Fernando 1994)

This history means that psychiatry and most of the allied mental health professions have very little to offer British citizens from populations that are not European.

Research evidence

There has now been sufficient research to show beyond all doubt that black people are more likely than white to be:

- removed by the police to a place of safety under section 136 of the Mental Health Act 1983
- retained in hospital under sections 2, 3 and 4 of the Mental Health Act
- diagnosed as suffering from schizophrenia or another form of psychotic illness
- detained in locked wards of psychiatric hospitals
- given higher dosages of medication.

They are less likely than white people to:

- receive appropriate and acceptable diagnosis or treatment for possible 'mental illness' at an early stage
- receive treatments such as psychotherapy or counselling. (MIND 1993*a*)

Implications for community care

The future of community care depends on the new services addressing these issues. This must be done primarily by listening to people from the black community, ensuring that they are represented at all levels of service provision and offering culturally sensitive resources. The discrimination that happens to staff must be addressed as well as that experienced by users. The promotion of a sufficient number of black nurses, doctors and managers to senior and powerful positions will begin to have a significant effect on services – both on what is offered and also on how willing people from those communities are to enter them.

User empowerment

The necessity for the direct involvement of users and carers both in their own treatment, the development of services and the training of professionals is gradually being recognized. This promotes a very real shift in power, from users and carers being oppressed by psychiatry to their taking their share of the power and authority. All MIND policies and some of the recent legislation and guidelines have promoted these changes. The professions are changing; for example,the mental health nursing review *Working in Partnership* (DoH 1994) recommends that users and their carers are involved in teaching as well as research, service planning and management. The Central Council for Education and Training in Social Work (CCETSW) has published guidelines on how to involve users in approved social worker (ASW) training (CCETSW 1994).

Implications for community care

The user groups and organizations are gathering strength in terms of being able to provide the input and consultancy and more importantly actively campaigning for change in their own right. There is a steadily increasing number of user groups around Britain which have been established by users, primarily as support and action groups but who are becoming involved in local training and consultation as well as developing much needed advocacy projects. The involvement of these individuals and the actions that they are prepared to take is beginning to have an impact on local services in some areas. At a national level the Department of Health is ever more willing to engage with users directly and to invite them to be represented on the various policy and decision-making groups that are established.

Bad Practice

Collusion with bad practice and abuse is an area that will continue to be difficult to tackle within community-based multidisciplinary teams. There is currently a feeling amongst users that staff, including nurses, will not actually stand up and confront abuse that they are fully aware of. Peter Campbell, in *Mental Health Care in Crisis*, states that:

> I have met a few staff who clearly despise the 'mentally ill' and will openly abuse you. Their colleagues may agree in private that it is disgusting but they will always, in my experience, rally behind them when it matters.
>
> (Campbell 1989)

Such experience is by no means unique and neither does it accuse all mental health professionals. This kind of collusion may become easier when staff are based in the community and their actions are even less open to the observation that is part of institutional life. It may be less painful to blame other professions within the team for the abuse or bad practice, rather than confront it.

Needs-led provision

The planning of services must be defined by assessed need rather than what buildings are available or what the current professionals can do. People involved in planning need to move away from the assumption that community care means a set of buildings and activities that people should be fitted into. Rather this is an opportunity to look at community care in the broadest sense, to link in to all the other resources within the community and reduce the stigma of specialist mental health services. This model would have the additional spin-off of educating the community, who would then be using the same resources, that people who have experienced mental distress are not two-headed axemen, or whatever the prevailing stereotype suggests.

There must also be some discussion about the difference between needs and wants. There is a tendency to dismiss what users say they want as if they were excessive and uninformed rather than a legitimate expression of a noticeable absence or lack of something that would make their lives better. The professionals' definition of the same person's needs is usually accepted as an objective description of what would change the current, presumably unacceptable, situation. The problems with this practice are manifest. First, the assumption is that the professional knows best, when in fact they know differently. The best outcome would be achieved by putting together the users' actual experience and knowledge about what is useful to them with the professional understanding of the situation and information about local resources. Second, it is assumed that professional understanding of mental distress, and the ways of curing or alleviating it, are based on good evidence Again this is not necessarily the case. Too many people are shuffled into day centres and social clubs when what they actually want is someone to visit them at home or to be able to get a job.

Implications for community care

The care programme approach offers a system within which this process should be easier to implement. The Social Services Inspectorate (SSI) guidelines on care management and assessment note that these processes are 'the corner stones of quality care in the community' (DoH 1992). The care programme approach should, if it were to be implemented create an integrated process for identifying and addressing needs by dealing with the person as a whole. People will be assessed for their needs for community care rather than their needs for social work, then their needs for housing, and then their needs for nursing, and so on. The plan must take account of the individuals' strengths and abilities and their current networks, as well as linking them into ordinary resources. Joint assessment protocols and good information about local services and resources will begin to make these outcomes easier to achieve.

Mixed economy of care

The NHS and Community Care Act promotes a model of a mixed economy of cam where the statutory services are purchasers of services after having first identified the needs of their particular population. These changes are not necessarily conducive to multidisciplinary work because it is likely that the number of agencies active within the networks of community care will increase, thus increasing the numbers of relationships that have to be made and the numbers of people that have to be consulted. However, the more positive outcomes of increased choice – better utilization of resources and the separation of assessment of needs from the delivery of services – may outweigh these disadvantages. It also means that contracts could be given to user-run groups as well as the more conventional service providers.

What could community care consist of?

Policies and principles

It is from this history and context that the implementation of community care, and the inevitable changes in working practices, mtust be viewed. Community care is a relatively new slogan which signals a whole new way of working in different places and involving different people within new power structures and new ways of talking about them.

Policies

MINDS's policy on community care identifies some of these patterns and ways of talking. It states that community care policy should:

• build services around people's needs

- transfer the focus of care from institutions to the community
- extend the range of services
- ensure a rights-based approach
- provide services on the basis of consent
- link users into ordinary opportunities. (MIND 1993*b*)

Each of these policy statements indicates an area for improvement, all of which will demand detailed local work to put into practice.

Principles

Fundamental to this is the principle that community care is only a means of retaining integration within society for people who experience mental distress. History makes this statement almost tautologous as it was seen as not to be possible, almost by definition, for people experiencing mental distress to be integrated.

Respect and rights

All services should be run on a basis of respect for individuals, protecting and promoting their rights and supporting their responsibilities. They should ensure that users are involved at every level and that all service evaluation and staff training has input from users.

Help with ordinary living

People consistently ask for help with ordinary life as well as more sophisticated professional help. This includes help with benefits and paying bills as well as practical help with ordinary domestic events which can easily turn into crises and so precipitate mental health problems. There can be little doubt that the drudgery of poverty exacerbates mental health problems. If you cannot afford to pay the bills, eat the food you enjoy, buy some clothes and go out from time to time, the quality of your life will not be high. Equally, the constant worry about bills and food, and not being able to keep up with your social networks, will erode your already battered self-confidence and lead to a crisis of some kind. This kind of support must be available from the network of community care.

Quality of relationships

The quality of these services will, as now, be dependent on the quality of the relationship with the user. This relationship should be predicated on honesty and respect and an acknowledgment of the power differentials. This honesty must be based on an openness about what is possible, about the professional understanding of the situation and above all on giving information. Service providers will need to find a way of responding to users in ways that do not degrade them and, most importantly, in ways that do not undermine people's self-confidence and destroy their existing networks.

The development of this kind of relationship between individuals will enable workers to use themselves as a resource and reduce the distance between 'us' and 'them'. This should contribute to the reduction of the stigma attached to mental distress and to the difficulties that many workers face, as they seem not to know how to work with users who have also been workers.

Standards and rights to a service

The lottery facing people who experience mental distress must be discredited. The fact that not only the quality of the service you receive but also the very existence of a service is a matter of luck and geography is not tolerable. Citizens should have a right to a service of an acceptable quality all over the UK.

MIND's 1994 *Breakthrough* campaign has begun this process by promoting a Bill to 'provide for comprehensive services for persons referred to specialist psychiatric services or discharged from hospital following treatment for mental disorder and for connected purposes'.

This Bill was presented to parliament in the autumn session of 1994 as a private member's Bill, not with any expectation of it reaching the statute book, but with the purpose of initiating a discussion about rights to a service. Until people have a right to a service any amount of tinkering with the quality and quantity of provision will remain only tinkering. Equally, standards of care in mental health services should be agreed and implemented nationally.

> MIND is convinced that the only answer to the current crisis of confidence in community care is to set up national care standards, so that everyone with mental health problems wherever they live knows they can expect help if they are in emotional crisis, and to make sure that the public has faith in the system. (MIND 1994)

Elements of community care

Services that are available in the community should function to prevent mental distress, support people currently experiencing it and offer help in a crisis for both users and their carers. They should ensure that people are not removed from their ordinary networks unless they want to be and that access back into their ordinary life is eased. This means influencing employers and other ordinary service providers to stop discrimination against people who have experienced mental health problems.

Community care must also be local, that is, provided by a network of local agencies on the basis of the identified needs of the community and the assessment of each individual asking for a service.

Community care should then consist of a network of resources including:

- asylum
- a 24-hour crisis service that is local and possibly run by users (certainly that has a lot of input from users)
- information about the range of services available and effects of the various treatments
- housing with a range of types of support from 24-hour, seven-day staffing

to peripatetic staff
• a reasonable income or access to employment at proper rates of pay
• supported activities during the day
• social activities in the evenings and weekends
• independent advocacy
• therapy and counselling and other forms of help
• integration of ordinary resources
• help with ordinary life.

Community care must also include the acceptance of crisis cards and support for local user groups, forums and patients councils.

Where does community care happen?

Community care is not a single service, a building or even a group of workers. It is a network of resources, integrating specialist services and ordinary community activities that people can move in and out of. As much of this as possible should be in ordinary surroundings. Resources like the local choir or allotment society should also be included in the development of care plans. It will often be much more useful to pay the rent on an allotment, buy someone a few tools and offer some support to others in the society if necessary, than to insist on the same individual attending a day centre.

Can this work ever be multidisciplinary?

Multidisciplinary work is an inevitable means to this end as none of the current professional groups or agencies could achieve this alone. It therefore simply has to be. The old barriers and problems have to be confronted and broken down.

One agent or profession or multidisciplinary work?

The more radical option would be to change the whole structure of the management of services. This would involve creating one government department to fund the whole range of community care services including housing and finance as well as ordinary leisure pursuits. As this option is unlikely in the foreseeable future and is in many other ways undesirable, this review will restrict itself to the best way of using the current structures.

This is possible at a local level if health and social services are prepared to pool their resources and integrate their mental health services into one agency. This solution would not address the need to integrate social security and housing to complete the package, but could at least mean that the local specialist services were not contaminated by the lack of cooperation that currently exists.

Common Concerns, MIND's manifesto for a new service in 1983, put forward the idea of community mental health workers as one solution to the difficulties of multidisciplinary work:

The suggestion is for the development of a new group or profession provided with specialist training that incorporates aspects of the training and skills of existing professional groups; this may, perhaps, be done by widening the community psychiatric nurse training. Community mental health workers could well become the largest group within the mental health service, their skills and responsibilities would be backed by the specialist skills of the psychiatrist, clinical psychologist and social worker.

(MIND 1983)

This suggestion has never been taken up seriously as it challenges some deeply held convictions about the difference and specialness of the separate professions. Whether this split is in the best interests of the users of the services and indeed the development of good community care is still open to question. The world that we currently have to work in is one which cherishes these differences and demands multidisciplinary work. The problem could be solved as well by a genuine partnership between skilled professionals who can identify needs and responses and manage the transition, so enabling people to get access to the right services.

There are now a couple of models developing of single agencies or joint purchasing and joint providing of services, between health and social services. The lessons are not clear yet, but the dangers experienced in Northern Ireland, where the predominance of the medical model over other ways of understanding and responding to mental distress is unhelpful to other developments, must be heeded. The potential advantages of joint work, less bureaucracy, economies of scale and most importantly a flexible response to individual need must be explored.

Who is included?

The word 'multidisciplinary' is used, even overused, to cover a multitude of things. This review is using the term in a very broad sense. Included within it, therefore, is the notion of equal working partnerships with users and carers, as well as the more usual work between professions either in established teams or in ad hoc units, and across agency boundaries. This inclusion of users as partners demands some very different ways of working based on the fundamentally different attitudes already outlined. It is also taken to include cooperation with all sectors of the community and in particular the importance of addressing the specific needs of people from black and minority ethnic communities.

The purpose of multidisciplinary work

The purpose of multidisciplinary work is to make the best use of the available resources and to ensure that the inevitable rationing decisions are made on the best possible information. This would harness all the contributions of the workers and agencies involved to create a dynamic, 'seamless' and flexible network of services that respond to individual needs. It would also eliminate replication and competition. Experience has shown that this is not how many people naturally work. Multidisciplinary work therefore needs to be managed and organized to make sure that it happens.

Lessons from child care

The need for agencies and professionals to work together has been endorsed by every child abuse report since that into the death of Maria Colwell in 1974 (DoH 1974). This report and most others since have recommended multidisciplinary coordination and effective communication between agencies. The Maria Colwell report went on to suggest the establishment of area review committees made up of all the relevant professionals. This structure was considered to be necessary to facilitate the coordination which had been so lacking in the particular situation under consideration. The difficulties facing agencies trying to provide community care for adults are not significantly different. It would seem that social welfare professions are being slow to learn these lessons and change their behaviour accordingly. The Ritchie Report into the case of the killing by Christopher Clunis (Ritchie *et al.* 1994) outlined many similar problems The litany of attempts to offer this young man a service and the inability to make any headway with him through failure to respond to his needs makes very sad reading. Christopher Clunis is quoted by the report as saying that at no point did he understand what was wrong with him, and nobody tried to explain his problems to him or tried to respond to his inability to ask for help. All he wanted, he said, was 'some help with settling down and finding a home of his own'.

Guidelines for fostering multidisciplinary work in community care

In this section those changes that need to be made positively to promote multidisciplinary work are outlined. Smith *et al.* (1993) quote Hudson's work on collaboration by noting her five factors that predispose agencies to work together. These are:

- interorganizational homogeneity (i.e. how similar in values and culture the collaborating agencies are)
- domain consensus (i.e. whether there is there agreement on roles and responsibilities)
- network awareness
- organizational exchange (i.e. with all the parties gaining from working together)
- the absence of alternative resources.

These elements are included and expanded on in the factors described below.

Personalities

Everybody who has experienced good multidisciplinary work will describe a range of factors that made working in that environment better or worse. They will always, at some point in the description, mention an individual or group of people who were willing to cooperate, who opened their work up to others confidently and who were willing to engage in debate and experimentation about developments and essentially set the tone for this style of working.

The model is often not dissimilar to the ideal type of higher education. That is where the professors and the 'experts' are available to people studying in their field, there are regular tutorials with those experts, and seminars and lectures are held that are open to all. The expectation is that people come to discuss ideas, to think things through and develop their own ideas. This ideal type is not always met and is dependent on the personalities of some of the participants. If the professor or the experts want to guard their particular specialty jealously or are insecure about their own work, there will be no multidisciplinary cooperation.

Clarity and competition

Consequences

One of the major difficulties facing multidisciplinary work is the lack of clarity about what particular agencies and professions actually provide, and the consequent competitiveness between professions. The lack of clarity means, in turn, that people cannot be sure about what services they will get when they approach a particular agency and that other referring agencies are not clear about what they are referring people on to.

Nursing and social work, two of the professions involved in providing community care, do not easily define the boundaries of their role. Without this professional self-confidence, workers find it difficult to collaborate because they are not clear about their professional role in relation to other local professionals (Hornby 1993).

Entry to services

As it is neither possible nor desirable to define a single point of access to community-based services, each entry point must respond to people in a similar way and have the appropriate information. Some, like youth services and ordinary community services, may simply send people on to more appropriate points in the system whilst others should have the full complement of information and support to enable users to get access to the full range of resources available locally. It is important to maintain this range of entry points as some people will feel unable to go to a social worker, but will have heard of MIND, whilst others will trust their GP enough to be able to ask them for help.

Assessment

Workers in each agency must not treat people as 'their' clients who will, therefore, receive whatever their particular skill is. Rather they must be able to carry out a full and comprehensive assessment of their needs and create a full care plan. Assessment and care planning are different skills and should be kept separate to ensure that resource constraints do not contaminate the process. This separation is identified as necessary by the SSI guidelines on care management and assessment (DoH 1992).

The competitiveness is exemplified by the lack of joint assessment procedures. One of the implications of this is that people have to repeat their story to each different professional that they come across and can be given a different label and different services each time. This is clearly not good use of time and is demeaning and irritating for users. It can lead to real problems as people often move between services and the appropriate information does not necessarily go with them. This was a major problem identified by the Ritchie Report. It also means that people may well end up being offered only the service that is available from the agency that they happen to approach first, rather than that which is most appropriate to their needs. They may not be offered the services of other agencies or even information about other agencies.

The Mental Health Act code of practice identifies the necessity for assessments to be made as independent decisions, based on a good working knowledge and understanding of each profession's roles and responsibilities and that they should be carried out jointly (DoH 1989).

Implications

The task is then for local workers to get to know what the others can realistically offer and define the boundaries of their own services. This will help professional self-confidence as well as giving out a clear message about what can be expected from any particular profession or agency.

Information

Lack of information

Information is a key factor in multidisciplinary work and is often not available. Ward-based nursing staff often do not know what their community-based colleagues do, still less what social workers or the voluntary sector have to offer. Inevitably, then, people leaving the ward are likely to be ill-informed and will find the transition back into community the more difficult.

Information about what?

Members of multidisciplinary teams must have information about the skills and abilities of their fellow professionals as well as about the other services available locally. They must take the time to find out about each other's skills, both on a personal level and across professions, and this must be seen as time well spent by all the team members. Equally, teams must make the effort to find out about other services available to people in their locality. This can be done in a variety of ways, including local mental health fora, regular liaison meetings and the publication and promotion of directories. There is little doubt that cooperation between agencies is improved where the individuals involved know and trust each other, and the information in directories, and indeed the process of collecting and up-dating that information, is a good-starting point. Agreed joint assessment protocols will also depend on this kind of information.

Structural differences

All the agencies and professions involved in mental health services have different career patterns, management structures, conditions of service and pay scales. Thus the members of multidisciplinary teams who meet together often have differing decision-making power and differing access to resources. This is even more apparent when professionals meet together from different agencies to plan services or assess someone's needs.

If there was one agency offering all the services, this would no longer be a problem. However, the different professions are here to stay for the foreseeable future and the development of the mixed economy of care is likely to mean that there are more agencies rather then fewer.

Acknowledging differences

The best solution will be to acknowledge the differences that do exist in particular groupings and then, where possible, to ensure that people of similar levels of decision-making power represent the agencies. Alternatively, individual workers could be delegated sufficient power for specific activities. The essential point is for all concerned to be clear about what is possible within particular settings and to use that effectively. It is not unknown for staff with less decision-making power to be sent to some meetings to ensure that they 'buy' thinking and negotiating time for their managers, by having to come back and discuss whatever was raised. This can be a time-consuming and irritating strategy, not least because it exemplifies a complete lack of trust and respect between the organizations. Such behaviour is conducive only to competition not to cooperation.

Quality of relationships

The quality of the relationship between workers in different agencies and between workers and users is the basis of effective multidisciplinary work.

Relationships between users and workers

There are numerous descriptions of this relationship in biographical accounts written by users. Some of the respondents in Rogers *et al.* (1993) described their experiences as follows:

> They [the health professionals] appear unconcerned about the problem. They come across as more interested in what they have to say about the problem than what the patient has to say.

> I felt I was treated too much as an object rather than a person.

> Nurses just wanted to comply with regulations or instructions. They didn't care about my needs.

Some of those who felt that they had experienced good medical practice described it as follows (Rogers *et al.* 1993):

When I was a day patient there was a very caring nurse. She never talked down to me. She always treated me as an equal and I always trusted her to tell me whether I was making progress or deteriorating. Basically I trusted her.

Warm empathy experienced when I was just coming out of psychosis. It was really nice to meet a caring nurse who I could talk to at this point.

They understand my problems and they have always given me an appointment when I've asked for one.

The theme that the researchers identified as running through the comments made was that what people valued most was contact which is respectful and empathic and where professionals are willing to share information. People did not like contact with workers who were distant and uninvolved or authoritarian and abusive.

Relationships between workers and between agencies

The relationship between workers within or between different agencies is also important to the development of multidisciplinary work. The traditional culture gap between field and residential social workers where the residential workers are considered to be little more than domestic helps and custodians, whilst the people with the real skills are the field workers, does not help the users caught between them. Equally, the assumption that workers in the voluntary sector are little more than 'do-gooding', often interfering, amateurs is not conducive to the development of trust and a 'seamless' network of services

In localities where there is good communication and information exchange between workers and agencies users always get a better service and the development of community care is improved. The effect is that resources are not wasted on duplication or the production of services that no one actually wants. It also means that all the skills and resources that are available are harnessed to the same, or at least similar, outcomes.

The fear in this is that agencies will lose their autonomy and independence. There is of course some truth in this. But, as in all relationships, the benefits outweigh the costs. Each individual agency can no longer just make a decision and put it into action. Rather they have to consult with others, modify their plans and maybe hand over complete pieces of work to others. Smith *et al.* (1993) note that trust is fundamental to effective working together, and this style of working depends on the development of trust.

If the mission of the agency is about the development of good-quality community-based services, these activities will be seen as an effective way of achieving that. If the mission is rather about promoting a particular interest group or raising the profile of one agency, then these activities will be seen as a complete waste of time.

All involved, therefore, have to understand the principle and purpose of good relationships and this has implications for recruitment, selection, training and development, as well as being committed to the time and resources to make them work. Abusive behaviour (towards clients) should always be the subject of a disciplinary enquiry to ensure that both staff and users really believe in the commitment to stamping it out and as proof that the management is actually prepared to enforce the rules. Equally, complaints procedures must be publicized and utilized as a source of management information.

Attitudes: who knows best?

Effective multidisciplinary work is based on honest and respectful relationships between all the partners. This assumes that all those involved have something to offer that is equal and different.

Respecting users' views

If workers think that they inevitably know better than users what is good for them and that they have the right to impose that view on both the individual and their carers, then community care is never going to be an effective partnership. This is the way to achieve mistrust and to waste resources. It should be accepted as a statement of the obvious that the person who knows best what is the most helpful to them in times of crisis is the person themselves. It may be that the views that they have expressed prior to the current episode have to be noted and honoured rather than putting one more demand on them in the middle of a crisis. The use of crisis cards, similar to donor cards, where people can describe what they want to happen to them in a crisis, as well as listing allergies to drugs, is a useful step towards achieving this.

Users commonly tell of their real physical problems going undiagnosed or the symptoms dismissed as part of their 'mental illness'. The doctors involved in mental health services need to take that part of their medical responsibility seriously and ensure that their colleagues in general medicine also treat people properly.

Who is responsible?

The notion of clinical responsibility is sometimes expanded to imply that psychiatrists always know best what would help an individual. It is true that there needs to be someone keeping an overview of the medical treatment that a person is receiving ensuring that cocktails of drugs are not prescribed and reviewing their physical progress. However, as it is better recognized that medication can only play a small part in the response to mental distress, then that responsibility, though important, is equally small. There will be other people with different skills and training who will have more to offer particular individuals and they should not have to be constrained by psychiatric decisions. Where psychiatrists have extended their training beyond the medical response this should also be recognized as part of the network of resources.

Empowerment

If users and carers are to become effective partners in multidisciplinary work and the development of community care then they must be empowered to do so. The mental health system as it is currently designed serves rather to shatter people's self-confidence and often treats adults as irresponsible children.

How can they be involved?

This demands a change in attitude and an acceptance of users as partners in the service. This can be exemplified by ensuring that users and carers are involved in professional training and curriculum development, as well as service planning, management and evaluation. Also the focus of research must move away from professionals' interests to start from the experience of users and their needs. Black and minority ethnic communities have had plenty of research done into them and the time has come to support research ideas that come from within those communities and look at the issues that are of importance to them.

Management support

All these factors are compounded by management attitudes within the organization. The management culture can block multidisciplinary work at all levels by not publishing information, not recognizing the time and resources that have to be put into cooperation and, above all, by seeing themselves as the main or the most important providers rather than as part of a network. This isolationist behaviour causes real problems for people seeking help from mental health services, as it denies them access to other resources and it means that information does not travel efficiently. In other words this is a major element of people 'falling through the net'.

How can management support be encouraged?

Managers must recognize and value the time that their staff put into multidisciplinary work. This will mean that workers have to spend time out at meetings, that they will have to do things like presentations on the work of their team and agency or that the multidisciplinary team has to spend some time getting to know one another and their respective roles and skills. This organizational support can also be enacted by negotiating common policies on issues like confidentiality and open files. If common policies are too difficult, then at least an agreement to recognize and support each other should be sought. It is easy to sabotage such a policy within another agency by tanking about individuals in public and marking all correspondence as confidential.

Advocacy

It must be remembered that professionals cannot be advocates in the accepted sense of the word, the inevitable conflict of interests are too great. The best definition of the process of advocacy is the notion of self-advocacy where individuals are enabled, if necessary, to stand up for themselves and play an active role in their own treatment.

Professionals do have a responsibility to fight for users' rights, particularly, of people who find it more difficult to stand up for themselves. This will best be done by ensuring that people know about advocacy services and by supporting them in very practical ways, like funding, making available office space and facilities, and the development of local projects. Local advocacy projects are as much a part of the network of services within a community as the health and social services. Recognition of the role these projects play facilitates the development of multidisciplinary work and can help prevent the development of services that are not wanted and the consequent waste of money.

What is mental distress?

Hudson's notion of interorganizational homogeneity is important here as the understanding of mental distress will profoundly affect the types of service offered. While it may not be necessary for every worker to hold exactly the same views about mental distress there should at least be a shared understanding of the role and function of community care.

Multi-factor model

If mental distress is mostly caused by social and psychological factors, it will be alleviated, primarily, by support that enables people to continue to live in their community with their preferred social networks. Local agencies need to spend some time clarifying and publicizing their own position on the function of community care and identifying common ground with other agencies. The more common ground there is, the easier collaboration will be.

Whose needs are being served?

Common Concerns' overview of staffing matters suggested that: 'Staff must be appointed to the mental health service as a whole, and be prepared to work flexibly within that service and to move appropriately to the needs of patient care' (MIND 1983). This model might well be the most appropriate for people's care but it will be difficult to manage in a mixed economy of care. The compromise must be that staff are prepared to move, that they are appointed to a service not a building, and that they will have to work 'unsocial hours'. Users are consistently asking for services that are available in the evenings and at weekends, as these are the times that they find hardest to manage at home alone. The fact that staff are often unwilling to work outside normal office hours must be challenged by management in the name of developing services that actually meet people's needs. Working rotas or shifts will also mean that more energy will have to be put into creating and maintaining the multidisciplinary team, as they will meet as a whole less often.

Joint training

Joint training is often cited as an important step towards better multidisciplinary work, but it still does not actually seem to happen all that often. There is a range of local initiatives where post-qualification training is done jointly but that only seems to happen where there is already a good relationship between agencies, and management support for the principle.

Local initiatives

Local joint training on the implementation of the Community Care Act, and in particular the care programme approach, could begin to shift some of the stumbling-blocks to cooperation. It may be possible to introduce some joint training at the qualifying level once the current pilot programmes are completed and evaluated, but until then it will be most effective to recognize that the different disciplines need a specific basic training, but that all-post qualification and local training should at least have some elements that are joint. The statutory services should open their training up to workers from the voluntary sector as well as users and carers, both as experts in their own field and as participants.

Incentives

Smith *et al.* (1993) note that external incentives, usually money or legislation, are important factors in the development of effective working together. There usually has to be a reason for the necessary time and money to be invested in the process. A lot of the failures have been where agencies with a history of mistrust suddenly take on a large project together. The shift in culture and expenence is just too large to be negotiated at one go. It also begs the question of how much of a self-fulfilling prophecy those managers with an investment in the mistrust wanted to create.

The spirit of the NHS and Community Care Act 1990 was that health and social services should work together closely and that they should involve users and carers as well as the private and voluntary sectors in their planning and assessments. The legislation, however, only encourages this kind of working, it does not prescribe it.

Anti-discriminatory practices

The evidence that mental health services are discriminatory and that the take-up is low from within the black and minority ethnic communities is overwhelming. Services should therefore be established that are accessible and responsive to the needs of these groups. There will need to be some separate services initially, as the currently established resources are not being used effectively. Also, staff from these communities are usually only apparent in the lower grades, as domestics and nursing assistants, and less often as managers and directors.

Multidisciplinary community care must then encompass the needs of the whole local population. If the numbers of people from minority ethnic communities within any one catchment area are small, there is even more need to ensure that their specific requirements are met, as it will be even easier to overlook a small group.

Supporting good practices

Collusion with bad practice must be stopped, wherever it occurs. There is growing support for the activities of 'whistle blowers' from managers and this must continue. The organizational culture should ideally be one of supporting good practice rather than preventing bad practice. A culture of development, of evaluation and of learning within a community mental health service will make it easier to establish good cooperation and certainly to develop good practice. This will necessitate managers never being satisfied with the status quo, always striving to improve the quality of what is available, and engaging the staff in this process without undermining what they currently do well. This culture needs be organization-specific but it can thread through the whole network of community care.

Who leads the team?

The prevailing practice is that multidisciplinary teams, especially those within hospitals, are led by psychiatrists. This pattern will be replicated in the community by default unless those involved take the time to think about the appropriate model for the new circumstances.

There needs to be someone providing clear leadership to the members and ensuring that the different skills and abilities do not get lost, that problems are solved efficiently and that medical responsibility is taken seriously. This management role could be taken on by any of the members as long as they have the skills and the respect of the other members. The important skill will be the management of the team and the implementation of its role within a network of resources. These networking skills are more often found in community-based workers. There is not an overwhelming argument for the leadership to be automatically in the hands of any one profession; rather it is a distinct role in itself and it should go to the person with the most appropriate skills.

Sims and Sims (1993) argue that the consultant psychiatrist should continue to lead the team. They state that the consultant is best placed to provide essential leadership because:

> their comprehensive biological, psychological and social training in medicine, and then in psychiatry best fits them for this role; other professional disciplines, medical referrers and patients will assume and prefer them to be in this role; remuneration rates imply responsibility; they will be the responsible medical officer at law; and their specialist training in diagnosis and the range of treatment methods which they can prescribe equip them uniquely.

The arguments are much less persuasive when the team is operating as part of a network of resources in the community and when it takes in a much wider selection of professions and includes users and carers.

The most difficult change to make will be to question the almost automatic assumption on both sides that the consultant will lead the team. This assumption is based on many years of experience and has worked well in a medically-led model of service. Community care should no longer be dominated by this model or by the assumption that mental distress is cured by medication. It must take on a much broader management base and a very new culture.

Conclusions

The implementation of the changes outlined would lead to the development of community care within a locality which made good use of the scarce resources that are available. The multidisciplinary work would be based on the development of trust and respect between the partners, the provision of good information to people within and outside the services, the empowerment and involvement of users and carers, and the implementation of anti-discriminatory practices, thus ensuring that the services were equally acceptable to and available to the whole community.

This demands a fairly high level of commitment from all the workers and agencies involved. The workers will have to take the time to get to know others and to consult on plans and ideas. On an individual level, they will have to take the risk of identifying both what they can do and more importantly what they cannot do. This will enable them to refer people on easily when it is clear that they would do better with a service from someone else, without feeling that this is a personal failure. The agencies may have to alter their planning process or development timetable to accommodate the views of others and the necessary changes. Joint policies will have to be developed to cover particular situations and joint assessment protocols will need to be agreed. This will not be achieved overnight and will be vulnerable to sabotage in its early days.

Financial incentives may have to be strengthened in order to persuade organizations to get involved in this work. If all the funding for new developments was dependent on the joint commitment of all agencies involved this might encourage agencies to work together. However, those who were committed to continuing on their individualistic path would always find ways round such directives. More optimistically, those who are committed to multidisciplinary work will continue to push forward, to create new models and to achieve far higher standards of care in the community.

These changes will help clear up some of the muddle that exists at the moment. The critical factor is actually the personalities in the various agencies. Organizations do not collaborate, people do, and people tend not to. There are some individual exceptions who can open up their work and their departments willingly and can create the environment described above. It is in these organizations that new models of service develop, that individual practice improves, and that users get the best service.

References

Campbell P (1989). Peter Campbell's story. In *Mental Health Care in Crisis* (eds. A Brackx and C Grimshaw). Pluto, London.

CCETSW (1994). *Involving Users in ASW Training*. HMSO, London.

Department of Health (1974). *Report of the Committee of Inquiry into the Care and Support in Relation to Maria Colwell*. HMSO, London.

DoH and Welsh Office (1989). *Mental Health Act Code of Practice*. HMSO, London.

DoH Social Services Inspectorate Scottish Office S W Service Group (1992). *Care Management and Assessment; Managers' Guide*. HMSO, London.

Department of Health (1994). *Working in Partnership: A Collaborative Approach to Care*. HMSO, London.

Fernando S (1993). *Roots of Racism*. Open MIND, London.
Hornby S (1993). *Collaborative Care: Interprofessional, Interagency and Interpersonal*. Blackwell, Oxford.
MIND (1983). *Common Concerns: MIND's Manifesto*. MIND, London.
MIND (1993). Policy on black and minority ethnic people and mental health. In *MINDfile 1 Policy*. MIND, London.
MIND (1993b). Policy on community care. In *MINDfile 1 Policy*. MIND, London.
MIND (1994). *Breakthrough; Making Community Care Work*. MIND Campaign pack, MIND, London.
Ritchie J H, Dick D and Lingham R (1994). *The Report of the Committee of Inquiry into the Care and Support of Christopher Clunis*. HMSO, London.
Rogers A, Pilgrim D and Lacey R (1993). *Experiencing Psychiatry*. Macmillan, Basingstoke.
Sims A and Sims D (1993). Top teams. *Health Service Journal*, **103**(5358), 28–30.
Smith *et al.* (1993). *Working Together for Better Community Care*. School of Advanced Urban Studies, Bristol University.

Index